Neuropsychiatric Symptoms of Neurological Disease

Series Editor
José M. Ferro
Serviço de Neurologia Stroke Unit
Hospital de Santa Maria
Lisboa
Portugal

Heinz Reichmann
Editor

Neuropsychiatric Symptoms of Movement Disorders

Springer

Editor
Heinz Reichmann, MD, PhD
Department of Neurology
Technische Universität Dresden
Dresden, Sachsen
Germany

ISBN 978-3-319-09536-3 ISBN 978-3-319-09537-0 (eBook)
DOI 10.1007/978-3-319-09537-0
Springer Cham Heidelberg New York Dordrecht London

Library of Congress Control Number: 2014951832

Printed on acid-free paper

Springer is part of Springer Science+Business Media (www.springer.com)

Preface

It has become obvious that the most common serious movement disorder, Parkinson's disease (PD), is more than a disease with motor symptoms such as bradykinesia, rigidity, tremor, and postural instability. While James Parkinson claims in his "assay on the shaking palsy" that "the senses and the intellect are uninjured," we know that PD starts with malfunction of the olfactory system and the nc. vagus which is underlined by the recent findings by Braak and colleagues who described that the first Lewy bodies in PD do not occur in the substantia nigra but in the olfactory bulb and in the nc. vagus. Besides olfaction and gastrointestinal malfunction, there is disturbance of sleep and of the autonomic nervous system. In addition, many patients present over the course of the disease with psychiatric problems such as anxiety, depression, dementia, hallucinations, addiction, and sexual abnormalities. Most recently it could be shown that depression and cognitive dysfunction lead to a major impairment of health-related quality of life.

This is just one example of the existing neuropsychiatric problems in movement disorders. This book addresses such problems in a variety of movement disorders and brings together current information on important topics such as PD, Huntington's disease, dystonia, tic, and ataxia. New topics, such as mild cognitive deficit and impulse control disorders, are included in this book. The authors are well-known experts in the field, and they succeed in giving us an up to date on these important issues.

I trust that this book will be able to inform on the prevalence, symptomatology, diagnosis, and treatment of these neuropsychiatric symptoms in movement disorders. This is a totally new approach, and thus we hope that the book will find many satisfied readers.

I would like to thank the authors and the representatives of the publishing company for their continuous support in putting together this exciting work, which may become an important reference to everyone who deals with such problems, including neurologists, geriatricians, and psychiatrists who take care of patients with movement disorders.

Dresden, Germany Heinz Reichmann, MD, PhD

Acknowledgements

I would like to thank the authors and contributors who have helped make this volume come to fruition. Their time, energy, and unwavering commitment to this project have made this a concise, up-to-date, and reliable volume on neuropsychiatric problems in movement disorders. I sincerely appreciate all their hard work and dedication and thank them for their contributions. Without them, this book would not have been possible.

I am also grateful to the Springer publishing team, and especially Stephanie Frost, for their continuous support in assembling, editing, and publishing this exciting medical work that may become an important reference to medical professionals dealing with patients with movement disorders, including neurologists, geriatricians, and psychiatrists. It has been a pleasure working with all of you on this excellent volume.

Contents

Contributors

Alberto Albanese, MD Department of Neurology, Catholic University, Milan, Italy

Movement Disorders Unit, IRCCS Istituto Neurologico Carlo Besta, Milan, Italy

Paolo Amami, PsyD Department of Psychology, Milano-Bicocca University, Milan, Italy

Movement Disorders Unit, IRCCS Istituto Neurologico Carlo Besta, Milan, Italy

Marianna Amboni, MD, PhD Neuroscience Section, Department of Medicine and Surgery, Center for Neurodegenerative Diseases, University of Salerno, Baronissi, Salerno, Italy

Department of Neurology, IDC Hermitage-Capodimonte, Naples, Italy

Paolo Barone, MD, PhD Neuroscience Section, Department of Medicine and Surgery, Center for Neurodegenerative Diseases, University of Salerno, Baronissi, Salerno, Italy

Başar Bilgiç, MD Behavioral Neurology and Movement Disorders Unit, Department of Neurology, Istanbul Faculty of Medicine, Istanbul University, Capa, Istanbul, Turkey

Beth Borowsky, PhD Department of Clinical Research and Development, CHDI Management/CHDI Foundation, Princeton, NJ, USA

Ilia Bountouni, MRCPsych, MD Department of Psychiatry, South London and Maudsley NHS Trust, Lewisham University Hospital, London, England, UK

Valerie C. Brandt, Dipl.-Psych, MPhil (CANTAB) Paediatric and Adult Movement Disorders and Neuropsychiatry, Institute of Neurogenetics, University of Lübeck, Lübeck, Germany

K. Ray Chaudhuri, DSc, MD, FRCP (Edin), FRCP (Lond) National Parkinson Foundation International Centre of Excellence, Kings College Hospital and Kings College, Kings Neuroscience Research and Development, DeNDroN, London South, UK

Movement Disorders Society Non Motor Study Group, London, UK

Dirk Dressler, MD, PhD Movement Disorders Section, Department of Neurology, Hanover Medical School, Hannover, Germany

Murat Emre, MD Behavioral Neurology and Movement Disorders Unit, Department of Neurology, Istanbul Faculty of Medicine, Istanbul University, Capa, Istanbul, Turkey

Haşmet A. Hanağası, MD Behavioral Neurology and Movement Disorders Unit, Department of Neurology, Istanbul Faculty of Medicine, Istanbul University, Capa, Istanbul, Turkey

Lucrezia Islam, MD Department of Psychiatry, University of Milan Medical School, Ospedale San Paolo, Milan, Italy

Thomas Klockgether, MD Department of Neurology, University Hospital Bonn, Bonn, Germany

Vladimir S. Kostić, MD, PhD Movement Disorders Department, Institute of Neurology CCS, School of Medicine, University of Belgrade, Belgrade, Serbia

Nikola Kresojević, MD Movement Disorders Department, Institute of Neurology CCS, Belgrade, Serbia

Jaime Kulisevsky, MD, PhD Movement Disorders Unit, Department of Neurology, Hospital de la Santa Creu i Sant Pau, Barcelona, Spain

Sant Pau Institute of Biomedical Research (IIB-Sant Pau), Barcelona, Spain

Centro Investigación Biomedica en Red-Enfermedades Neurodegenerativas (CIBERNED), Barcelona, Spain

Universitat Oberta de Catalunya (UOC), Barcelona, Spain

Matthias Löhle, MD Department of Neurology, Dresden University of Technology, Dresden, Germany

Saul Martínez-Horta, PhD Movement Disorders Unit, Department of Neurology, Hospital de la Santa Creu i Sant Pau, Barcelona, Spain

Sant Pau Institute of Biomedical Research (IIB-Sant Pau), Barcelona, Spain

Centro Investigación Biomedica en Red-Enfermedades Neurodegenerativas (CIBERNED), Barcelona, Spain

Alexander Münchau Paediatric and Adult Movement Disorders and Neuropsychiatry, Institute of Neurogenetics, University of Lübeck, Lübeck, Germany

Christiana Ossig, MD Division of Neurodegenerative Diseases, Department of Neurology, Dresden University of Technology, Dresden, Germany

Heinz Reichmann, MD, PhD Department of Neurology, Dresden University of Technology, Dresden, Germany

Cristina Sampaio, MD, PhD Department of Clinical Research and Development, CHDI Management/CHDI Foundation, Princeton, NJ, USA

Gabriella Santangelo, PhD Department of Psychology, Second University of Naples, Caserta, Italy

Ludger Schöls, MD Department of Neurology, University Hospital Tübingen, Tübingen, Germany

Anette Schrag, FRCP, PhD Department of Clinical Neurosciences, Institute of Neurology, Royal Free Campus, University College London, London, UK

Iva Stankovic, MD Movement Disorders Department, Neurology Clinic, Clinical Center of Serbia, Belgrade, Serbia

Alexander Storch, MD Division of Neurodegenerative Diseases, Department of Neurology, Dresden University of Technology, Dresden, Germany

Marina Svetel, MD, PhD Movement Disorders Department, Institute of Neurology CCS, School of Medicine, University of Belgrade, Belgrade, Serbia

Aleksandra Tomić, MD Movement Disorders Department, Institute of Neurology CCS, Belgrade, Serbia

Valerie Voon, MD, PhD Department of Psychiatry, University of Cambridge, Addenbrookes Hospital, Cambridge, UK

Gregor K. Wenning, MD, PhD, MSc Division of Neurobiology, Department of Neurology, Innsbruck Medical University, Innsbruck, Austria

Panagiotis Zis, MRCPsych, MSc, PhD Department of Neurology, National Parkinson Foundation International Centre of Excellence, King's College Hospital, London, UK

Chapter 1
Depression, Apathy, Anhedonia, and Fatigue in Parkinson's Disease

Marianna Amboni, Gabriella Santangelo, and Paolo Barone

Depression in PD

Definition and Pathophysiology

Definition

Depression is a common neuropsychiatric disorder characterized by the persistence and pervasiveness of a spectrum of symptoms that can variously aggregate. These symptoms include: depressed mood, loss of interest/pleasure, loss or gain in weight or appetite, insomnia or hypersomnia, psychomotor agitation, fatigue, feelings of worthlessness or guilt, diminished ability to think or concentrate, indecisiveness, thoughts of death, and suicidal ideation.

M. Amboni, MD, PhD
Neuroscience Section, Department of Medicine and Surgery, Center for Neurodegenerative Diseases, University of Salerno Via S. Allende, 1, Baronissi, Salerno 84081, Italy

Division of Neurology, IDC Hermitage-Capodimonte, Via Cupa Delle Tozzole, 2, Naples 80131, Italy
e-mail: marianna.amboni@libero.it

G. Santangelo, PhD
Department of Psychology, Second University of Naples, Viale Ellittico 31, Caserta 81100, Italy
e-mail: gabriella.santangelo@unina2.it

P. Barone, MD, PhD (✉)
Neuroscience Section, Department of Medicine and Surgery, Center for Neurodegenerative Diseases, University of Salerno Via S. Allende, 1, Baronissi, Salerno 84081, Italy
e-mail: pbarone@unisa.it

H. Reichmann (ed.), *Neuropsychiatric Symptoms of Movement Disorders*, Neuropsychiatric Symptoms of Neurological Disease,
DOI 10.1007/978-3-319-09537-0_1

Depressive disorders are common in Parkinson's disease (PD) (see section "Epidemiology") and impact negatively on disability [1, 2] and quality of life [3], accounting for approximately 40 % of the variability in quality of life scores [4]. Symptoms of depressive disorders in PD span across a spectrum of severity and of variety, but no distinctive profile has been identified [5]; nevertheless guilt or feelings of failure are not common, and the risk to commit suicide is low despite the frequent suicidal ideation [6]. Mood disorders in PD include major depression, minor depression, dysthymic disorders, and subthreshold depression [7, 8]; subthreshold (or subsyndromal) depression in PD identifies a clinical picture of depressive symptoms that does not meet the criteria for major depression, minor depression, or dysthymic disorder but nonetheless has a clinical relevance; furthermore patients with PD suffering from depressive symptoms only during off states may be diagnosed as having subthreshold depression [9].

Despite the importance of recognizing mood disorders in PD, their diagnosis is greatly complicated since physical or cognitive symptoms of the neurological disorder overlap with symptoms of depression. The application of the criteria of the Diagnostic and Statistical Manual of Mental Disorders IV (DSM-IV) [10] (Table 1.1) for the diagnosis of depression in PD might generate an overdiagnosis, due to the overlapping of the DSM-IV criteria with somatic and cognitive symptoms of PD. Furthermore, little is known about the contribution of either apathy or anhedonia or their association in the diagnosis of depression in PD. The diagnostic criteria for depression in PD were reviewed by the workgroup established by the National Institute for Neurological Disease and Stroke and the National Institute of Mental Health in 2006 [7]. The workgroup recommended using an inclusive approach in assessing symptoms when using the DSM criteria to diagnose depression to enhance reliability. An inclusive approach means considering all symptoms as related to depression, regardless of their overlap with PD or other medical conditions. Briefly, the workgroup recommended:

I. The diagnosis of depression in PD should be made according to DSM-IV criteria using an inclusive approach. Subthreshold depression should be included.
II. The timing of assessing should be specified (on versus off periods).
III. Informants should be used for cognitively impaired patients.
IV. Decreased interest should be omitted as core affective symptom when diagnosing minor or subthreshold depression.

The workgroup concluded that the recommended guidelines for diagnosing depression in PD require further assessment and validation as research tools and in clinical practice.

Pathophysiology

Two major pathophysiological and not mutually exclusive mechanisms have been proposed for depression in PD: (1) a nonspecific reactive comorbid depression in PD, patients develop depression as a reaction to a chronic debilitating illness, and (2) specific comorbid depression in PD, depression is related to the pathophysiology of PD.

Table 1.1 Diagnostic and statistical manual of mental disorders 4th edition criteria for major and minor depression

Major depressive episode
A. Persistence and general pervasiveness of five or more of nine potential symptoms during the same 2-week period that represent a change from previous functioning; at least one of the symptoms is either (1) depressed mood or (2) loss of interest or pleasure that is present most of the day, nearly every day, as indicated by either subjective report or observation made by others
1. Depressed mood
2. Markedly diminished interest or pleasure in all, or almost all, activities
3. Loss or gain in weight or appetite
4. Insomnia or hypersomnia
5. Psychomotor agitation or retardation
6. Fatigue or loss of energy
7. Feelings of worthlessness or excessive or inappropriate guilt
8. Diminished ability to think or concentrate or indecisiveness
9. Recurrent thoughts of death, recurrent suicidal ideation without a specific plan, or a suicide attempt or a specific plan for committing suicide
B. Symptoms do not meet criteria for a DSM mixed episode (presence of phenomena of both a manic and a depressed episode)
C. Symptoms cause clinically significant distress or functional impairment
D. Symptoms are not due to the direct physiological effects of a substance or a general medical condition
E. Symptoms are not better accounted for by bereavement
Minor depressive episode
Requires only two of the nine symptoms above, but one must be either depression/sadness or loss of interest/pleasure

The finding that depression can develop in any stage of PD and even may antecede the onset of motor symptoms [11] would not support the first hypothesis; in addition, when compared with subjects affected by other chronic conditions matched for disability, PD patients show more severe depressive symptoms [12]. Therefore, even if motor and nonmotor disability in PD might contribute to depression, it cannot be considered the unique determinant, suggesting that the cause of depression is intrinsic to the pathophysiology of PD. A combination of dopaminergic, noradrenergic, and serotoninergic system dysfunction has been thought to underlie the development of depression in PD [13, 14].

Studies on dopamine transporter (DAT) availability in depressed PD patients have produced conflicting results. Depression in PD has been associated with higher loss of striatal dopamine transporter availability [15, 16] maybe due to greater dopaminergic degeneration in PD patients with depressive symptoms as compared with PD patients without. Other studies have found an association between depressive symptoms and increased dopamine transporter availability [17, 18]. These inconsistencies might be due to methodological heterogeneities among studies and/or to the finding that striatal dopaminergic dysfunction in PD may be itself heterogeneous, related with some depressive symptoms but not all [19]. Apart from such discrepancies, these results confirm the pivotal role exerted by dopaminergic pathways in the occurrence of depression in PD.

In addition to dopamine, other monoamines seem to have a role in the pathogenesis of depression in PD. In a recent positron emission tomography (PET) study, serotonin transporter binding was found increased in PD patients with depressive symptoms in limbic structures and caudal raphe nuclei, suggesting a lower serotonin availability [20]. Accordingly, another study, using transcranial sonography, has shown reduced echogenicity of the dorsal raphe in subjects with depression preceding PD motor onset [21]. Finally, in regard to noradrenergic contribution, another PET study found loss of dopamine and noradrenaline innervations in the locus coeruleus and in limbic areas in depressed PD patients [22], and, consistently, a neuropathological study demonstrated neuronal loss and gliosis in the noradrenergic locus coeruleus [23].

In line with this model of dysfunctional monoamine pathways projecting to cortical areas, altered brain metabolism or blood flow in the frontal cortex has been associated with depression in PD [24–27]. Accordingly, structural neuroimaging techniques have shown gray matter loss and white matter abnormalities in the prefrontal, temporal, and some limbic regions in depressed PD patients [28, 29]. Finally a very recent resting-state functional magnetic resonance study (RS fMRI) revealed reduced functional connectivity in the prefrontal-limbic network in PD patients with depression as compared with PD patients without [30].

Epidemiology

Depressive disorders are common in PD and may even precede the diagnosis of PD in up to 30 % of patients [31–33]. In addition, subjects with depression were found to be 3.14 times more likely to develop PD [34]. Estimates of prevalence of depression in PD vary considerably in published studies mostly due to the heterogeneity of population included and to the criteria used for defining depression in PD (e.g., DSM-IV criteria, clinical rating scales, etc.). In a large systematic review of the prevalence of depression in PD including 36 studies, the weighted prevalence of major depressive disorder was 17 %, minor depression 22 %, dysthymia 13 %, and clinically significant depression 35 % [35]. Prevalence of depressive symptoms and of major depression of more recent studies is reported in Table 1.2. Depressive disorders in PD patients as well as in the general population develop in the context of multiple interacting risk factors. PD-specific risk factors for depression include more severe motor symptoms, greater PD-related disability, more advanced disease stage, longer disease duration, higher levodopa equivalent dosage, presence of hallucinations, cognitive impairment, sleep disorders, and dysautonomia [44–48]. In addition, older age, longer duration, and increased severity of PD were found to contribute to care dependency in patients with untreated depression [49].

A recent cross-sectional study, aimed at building a model for risk factors of depression in PD, found that three PD-specific factors (longer disease duration, more severe motor symptoms, levodopa use) and six nonspecific factors (female gender,

Table 1.2 Frequency rates of depressive symptoms/depression in PD [36–43]

Study	Population	Depressive symptom frequency (%)	Major depression frequency (%)	Scale/criteria used for assessing depressive symptoms/depression
Barone et al. (2007) [36]	1,023 PD patients	27.8	9.2	BDI, HAM/DSM IV
Farabaugh et al. (2009) [37]	158 PD patients	58	NA	HANDS
Riedel et al. (2010) [38]	1,449 PD patients	33.6	NA	MADRS
Inoue et al. (2010) [39]	105 PD patients	38	4.7	BDI/DSM IV
Nègre-Pagès et al. (2010) [40]	450 PD patients	40	NA	HADS
van der Hoek et al. (2011) [41]	256 PD patients	36.3	12.9	BDI
Yamanishi et al. (2013) [42]	117 PD patients	56	NA	BDI
Weerkamp et al. (2013) [43]	73 nursing home residents with PD	45	NA	BDI

BDI Beck Depression Inventory, *HAM* Hamilton Depression Rating scale, *DSM IV* Diagnostic and Statistical Manual of Mental Disorders 4th edition, *NA* not assessed, *HANDS* Harvard Department of Psychiatry/National Depression Screening Day Scale, *MADRS* Montgomery-Asberg Depression Rating Scale, *HADS* Hospital Anxiety and Depression Scale

personal or family history of depression, worse disability, and more affected cognition) were significantly associated with depression; interestingly, nonspecific factors were more strongly related to depression than PD-specific factors [50].

Assessment Tools

In clinical practice, the use of depressive symptom rating scales can improve identification of depression in parkinsonian patients without substituting clinical criteria [51]. Clinician-rated depression scales such as the 24-item and 17-item Hamilton Depression Rating Scale (HAM-D), the Montgomery-Asberg Depression Rating Scale (MADRS), and item depression of the Unified Parkinson's Disease Rating Scale (UPDRS) and self-reported scales such as the Beck Depression Inventory (BDI) and 30-item and 15-item Geriatric Depression Scale (GDS) are considered to be valid in PD [52–64].

Recently, the Patients Health Questionnaire-9 has shown to be an adequate instrument for screening depression in PD [65, 66].

A recent study compared the performance of six self-reported (BDI-II, GDS-30, Center for Epidemiologic Studies Depression Rating Scale-Revised, Inventory of Depressive Symptoms Self Report (IDS-SR), PHQ-9, part I of UPDRS) and three clinician-rated (HAMD-17, Inventory of Depressive Symptomatology-Clinician-Rated, and MADRS) depression scales in community-based parkinsonian patients against psychiatric diagnosis based on DSM-IV-TR criteria [51]. The finding revealed that all self-reported scales, mainly BDI-II, and clinician-rated scales had strong psychometric properties and thus may be useful for depression screening with their cutoff. The study also provided information about the time needed to complete self-report depression scales in PD, and therefore it is a useful guide for the clinician to choose the most appropriate depression rating scale [51].

PD Nonmotor-Associated Features

There is controversy about the relationship between depression and cognitive dysfunctions in PD patients. Three possible patterns emerge: (1) depression influences cognition in PD, in this case depression would influence the severity of cognitive impairment [44, 67–76]; (2) depression and cognition are independent, although many symptoms of the two conditions might overlap in PD [31, 77–80]; and (3) cognitive dysfunctions, that are related to PD neuropathology, are the substrate of a depressive disorder in PD, in this case a distinct pattern of cognitive impairment (quality) would be associated with depression.

The relationship between depression and executive dysfunctions is generally considered as depression affecting severity of cognition. However, frontal dysfunctions related to neuropathology of PD might be responsible for depressive symptoms, especially considering that DSM-IV criteria for major depression diagnosis do not separate anhedonia from apathy. Santangelo et al. [81] found that depressed PD patients with high level of apathy and/or anhedonia scored significantly lower on frontal tasks than patients with depressed mood (DSM-IV, criterion 1) and nondepressed patients. These findings suggest that the combination of apathy, anhedonia, and frontal lobe dysfunctions might contribute to the overdiagnosis of depression in PD. Varanese et al. [82] found that apathy was not associated with executive impairment in PD patients. These findings support the idea that apathy and depression are two independent nonmotor symptoms of PD.

Management

Treatment options for depressive symptoms in PD should be based on the specific characteristics of the patient. The first step should include a review of all drugs taken by the patient in order to identify and possibly eliminate those medications that could contribute to affective symptoms; then, the optimization of dopaminergic treatment should be considered, since this strategy is often effective in cases of subthreshold (e.g., "off"-related nonmotor fluctuations including depression) and mild depression. In regard to dopaminergic treatment, a number of open-label studies have suggested that both pramipexole and ropinirole exert antidepressant effect in PD patients [83–86]. A recent large 12-week randomized, double-blind, placebo-controlled study in PD, enrolling patients with depressive symptoms (15-item GDS score ≥ 5 or UPDRS Part I depression item score ≥ 2), compared pramipexole (0.375–3 mg/day, $N=139$) and placebo ($N=148$) and showed that pramipexole significantly improved BDI scores ($p=0.01$) and UPDRS motor scores ($p=0.003$); statistical analysis, adjusting for UPDRS, suggested a direct effect of pramipexole on depression [87]. A randomized, placebo-controlled, double-blind study of ropinirole extended-release preparation [88] also showed improvement on BDI scores as compared to placebo; nevertheless, the primary outcomes of this study were motor fluctuations; therefore, patients were not selected according to criteria for depression. Similarly, a double-blind, randomized, placebo-controlled study aimed at assessing rotigotine efficacy on early motor dysfunction and sleep problems in PD [89] found, as additional efficacy outcome, greater improvement with rotigotine than placebo on BDI-II scores and on mood/cognition domain score of nonmotor symptoms scale (NMS).

The evidence-based data regarding the therapeutic efficacy of antidepressants for treating depression in PD are still equivocal. A systematic review and meta-analysis of ten studies showed uncertainty and lack of strong evidence supporting the clinical efficacy of selective serotonin reuptake inhibitors (SSRIs) for depression in PD [90]. A successive evidence-based review concluded that tricyclic antidepressants (TCA) are likely efficacious and possibly useful; nevertheless side effects are common [91]. Recently, a large randomized, double-blind, placebo-controlled trial of antidepressants in PD has provided Class I evidence that both paroxetine (SSRI) and venlafaxine (a serotonin and norepinephrine reuptake inhibitor, SNRI) significantly improve depression in subjects with PD without worsening motor function [92]. Double-blind, placebo-controlled studies of antidepressant drugs in PD are summarized in Table 1.3.

Non-pharmacological interventions for depression in PD include cognitive behavior therapy (CBT) and repetitive transcranial magnetic stimulation (rTMS). The largest study on CBT for depression in PD was a 10-week randomized controlled trial of 80 patients that showed significant improvement in the treated group as compared with the control group [98]. rTMS has been proposed as a technique to improve mood in PD, but results are still preliminary and potentially confounded by the possible effect on motor and cognitive function. A double-blind sham-controlled study of the left prefrontal rTMS showed significant improvement on depression scales [99]. In double-blind studies, comparing dorsolateral prefrontal cortex (DLPFC) rTMS and fluoxetine (using placebo and sham rTMS, respectively), both interventions resulted comparably efficacious in improving depressive symptoms [100, 101].

Table 1.3 Antidepressants in PD: double-blind, placebo-controlled studies [92–97]

Study	*N*	Drug	Daily dose (mg)	Results	Worsening parkinsonism
Wermuth et al. (1998) [93]	18/19	Citalopram/placebo	10	Citalopram = placebo	No
Leentjens et al. (2003) [94]	6/6	Sertraline/placebo	50	Sertraline = placebo	No
Weintraub et al. (2010) [95]	28/27	Atomoxetine/placebo	80	Atomoxetine = placebo	No
Devos et al. (2008) [96]	16/15/17	Desimipramine/citalopram/placebo	75	Improvement for both drugs	No
			20		
Menza et al. (2009) [97]	18/17/17	Paroxetine/nortriptyline/placebo	37.5	Improvements for nortriptyline but not for paroxetine	No
			75		
Richard et al. (2012) [92]	42/34/39	Paroxetine/venlafaxine/placebo	40	Improvement for both drugs	No
			225		

Apathy in PD

Definition and Pathophysiology

Definition

Apathy refers to a combination of behavioral, emotional, and cognitive features that originate from reduced interest/motivation in goal-directed behaviors and from lack of emotional responsiveness. The clinical picture of apathy is characterized by loss of self-activation or self-initiated behavior, indifference, impassibility, and flattened affect.

Apathy is one of the most common nonmotor symptoms in PD, occurring since early stages of disease, and increasing in frequency as the disease progresses (see section "Epidemiology"). It has been associated with decreased quality of life and poor performances on activity of daily living [102]. The diagnosis of apathy in PD is challenging since it is commonly associated with disorders such as depression, cognitive impairment, and fatigue; in addition, many features of such disorders overlap with symptoms of apathy.

Recently two sets of diagnostic criteria have been validated in PD [103, 104]. The criteria used in these two studies are similar and include: (1) diminished motivation compared to baseline level of functioning; (2) reduction of goal-directed behavior, goal-directed cognitive activity, and emotion; (3) symptoms sufficiently severe to cause significant impairment of personal, social, or occupational function; and (4) symptoms not attributable to the effects of physical disability, level of consciousness, or medication.

Pathophysiology

The pathophysiological mechanism underlying apathy in PD is still not fully understood. Apathy is probably related with a dysfunction in the mesocorticolimbic circuit including the ventral striatum, anterior and posterior cingulate (AC, PC), and inferior prefrontal gyrus since these structures are key components of the brain motivational and reward system [105]. Recently, a morphological magnetic resonance imaging (MRI) study on 55 PD patients [106] showed that high apathy scores were correlated with low gray matter (GM) density in the right PC gyrus and the bilateral inferior frontal gyrus; based on the involvement of the cingulate and premotor cortices, the authors suggested that "autoactivation" processing deficits could be associated with apathy in PD. Consistently, in an 11C-raclopride PET study, apathy scores after deep brain stimulation of the subthalamic nucleus (STN-DBS) in PD patients correlated with a decreased dopamine transmission particularly in the dorsolateral and orbitofrontal cortex, AC and PC [107], suggesting that apathy in PD would be underlied by greater mesocorticolimbic dopaminergic denervation. The involvement of mesocorticolimbic networks in apathy has been further corroborated by a recent fluorodeoxyglucose PET study on 45 PD patients neither depressed nor demented [108]; in addition, this study found a negative correlation between metabolism within the bilateral posterior lobe of the cerebellum and apathy scores on AES, supporting the view of a topographic segmentation of the cerebellum, with some structures implicated in motivation and behavioral regulation. Finally, further evidence suggesting that mesocorticolimbic dopaminergic denervation would have a key role in the pathogenesis of apathy derived from studies on DBS in PD patients. STN-DBS can induce or worsen apathy in some parkinsonian patients [107, 109]: reduction of dopaminergic agents and/or stimulation of the associative and limbic regions has been proposed as mechanisms underlying apathy after surgery [110].

Epidemiology

Apathy is one of the most common nonmotor symptoms of PD, with prevalence rates ranging from 13.9 to 70 % and a mean prevalence of 35 % (for a recent review see Santangelo et al. [111]). Several factors may contribute to variable prevalence rates found across studies. First, apathy frequently occurs with depression and with cognitive impairment, particularly dysexecutive syndromes; thus, studies not excluding depression and/or dementia could overestimate its frequency. Second, apathy rate can vary based on the PD population studied (e.g., community sample versus tertiary movement disorders clinic sample). Finally, apathy frequency might be biased by the different tools used for diagnosis (e.g., specific, nonspecific scales, clinical criteria, etc.).

Apathy is common in PD since early stages. Recently, Pedersen and colleagues [112] reported an apathy prevalence rate of 22.9 % in 175 newly diagnosed PD patients with a prevalence of "pure apathy" (i.e., apathy without comorbid depression and dementia) of 14.3 %.

In regard to the mutual relationship among apathy, motor symptoms, and nonmotor symptoms in PD, a recent 4-year longitudinal study showed that at follow-up, apathetic PD patients were more frequently depressed and demented than never-apathetic patients; moreover, dementia at baseline and a more rapid decline in speech and axial symptoms during follow-up were independent risk factors for incident apathy [113] (see also section "PD nonmotor-associated features"). Finally, two recent studies found that patients with right predominant PD motor laterality were at higher risk of suffering from apathy as compared with those with left predominant motor symptoms [114, 115].

Assessment Tools

In clinical practice and research, several rating scales are available to identify and measure severity of apathy in PD patients. Among questionnaires, Apathy Evaluation Scale (AES) [116], Apathy Scale (AS) [117], Lille Apathy Rating Scale (LARS) [118],

Apathy Inventory (AI) [119], Item 7 of the Neuropsychiatric Inventory (NPI) [120], and Item 4 (motivation/initiative) of the UPDRS [121] can be used in PD patients.

Recently, a task force commissioned by the Movement Disorders Society (MDS) [122] reviewed the psychometric properties of the abovementioned scales and reported that both AS and apathy items of UPDRS fulfilled criteria for "recommended scale" for screening apathy, but Item 4 of the UPDRS can be only used as a screening question with caution because it consists of a single item [52]. The AES has good internal consistency [123], and it has been classified as "suggested scale" because only information on reliability but not on validity is now available. The AI has been poorly studied, and it has been classified as "listed scale"; its brevity may make it an attractive and useful instrument to measure apathy in PD. The LARS was developed for PD patients; it has good internal consistency, adequate test-retest, inter-rater reliability, good sensitivity, and specificity in PD population [124]. It is the longest of the all available apathy rating scales, and it was classified as a "suggested scale" by MDS review. The Item 7 of the NPI showed good inter-rater agreement, but other clinimetric properties were not investigated in PD; therefore, it can be considered as a "suggested scale."

PD Nonmotor-Associated Features

Three prospective studies found a close relationship between cognitive dysfunction and apathy. In particular, dementia [113] and reduced inhibitory control assessed by means of Stroop Test [125] were found to be independent risk factors for incident apathy, whereas apathy may be a predictive factor for cognitive decline over time in non-demented, nondepressed PD patients [126]. The association between apathy and executive/frontal dysfunction is consistently found in PD patients at early and advanced stages of disease [82, 112, 117, 123, 125, 127–129]. Few studies investigated other cognitive domains such as memory and visuospatial functions in apathetic PD patients yielding discordant results: some authors found that apathetic patients performed worse than non-apathetic patients on the memory subtest of the Cambridge Cognitive Examination (CAMCOG) [123], on Grober and Buschke 16-item recall test [126], and on paired associative learning test [117], silhouette recognition task [112], and praxis subtest of CAMCOG [123]. Other studies did not find similar results [128]. A recent study showed a significant association between the apathy and affective component of Theory of Mind (ToM) [130], which is the ability of processing inferences about other people's emotions and feelings.

Management

There are no approved drugs for managing apathy. Since apathy is closely related to depression and cognitive impairment, first, possible comorbid depression should be treated in patients with apathy. Because of the association with depression and cognitive impairment, pharmacologic agents most frequently administered to apathetic patients include dopaminergic drugs and acetylcholinesterase inhibitors.

Previous small open-label trials have suggested that dopaminergic agents could be effective in improving apathy in PD patients [131, 132]. A recent meta-analysis of seven randomized, double-blind, placebo-controlled trials of pramipexole, using the UPDRS Part I as a secondary outcome measure, showed that patients who had a baseline UPDRS Part I Item 4 score >0 (motivation, $N=570$), motivational symptoms improved in 63.2 % of patients taking pramipexole compared to 45.0 % of those taking placebo (weighted OR 2.06; $p<0.001$) [133]. Very recently, in a post hoc analysis of RECOVER study ($N=287$), Chaudhuri and collaborators [134] found significant improvement from baseline on apathy items of NMSS ("lost interest in surroundings," "lost interest in doing things") in the rotigotine group as compared with the placebo group. In addition, in a randomized, placebo-controlled trial ($N=37$, PD patients treated with STN-DBS), Thobois and collaborators [135] found that the dopamine agonist piribedil is effective in treating apathy.

Apart from dopaminergic agents, a randomized controlled trial evaluating efficacy of atomoxetine, a selective norepinephrine reuptake inhibitor, for treatment of clinically significant depressive symptoms in PD patients and with apathy as a secondary outcome measure, showed no benefit for either depression or apathy [95].

In regard to acetylcholinesterase inhibitors, an open-label controlled study of galantamine ($N=41$) in PD patients with dementia found significant improvement in the primary cognitive outcome measures but also in the apathy section of the NPI ($p=0.006$) [136]. Nevertheless, a subsequent double-blind, placebo-controlled study in nondemented PD subjects ($N=54$) designed to assess cognitive improvement as primary outcome did not find significant difference in apathy measures [137].

Finally, two ongoing randomized, placebo-controlled trials are evaluating efficacy of acetylcholinesterase (rivastigmine) [ClinicalTrials. gov identifier: NCT00767091; http://clinicaltrials.gov/ct2/show/NCT00767091] and MAO-B inhibitors (rasagiline) [ClinicalTrials.gov identifier: NCT00755027; http://clinicaltrials.gov/ct2/show/NCT00755027] on apathetic symptoms in PD patients.

Anhedonia in PD

Definition and Pathophysiology

Definition

Anhedonia is defined as a lowered ability to experience physical and social pleasure. It is recognized to be a core symptom of major depression [10] and is frequent in several psychiatric diseases including abstinence/intoxication with substances of abuse and schizophrenia [138, 139].

Anhedonia includes two types of pleasure deficits: anticipatory and consummatory [140]. Anticipatory anhedonia refers to the inability to experience pleasure at the thought of a future reward ("wanting"), whereas consummatory anhedonia reflects the inability to experience pleasure while the subject is engaged in an enjoyable experience ("liking").

In PD anhedonia has been seen as a symptom that can be part of various syndromes, such as depression, dementia, or apathy [122, 141]. To date, anhedonia in PD lacks an unambiguous and generally accepted definition, and its identification is based on specific rating scales (see section "Assessment tools"). Recent studies [142, 143] suggest that PD patients may have intact "consummatory" pleasure and altered "anticipatory" pleasure that has been frequently found associated with apathy.

Pathophysiology

Some recent studies have suggested that distinct neural networks would be involved in anticipatory and consummatory anhedonia in PD; the former type might be underlied by a dysfunction in the dopaminergic mesolimbic system including the ventral striatum and anterior cingulate cortex [22], whereas the latter one might be associated with alteration in the dopaminergic prefrontal cortex circuits [142, 144]. It is worth noting that the neural circuit involved in anticipatory anhedonia is the same that has been linked to apathy (see section "Pathophysiology of apathy") maybe suggesting that anticipatory anhedonia could be a symptom of apathy (reduced "wanting").

Epidemiology

Anhedonia is common in PD with a prevalence ranging from 15 % up to 79.7 % in PD patients with depression [84, 145–148]. As for depression and apathy, most prevalence differences across studies depend on methodological issues (e.g., tool and cutoff used for defining anhedonia, overlapping with other neuropsychiatric disorders, type of PD population studied).

Most studies conducted in PD patients [81, 84, 142–145, 147, 148] with the exception of one [146] suggest a significant relationship between anhedonia and other neuropsychiatric symptoms, namely, depression, apathy, and, to a less extent, cognitive dysfunction (see section "PD nonmotor-associated features").

In regard to the possible relationship between anhedonia and motor symptom severity, some studies reported an association [84, 145] and others did not [144, 146]; this inconsistency might be due to the different PD stages of the population included in these studies.

Assessment Tools

The identification of anhedonia is difficult since it may occur on its own or as part both of depression and apathetic syndrome [122]. However, in clinical practice and research, the clinician may use several questionnaires developed for measuring severity of anhedonia in patients with psychiatric diseases. The Chapman Scales for Physical and Social Anhedonia were used in one study on PD patients and were considered to have several shortcomings for this type of patients: the scales include items characterized by a very complex syntactic structure and were too long for patients with bradyphrenia [146]. Moreover, their clinimetric properties have not been fully investigated. The Chapman Scales were classified as listed by MDS task force [122]. To provide a short scale validated and easily applicable in clinical setting, Santangelo et al. [144] explored the clinimetric properties of the Snaith-Hamilton Pleasure Scale (SHAPS) and found it to be a reliable tool to evaluate apathy in patients with PD and other forms of parkinsonism. More recently, the psychometric properties of the Japanese version of SHAPS were also investigated [149].

PD Nonmotor-Associated Features

Several studies evidenced a strong association between anhedonia and apathetic or depressive syndromes in PD patients, indicating that reduced hedonic tone may be considered a feature of apathy [123] and of depression [81, 84, 145, 147]. Conversely, Isella et al. [146] did not find relationship between anhedonia, depression, and apathy. Increasing age, apathy, and cognitive dysfunctions were found contributing factors to anhedonia severity [144]. Recently, significant association between apathy and anxiety trait was reported [148].

As for association between anhedonia and cognitive deficits, one study on a small sample of PD patients revealed no significant correlation between anhedonia and score on frontal tasks [146]. Otherwise, Santangelo et al. [81] reported that patients with anhedonia performed worse than nondepressed patients without apathy or anhedonia on cognitive tasks tapping visuoconstructional and frontal functions. In addition, significant correlations were found between anhedonia and score on Frontal Assessment Battery (FAB) in patients with PD and other forms of parkinsonism [144]. The relationship between anhedonia and frontal dysfunctions might support the idea that anhedonia may depend on frontal lobe dysfunctions arising from alteration of prefrontal dopamine circuits.

Management

A number of open-label studies suggest that dopaminergic agents may be effective in improving hedonic tone (for a recent review see Assogna et al. [141]). Most trials focused on pramipexole may be due to its preferential action on D_3 dopaminergic receptors in the mesolimbic and prefrontal neural circuits; overall, such studies [84, 145, 147, 150] found that pramipexole was effective on depression, anhedonia, and motor symptoms. In particular, Reichmann and collaborators [150] found that PD patients switched from other dopamine agonists to pramipexole had a significant improvement on depression and anhedonia thus suggesting that such beneficial effects would not be simply reactive responses to motor improvement but specific effects of the treatment. Nevertheless, since these studies were open label, further randomized, double-blind, placebo-controlled trials are needed to confirm these results.

Finally, very recently, in a post hoc analysis of RECOVER study ($N=287$), Chaudhuri and collaborators [134] found significant improvement from baseline on the anhedonia item of NMSS ("difficulty experiencing pleasure") in the rotigotine group as compared with the placebo group.

Fatigue in PD

Definition and Pathophysiology

Definition

Fatigue has been commonly defined as an overwhelming sense of tiredness, lack of energy, and feeling of exhaustion. It is characterized by difficulty in initiating and sustaining mental and physical activities. Despite fatigue is one of the most common and disabling symptoms in neurological disorders, its identification and understanding is hampered by the lack of standard definition [151].

Fatigue is common in PD (see section "Epidemiology"). Although several features of fatigue in PD have been described, it is still unclear whether fatigue can be considered either a motor or nonmotor symptom [152]. Its identification is challenging due to the overlap with other common symptoms of PD like depression, apathy, sleep problems, and autonomic dysfunction. In addition, the presence of different components of fatigue (mental, physical) further complicates its recognition. Based on the fact that PD patients generally describe their fatigue as different from the fatigue, they had experienced prior PD onset, and Brown et al. [153] proposed an operational definition of fatigue in PD as a "feeling of abnormal and overwhelming tiredness and lack of energy, distinct both qualitatively and quantitatively from normal tiredness." To date, identification of fatigue in PD is based on specific rating scales (see section "Assessment tools").

Pathophysiology

The pathophysiology of fatigue in PD is still poorly understood [154]. Fatigue is commonly subdivided into a peripheral and a central component; peripheral fatigue is commonly observed in diseases involving the peripheral nervous system like myasthenia gravis, whereas central fatigue is frequently observed in several chronic diseases of the central nervous system including PD. Several findings suggest that fatigue in PD might have a minor peripheral contribution and a major component underlied by central mechanisms [154]. It is worth noting that central fatigue features in PD may overlap with a number of nonmotor symptoms like depression, apathy, and sleep problems thus complicating the understanding of its pathophysiology. Few neuroimaging studies have addressed the pathophysiological mechanisms of central fatigue. By means of a single-photon emission computed tomography (SPECT) study, Abe and collaborators [155] reported that fatigue in PD correlated with reduced cerebral blood flow in the frontal lobe in absence of significant correlation between fatigue and depression. More recently, a PET study aimed at evaluating the dopaminergic and serotonergic contribution to fatigue in PD [156] showed that fatigue was mainly associated with denervation of serotonergic terminals in both dorsal and ventral striatum and in the thalamus; furthermore fatigue was associated with reduced dopaminergic transmission in the extra-striatal region, namely, the insula. Taken together these results could suggest that fatigue in PD would be associated with dysfunction in striatal serotonergic and extra-striatal dopaminergic neural circuits and in their projections to the frontal lobe.

Finally, fatigue in PD has been associated with abnormal primary motor cortex excitability [157], suggesting that altered cortical plasticity might be responsible for physical fatigue that would share both clinical features and pathophysiological mechanisms with bradykinesia and sequence effect.

Epidemiology

Fatigue in PD is a frequent symptom with a prevalence rate ranging from 28 to 77.6 % (Table 1.4). Most variability on frequency rates is due to methodological issues (e.g., different assessment tools, overlap with other PD symptoms, PD population studied). Fatigue can be present in every stage of disease and even may antecede the onset of motor symptoms in approximately one third of patients [164]. Fatigue has been identified as one of the most disabling symptoms in PD and has been found as an important determinant of worse quality of life [165].

Several factors have been variably associated with fatigue: female gender, postural instability gait difficulties (PIGD) phenotype, and many nonmotor symptoms like depression, anxiety, apathy, sleep disturbances, and autonomic impairment [163–165]. In addition, fatigue has been associated with reduced physical activity [166], though it is still not clear whether fatigue determines reduced physical activity or a sedentary lifestyle can favor the onset of fatigue.

Finally, available data in literature do not allow to find a definite relationship between fatigue and disease severity due to the controversial results.

Assessment Tools

Since fatigue has a multidimensional character, it is difficult to measure [167]. In clinical setting, it is possible to use several questionnaires from those generic which evaluate fatigue in a holistic manner to those specifically designed for PD [168].

Table 1.4 Frequency rates of fatigue in PD [158–163]

Study	Population	Fatigue frequency	Scale used for assessing fatigue
Friedman and Friedman (1993) [158]	58 PD patients	67 %	Fatigue severity questionnaire
Karlsen et al. (1999) [159]	233 PD patients	44.2 %	Rating scale for low energy in the NHP, 7-point scale devised to evaluate fatigue
Herlofson and Larsen (2003) [160]	66 PD patients	50 %	Fatigue severity scale
Alves et al. (2004) [161]	233 PD patients followed over a period of 8 years (from 1993 to 2001)	35.7 % at baseline 55.7 % at last follow-up	Rating scale for low energy in the NHP, 7-point scale devised to evaluate fatigue, fatigue severity scale
Skorvanek et al. (2013) [162]	165 PD patients	77.6 %	Multidimensional fatigue inventory
Beiske et al. (2013) [163]	176 PD patients	28 %	Fatigue questionnaire

NHP Nottingham Health Profile

Recently, a task force commissioned by MDS revealed that only four scales are recommended to use for PD patients [169]: the Fatigue Severity Scale (FSS) [170], the PD-specific 16-item Parkinson Fatigue Scale (PFS-16) [153], the Functional Assessment of Chronic Illness Therapy-Fatigue Scale (FACIT-F) [171], and the Multidimensional Fatigue Inventory (MFI) [172].

The FSS includes physical and mental aspects of fatigue, was validated for PD populations, and is useful to screen and measure severity of fatigue [169, 173].

The PFS-16 is the first specific scale for measuring fatigue in PD. This scale evaluates only physical aspects of fatigue and has very good internal consistency and discriminant and convergent validity [174].

The FACIT-F was designed for assessing anemia-associated fatigue in oncological patients; it seems to be able to discriminate between fatigued and non-fatigued PD patients [173] and shows promise in PD as reported in a recent systematic review of measurement properties of self-report fatigue questionnaires [175].

The MFI was recently validated in PD and is reliable and valid to assess fatigue [176].

More recently, other questionnaires have been investigated. The Fatigue Impact Scale for Daily Use (D-FIS) [177] is a unidimensional scale of fatigue impact, and it was validated in PD; its psychometric properties were good: it showed adequate internal consistency and no floor and ceiling effect [178]. The Modified Fatigue Impact Scale (MFIS) was validated in PD patients without dementia: it showed high internal consistency, strong convergent validity, and adequate divergent validity [179].

In conclusion, although fatigue is a nonmotor symptom reducing quality of life in PD at several stages of disease, until now no multidimensional questionnaire was validated in PD. Future studies should investigate specific aspects of fatigue in PD to allow the development of questionnaires that reflect both generic and PD-specific symptoms of fatigue.

PD Nonmotor-Associated Features

Several studies reported a relationship of fatigue with depression [158, 159, 180, 181], whereas others found high level of fatigue in nondepressed PD patients [161, 182]. Fatigue is associated with anxiety (both trait and state) [164, 183] and with sleep disorders [184]. However, some studies revealed that fatigue could not be attributable to excessive daytime sleepiness or poor sleep [164]. In a study, fatigue was related to cardiovascular sympathetic dysfunctions and with orthostatic hypotension [185]. The abovementioned associations might suggest that fatigue in PD is a nonmotor symptom. Finally fatigue was found to be associated with poor decision making evaluated by Iowa Gambling Task [186], with high level of apathy [182, 187] and to reduce quality of life in PD patients as evidenced in several studies [160, 182, 188]. More recently, fatigue was investigated in drug-naïve PD patient and was found to be associated with high level of depression and difficulties with activities of daily living (ADL) [189].

Management

Management of fatigue in PD is often complicated by the coexistence of several contributing factors like depression, anxiety, sleep disorders, and autonomic dysfunction; thus, the first treatment option should be identifying and possibly treating such symptoms.

In regard to medications with a specific action on fatigue in PD, most studies have evaluated the effect of dopaminergic drugs. Previous studies have suggested beneficial effect of levodopa and pergolide [190, 191]. More recently, methylphenidate, a dopamine transporter blocker, at a dose of 10 mg three times a day, has been found to be effective in improving fatigue in a randomized, placebo-controlled study ($N=36$) [192]. In addition, in a post hoc analysis of RECOVER study ($N=287$), Chaudhuri and collaborators [134] found significant improvement from baseline on the fatigue item of NMSS ("fatigue or lack of energy") in the rotigotine group as compared with the placebo group, though such benefit was associated with improvement also on depression, apathy, and anhedonia not allowing to support a specific action of rotigotine on fatigue. Finally, a sub-study of ADAGIO ($N=1105$) has shown that rasagiline was associated with significantly less progression of fatigue compared with placebo over a 9-month period [193].

References

1. Kuhn W, Heye N, Muller TH, et al. The motor performance test series in Parkinson's disease is influenced by depression. J Neural Transm. 1996;103:349–54.
2. Weintraub D, Moberg PJ, Duda JE, Katz IR, Stern MB. Effect of psychiatric and other non-motor symptoms on disability in Parkinson's disease. J Am Ger Soc. 2004;52:784–8.
3. Schrag A, Jahanshahi M, Quinn N. What contributes to quality of life in patients with Parkinson's disease? J Neurol Neurosurg Psychiatry. 2000;69:308–12.
4. Global Parkinson's Disease Survey Steering Committee. Factors impacting on quality of life in Parkinson's disease: results from an international study. Mov Disord. 2002;17:60–7.
5. Leentjens AF. Depression in Parkinson's disease: conceptual issues and clinical challenges. J Geriatr Psychiatry Neurol. 2004;17:120–6.
6. Kummer A, Cardoso F, Teixeira AL. Suicidal ideation in Parkinson's disease. CNS Spectr. 2009;14:431–6.
7. Marsh L, McDonald WM, Cummings J, Ravina B. Provisional diagnostic criteria for depression in Parkinson's disease: report of an NINDS/NIMH Work Group. Mov Disord. 2006;21:148–58.
8. Starkstein SE, Merello M, Jorge R, Brockman S, Bruce D, Petracca G, Robinson RG. A validation study of depressive syndromes in Parkinson's disease. Mov Disord. 2008;23:538–46.
9. Chen JJ, Marsh L. Depression in Parkinson's disease: identification and management. Pharmacotherapy. 2013;33:972–83.
10. American Psychiatric Association. Diagnostic and statistical manual of mental disorder. 4th ed. Washington: American Psychiatry Association; 1994.
11. Leentjens AF, Van den Akker M, Metsemakers JF, Lousberg R, Verhey FR. Higher incidence of depression preceding the onset of Parkinson's disease: a register study. Mov Disord. 2003;18:414–8.
12. Ehmann TS, Beninger RJ, Gawel MJ, Riopelle RJ. Depressive symptoms in Parkinson's disease: a comparison with disabled control subjects. J Geriatr Psychiatry Neurol. 1990;3:3–9.
13. Brooks DJ, Piccini P. Imaging in Parkinson's disease: the role of monoamines in behavior. Biol Psychiatry. 2006;59:908–18.
14. Eskow Jaunarajs KL, Angoa-Perez M, Kuhn DM, Bishop C. Potential mechanisms underlying anxiety and depression in Parkinson's disease: consequences of L-DOPA treatment. Neurosci Biobehav Rev. 2011;35:556–64.
15. Hesse S, Meyer PM, Strecker K, Barthel H, Wegner F, Oehlwein C, et al. Monoamine transporter availability in Parkinson's disease patients with or without depression. Eur J Nucl Med Mol Imaging. 2009;36:428–35.
16. Weintraub D, Newberg AB, Cary MS, Siderowf AD, Moberg PJ, Kleiner-Fisman G, et al. Striatal dopamine transporter imaging correlates with anxiety and depression symptoms in Parkinson's disease. J Nucl Med. 2005;46:227–32.
17. Felicio AC, Moriyama TS, Godeiro-Junior C, Shih MC, Hoexter MQ, Borges V, et al. Higher dopamine transporter density in Parkinson's disease patients with depression. Psychopharmacology (Berl). 2010;211:27–31.
18. Ceravolo R, Frosini D, Poletti M, Kiferle L, Pagni C, Mazzucchi S, Volterrani D, Bonuccelli U. Mild affective symptoms in de novo Parkinson's disease patients: relationship with dopaminergic dysfunction. Eur J Neurol. 2013;20:480–5.
19. Koerts J, Leenders KL, Koning M, Portman AT, van Beilen M. Striatal dopaminergic activity (FDOPA-PET) associated with cognitive items of a depression scale (MADRS) in Parkinson's disease. Eur J Neurosci. 2007;25:3132–6.
20. Politis M, Wu K, Loane C, Turkheimer FE, Molloy S, Brooks DJ, et al. Depressive symptoms in PD correlate with higher 5-HTT binding in raphe and limbic structures. Neurology. 2010;75:1920–7.

21. Walter U, Hoeppner J, Prudente-Morrissey L, et al. Parkinson's disease-like midbrain sonography abnormalities are frequent in depressive disorders. Brain. 2007;130:1799–807.
22. Remy P, Doder M, Lees A, Turjanski N, Brooks D. Depression in Parkinson's disease: loss of dopamine and noradrenaline innervation in the limbic system. Brain. 2005;128:1314–22.
23. Frisina PG, Haroutunian V, Libow LS. The neuropathological basis for depression in Parkinson's disease. Parkinsonism Relat Disord. 2009;15:144–8.
24. Mayberg HS, Starkstein SE, Sadzot B, et al. Selective hypometabolism in the inferior frontal lobe in depressed patients with Parkinson's disease. Ann Neurol. 1990;28:57–64.
25. Ring HA, Bench CJ, Trimble MR, et al. Depression in Parkinson's disease. A positron emission study. Br J Psychiatry. 1994;165:333–9.
26. Cardoso EF, Maia FM, Fregni F, et al. Depression in Parkinson's disease: convergence from voxel-based morphometry and functional magnetic resonance imaging in the limbic thalamus. Neuroimage. 2009;47:467–72.
27. Matsui H, Nishinaka K, Oda M, et al. Minor depression and brain perfusion images in Parkinson's disease. Mov Disord. 2006;21:1169–74.
28. Feldmann A, Illes Z, Kosztolanyi P, et al. Morphometric changes of gray matter in Parkinson's disease with depression: a voxel-based morphometry study. Mov Disord. 2008;23:42–6.
29. Kostic VS, Agosta F, Petrovic I, et al. Regional patterns of brain tissue loss associated with depression in Parkinson disease. Neurology. 2010;75:857–63.
30. Luo C, Chen Q, Song W, Chen K, Guo X, Yang J, Huang X, Gong Q, Shang HF. Resting-state fMRI study on drug-naïve patients with Parkinson's disease and with depression. J Neurol Neurosurg Psychiatry. 2013;260(11):2754–60.
31. Santamaria J, Tolosa E, Valles A. Parkinson's disease with depression: a possible subgroup of idiopathic parkinsonism. Neurology. 1986;36:1130–3.
32. Ishihara L, Brayne C. A systematic review of depression and mental illness preceding Parkinson's disease. Acta Neurol Scand. 2006;113:211–20.
33. Lieberman A. Depression in Parkinson's disease – a review. Acta Neurol Scand. 2006;113:1–8.
34. Shen CC, Tsai SJ, Perng CL, Kuo BI, Yang AC. Risk of Parkinson disease after depression: a nationwide population-based study. Neurology. 2013;81:1538–44.
35. Reijnders JS, Ehrt U, Weber WE, et al. A systematic review of prevalence studies of depression in Parkinson's disease. Mov Disord. 2008;23:183–9.
36. Barone P, et al. Depression and antidepressant use in Parkinson's disease: results from the PRODEST-PD study. Abstract P1122 poster presented at 11th Congress of EFNS, Brussels. 26 Aug 2007.
37. Farabaugh AH, Locascio JJ, Yap L, Weintraub D, McDonald WM, Agoston M, Alpert JE, Growdon J, Fava M. Pattern of depressive symptoms in Parkinson's disease. Psychosomatics. 2009;50:448–54.
38. Riedel O, Klotsche J, Spottke A, et al. Frequency of dementia, depression, and other neuropsychiatric symptoms in 1,449 outpatients with Parkinson's disease. J Neurol. 2010;257:1073–82.
39. Inoue T, Kitagawa M, Tanaka T, Nakagawa S, Koyama T. Depression and major depressive disorder in patients with Parkinson's disease. Mov Disord. 2010;25:44–9.
40. Nègre-Pagès L, Grandjean H, Lapeyre-Mestre M, Montastruc JL, Fourrier A, Lépine JP, Rascol O, DoPaMiP Study Group. Anxious and depressive symptoms in Parkinson's disease: the French cross-sectional DoPaMiP study. Mov Disord. 2010;25:157–66.
41. van der Hoek TC, Bus BA, Matui P, van der Marck MA, Esselink RA, Tendolkar I. Prevalence of depression in Parkinson's disease: effects of disease stage, motor subtype and gender. J Neurol Sci. 2011;310:220–4.
42. Yamanishi T, Tachibana H, Oguru M, Matsui K, Toda K, Okuda B, Oka N. Anxiety and depression in patients with Parkinson's disease. Intern Med. 2013;52:539–45.
43. Weerkamp NJ, Tissingh G, Poels PJ, Zuidema SU, Munneke M, Koopmans RT, Bloem BR. Nonmotor symptoms in nursing home residents with Parkinson's disease: prevalence and effect on quality of life. J Am Geriatr Soc. 2013;61:1714–21.

44. Starkstein SE, Preziosi TJ, Berthier ML, Bolduc PL, Mayberg HS, Robinson RG. Depression and cognitive impairment in Parkinson's disease. Brain. 1989;112:1141–53.
45. Dissanayaka NNW, Sellbach A, Silburn PA, O'Sullivan JD, Marsh R, Mellick GD. Factors associated with depression in Parkinson's disease. J Affect Disord. 2011;132:82–8.
46. Becker C, Brobert GP, Johansson S, Jick SS, Meier CR. Risk of incident depression in patients with Parkinson disease in the UK. Eur J Neurol. 2011;18:448–53.
47. Gallagher DA, Schrag A. Psychosis, apathy, depression and anxiety in Parkinson's disease. Neurobiol Dis. 2012;46:581–9.
48. Riedel O, Heuser I, Klotsche J, Dodel R, Wittchen HU, GEPAD Study Group. Occurrence risk and structure of depression in Parkinson disease with and without dementia: results from the GEPAD Study. J Geriatr Psychiatry Neurol. 2010;23:27–34.
49. Riedel O, Dodel R, Deuschl G, Klotsche J, Förstl H, Heuser I, Oertel W, Reichmann H, Riederer P, Trenkwalder C, Wittchen HU. Depression and care-dependency in Parkinson's disease: results from a nationwide study of 1,449 outpatients. Parkinsonism Relat Disord. 2012;18:598–601.
50. Leentjens AF, Moonen AJ, Dujardin K, Marsh L, Martinez-Martin P, Richard IH, Starkstein SE, Köhler S. Modeling depression in Parkinson disease: disease-specific and nonspecific risk factors. Neurology. 2013;81:1036–43.
51. Williams JR, Hirsch ES, Anderson K, Bush AL, Goldstein SR, Grill S, Lehmann S, Little JT, Margolis RL, Palanci J, Pontone G, Weiss H, Rabins P, Marsh L. A comparison of nine scales to detect depression in Parkinson disease: which scale to use? Neurology. 2012;78:998–1006.
52. Starkstein SE, Merello M. The unified Parkinson's disease rating scale: validation study of the mentation, behavior, and mood section. Mov Disord. 2007;22:2156–61.
53. Hamilton M. A rating scale for depression. J Neurol Neurosurg Psychiatry. 1960;23:56–62.
54. Montgomery SA, Åsberg M. A new depression scale designed to be sensitive to change. Br J Psychiatry. 1979;134:382–9.
55. Leentjens AF, Verhey FR, Lousberg R, Spitsbergen H, Wilmink FW. The validity of the Hamilton and Montgomery-Åsberg depression rating scales as screening and diagnostic tools for depression in Parkinson's disease. Int J Geriatr Psychiatry. 2000;15:644–9.
56. Kroenke K, Spitzer RL, Williams JB. The PHQ-9: validity of a brief depression severity measure. J Gen Intern Med. 2001;16:606–13.
57. Leentjens AF, Verhey FRJ, Luijckx GJ, Troost J. The validity of the Beck Depression Inventory as a screening and diagnostic instrument for depression in patients with Parkinson's disease. Mov Disord. 2000;15:1221–4.
58. Naarding P, Leentjens AFG, van Kooten F, Verhey FRJ. Disease-specific properties of the Hamilton Rating Scale for depression in patients with stroke, Alzheimer's disease, and Parkinson's disease. J Neuropsychiatry Clin Neurosci. 2002;14:329–48.
59. McDonald WM, Holtzheimer PE, Haber M, Vitek JL, McWhorter K, Delong M. Validity of the 30-item geriatric depression scale in patients with Parkinson's disease. Mov Disord. 2006;21:1618–22.
60. Silberman CD, Laks J, Capitao CF, Rodrigues CS, Moreira I, Engelhardt E. Recognizing depression in patients with Parkinson's disease: accuracy and specificity of two depression rating scale. Arq Neuropsiquiatr. 2006;64:407–11.
61. Weintraub D, Oehlberg KA, Katz IR, Stern MB. Test characteristics of the 15-item geriatric depression scale and Hamilton depression rating scale in Parkinson disease. Am J Geriatr Psychiatry. 2006;14:169–75.
62. Yesavage JA, Brink TL, Rose TL, et al. Development and validation of a geriatric depression screening scale: a preliminary report. J Psychiatr Res. 1983;17:37–49.
63. Visser M, Leentjens AF, Marinus J, Stiggelbout AM, van Hilten JJ. Reliability and validity of the Beck depression inventory in patients with Parkinson's disease. Mov Disord. 2006;21:668–72.
64. Ertan T, Kiziltan G, Uygucgil H. Reliability and validity of the Geriatric Depression Scale in depression in Parkinson's disease. J Neurol Neurosurg Psychiatry. 2005;76:1445–7.

65. Thompson AW, Liu H, Hays RD, et al. Diagnostic accuracy and agreement across three depression assessment measures for Parkinson's disease. Parkinsonism Relat Disord. 2011;17:40–5.
66. Chagas MH, Tumas V, Rodrigues GR, Machado-de-Sousa JP, Filho AS, Hallak JE, Crippa JA. Validation and internal consistency of Patient Health Questionnaire-9 for major depression in Parkinson's disease. Age Ageing. 2013;42:645–9.
67. Mayeux R, Stern Y, Rosen J, Leventhal J. Depression, intellectual impairment, and Parkinson disease. Neurology. 1981;31:645–50.
68. Starkstein SE, Bolduc PL, Mayberg HS, et al. Cognitive impairments and depression in Parkinson's disease: a follow up study. J Neurol Neurosurg Psychiatry. 1990;53:597–602.
69. Kuzis G, Sabe L, Tiberti C, Leiguarda R, Starkstein SE. Cognitive functions in major depression and Parkinson disease. Arch Neurol. 1997;54:982–6.
70. Cubo E, Bernard B, Leurgans S, Raman R. Cognitive and motor function in patients with Parkinson's disease with and without depression. Clin Neuropharmacol. 2000;23:331–4.
71. Anguenot A, Loll PY, Neau JP, Ingrand P, Gil R. Depression and Parkinson's disease: study of a series of 135 Parkinson's patients can. J Neurol Sci. 2002;29:139–46.
72. Norman S, Troster AI, Fields JA, Brooks R. Effects of depression and Parkinson's disease on cognitive functioning. J Neuropsychiatry Clin Neurosci. 2002;14:31–6.
73. Uekermann J, Daum I, Peters S, Wiebel B, Przuntek H, Müller T. Depressed mood and executive dysfunction in early Parkinson's disease. Acta Neurol Scand. 2003;107:341–8.
74. Stefanova E, Potrebic A, Ziropadja L, Maric J, Ribaric I, Kostic VS. Depression predicts the pattern of cognitive impairment in early Parkinson's disease. J Neurol Sci. 2006;248:131–7.
75. Tröster AI, Paolo AM, Lyons KE, Glatt SL, Hubble JP, Koller WC. The influence of depression on cognition in Parkinson's disease: a pattern of impairment distinguishable from Alzheimer's disease. Neurology. 1995;45:672–6.
76. Tröster AI, Stalp LD, Paolo AM, Fields JA, Koller WC. Neuropsychological impairment in Parkinson's disease with and without depression. Arch Neurol. 1995;52:1164–9.
77. Beliauskas LA, Glantsz RH. Depression type in Parkinson's disease. J Clin Exp Neuropsychol. 1989;11:597–604.
78. Taylor AE, Saint-Cyr JA, Lang AE, Kenny FT. Parkinson's disease and depression: a critical reevaluation. Brain. 1986;109:279–92.
79. Huber SJ, Paulson GW, Shuttleworth EC. Relationship of motor symptoms, intellectual impairment, and depression in Parkinson's disease. J Neurol Neurosurg Psychiatry. 1988;51:855–8.
80. Silberman CD, Laks J, Capitão CF, et al. Frontal functions in depressed and nondepressed Parkinson's disease patients: impact of severity stages. Psychiatry Res. 2007;149:285–9.
81. Santangelo G, Vitale C, Trojano L, Longo K, Cozzolino A, Grossi D, Barone P. Relationship between depression and cognitive dysfunctions in Parkinson's disease without dementia. J Neurol. 2009;256:632–8.
82. Varanese S, Perfetti B, Ghilardi MF, Di Rocco A. Apathy, but not depression, reflects inefficient cognitive strategies in Parkinson's disease. PLoS ONE. 2011;6:e17846.
83. Rektorova I, Rektor I, Bares M, et al. Pramipexole and pergolide in the treatment of depression in Parkinson's disease: a national multicentre prospective randomized study. Eur J Neurol. 2003;10:399–406.
84. Lemke MR, Brecht HM, Koester J, Kraus PH, Reichmann H. Anhedonia, depression, and motor functioning in Parkinson's disease during treatment with pramipexole. J Neuropsychiatry Clin Neurosci. 2005;17:214–20.
85. Barone P, Scarzella L, Marconi R, Antonini A, Morgante L, Bracco F, Zappia M, Musch B, Depression/Parkinson Italian Study Group. Pramipexole versus sertraline in the treatment of depression in Parkinson's disease: a national multicenter parallel-group randomized study. J Neurol. 2006;253:601–7.
86. Rektorova I, Balaz M, Svatova J, et al. Effects of ropinirole on nonmotor symptoms of Parkinson's disease: a prospective multicenter study. Clin Neuropharmacol. 2008;31:261–6.

87. Barone P, Poewe W, Albrecht S, et al. Pramipexole for the treatment of depressive symptoms in patients with Parkinson's disease: a randomised, double-blind, placebo-controlled trial. Lancet Neurol. 2010;9:573–80.
88. Pahwa R, Stacy MA, Factor SA, Lyons KE, Stocchi F, Hersh BP, Elmer LW, Truong DD, Earl NL, EASE-PD Adjunct Study Investigators. Ropinirole 24-h prolonged release: randomized, controlled study in advanced Parkinson disease. Neurology. 2007;68:1108–15.
89. Trenkwalder C, Kies B, Rudzinska M, Fine J, Nikl J, Honczarenko K, et al. Rotigotine effects on early morning motor function and sleep in Parkinson's disease: a double-blind, randomized, placebo-controlled study (RECOVER). Mov Disord. 2011;26:90–9.
90. Skapinakis P, Bakola E, Salanti G, Lewis G, Kyritsis AP, Mavreas V. Efficacy and acceptability of selective serotonin reuptake inhibitors for the treatment of depression in Parkinson's disease: a systematic review and meta-analysis of randomized controlled trials. BMC Neurol. 2010;10:49.
91. Seppi K, Weintraub D, Coelho M, et al. The movement disorder society evidence-based medicine review update: treatments for the non-motor symptoms of Parkinson's disease. Mov Disord. 2011;26 Suppl 3:S42–80.
92. Richard IH, McDermott MP, Kurlan R, et al. A randomized, double-blind, placebo-controlled trial of antidepressants in Parkinson disease. Neurology. 2012;78:1229–36.
93. Wermuth L, Sorensen PS, Timm B, et al. Depression in idiopathic Parkinson's disease treated with citalopram: a placebo-controlled trial. Nordic J Psychiatry. 1998;52:163–9.
94. Leentjens AF, Vreeling FW, Luijckx GJ, Verhey FRJ. SSRIs in the treatment of depression in Parkinson's disease. Int J Geriatr Psychiatry. 2003;18:552–4.
95. Weintraub D, Mavandadi S, Mamikonyan E, et al. Atomoxetine for depression and other neuropsychiatric symptoms in Parkinson disease. Neurology. 2010;75:448–55.
96. Devos D, Dujardin K, Poirot I, et al. Comparison of desipramine and citalopram treatments for depression in Parkinson's disease: a double-blind, randomized, placebo-controlled study. Mov Disord. 2008;23:850–7.
97. Menza M, Dobkin RD, Marin H, et al. A controlled trial of antidepressants in patients with Parkinson disease and depression. Neurology. 2009;72:886–92.
98. Dobkin RD, Menza M, Allen LA, et al. Cognitive-behavioral therapy for depression in Parkinson's disease: a randomized, controlled trial. Am J Psychiatry. 2011;168:1066–74.
99. Pal E, Nagy F, Aschermann Z, Balazs E, Kovacs N. The impact of left prefrontal repetitive transcranial magnetic stimulation on depression in Parkinson's disease: a randomized, double-blind, placebo-controlled study. Mov Disord. 2010;25:2311–7.
100. Boggio PS, Fregni F, Bermpohl F, et al. Effect of repetitive TMS and fluoxetine on cognitive function in patients with Parkinson's disease and concurrent depression. Mov Disord. 2005;20:1178–84.
101. Fregni F, Santos CM, Myczkowski ML, et al. Repetitive transcranial magnetic stimulation is as effective as fluoxetine in the treatment of depression in patients with Parkinson's disease. J Neurol Neurosurg Psychiatry. 2004;75:1171–4.
102. Pedersen KF, Larsen JP, Alves G, Aarsland D. Prevalence and clinical correlates of apathy in Parkinson's disease: a community-based study. Parkinsonism Relat Disord. 2009;15:295–9.
103. Starkstein SE, Merello M, Jorge R, Brockman S, Bruce D, Power B. The syndromal validity and nosological position of apathy in Parkinson's disease. Mov Disord. 2009;24:1211–6.
104. Drijgers RL, Dujardin K, Reijnders JS, Defebvre L, Leentjens AF. Validation of diagnostic criteria for apathy in Parkinson's disease. Parkinsonism Relat Disord. 2010;16:656–60.
105. Duffy JD. The neural substrates of motivation. Psychiatr Ann. 1997;27:24.
106. Reijnders JS, Scholtissen B, Weber WE, Aalten P, Verhey FR, Leentjens AF. Neuroanatomical correlates of apathy in Parkinson's disease: a magnetic resonance imaging study using voxel-based morphometry. Mov Disord. 2010;25:2318–25.
107. Thobois S, Ardouin C, Lhommee E, Klinger H, Lagrange C, Xie J, et al. Non-motor dopamine withdrawal syndrome after surgery for Parkinson's disease: predictors and underlying mesolimbic denervation. Brain. 2010;133(Pt 4):1111–27.

108. Robert G, Le Jeune F, Lozachmeur C, Drapier S, Dondaine T, Péron J, Travers D, Sauleau P, Millet B, Vérin M, Drapier D. Apathy in patients with Parkinson disease without dementia or depression: a PET study. Neurology. 2012;79:1155–60.
109. Lhommèe E, Klinger H, Thobois S, Schmitt E, Ardouin C, Bichon A, Kistner A, Fraix V, Xie J, AyaKombo M, Chabard'es S, Seigneuret E, Benabid AL, Mertens P, Polo G, Carnicella S, Quesada JL, Bosson JL, Broussolle E, Pollak P, Krack P. Subthalamic stimulation in Parkinson's disease: restoring the balance of motivated behaviours. Brain. 2012;135(Pt 5):1463–77.
110. Starkstein SE. Apathy in Parkinson's disease: diagnostic and etiological dilemmas. Mov Disord. 2012;27:174–8.
111. Santangelo G, Trojano L, Barone P, Errico D, Grossi D, Vitale C. Apathy in Parkinson's disease: diagnosis, neuropsychological correlates, pathophysiology and treatment. Behav Neurol. 2013;27:501–13.
112. Pedersen KF, Alves G, Brønnick K, Aarsland D, Tysnes OB, Larsen JP. Apathy in drug-naïve patients with incident Parkinson's disease: the Norwegian ParkWest study. J Neurol. 2010;257:217–23.
113. Pedersen KF, Alves G, Aarsland D, Larsen JP. Occurrence and risk factors for apathy in Parkinson disease: a 4-year prospective longitudinal study. J Neurol Neurosurg Psychiatry. 2009;80:1279–82.
114. Cubo E, Benito-Leo'n J, Coronell C, Armesto D, ANIMO Study Group. Clinical correlates of apathy in patients recently diagnosed with Parkinson's disease: the ANIMO study. Neuroepidemiology. 2012;38:48–55.
115. Harris E, McNamara P, Durso R. Apathy in patients with Parkinson disease as a function of side of onset. J Geriatr Psychiatry Neurol. 2013;26:95–104.
116. Marin RS, Biedrzycki RC, Firinciogullari S. Reliability and validity of the Apathy Evaluation Scale. Psychiatry Res. 1991;38:143–62.
117. Starkstein SE, Mayberg HS, Preziosi TJ, Andrezejewski P, Leiguarda R, Robinson RG. Reliability, validity, and clinical correlates of apathy in Parkinson's disease. J Neuropsychiatry Clin Neurosci. 1992;4:134–9.
118. Sockeel P, Dujardin K, Devos D, Deneve C, Destee A, Defebvre L. The Lille apathy rating scale (LARS), a new instrument for detecting and quantifying apathy: validation in Parkinson's disease. J Neurol Neurosurg Psychiatry. 2006;77:579–84.
119. Robert PH, Clairet S, Benoit M, et al. The apathy inventory: assessing apathy and awareness in Alzheimer's disease, Parkinson's disease and mild cognitive impairment. Int J Geriatr Psychiatry. 2002;17:1099–105.
120. Cummings JL, Mega M, Gray K, Rosenburg-Thompson S, Carusi DA, Gornbein J. The neuropsychiatric inventory: comprehensive assessment of psychopathology in dementia. Neurology. 1994;44:2308–14.
121. Fahn S, Elton RL, members of the UPDRS committee. Unified Parkinson's disease rating scale. In: Fahn S, Marsden CD, Goldstein M, Calne DB, editors. Recent developments in Parkinson's disease. Florham Park: McMillan Health Care; 1987. p. 153—63.
122. Leentjens AF, Dujardin K, Marsh L, Martinez-Martin P, Richard IH, Starkstein SE, Weintraub D, Sampaio C, Poewe W, Rascol O, Stebbins GT, Goetz CG. Apathy and anhedonia rating scales in Parkinson's disease: critique and recommendations. Mov Disord. 2008;23:2004–14.
123. Pluck GC, Brown RG. Apathy in Parkinson's disease. J Neurol Neurosurg Psychiatry. 2002;73:636–42.
124. Zahodne LB, Young S, Kirsch-Darrow L, Nisenzon A, Fernandez HH, Okun MS, Bowers D. Examination of the Lille Apathy Rating Scale in Parkinson disease. Mov Disord. 2009;24:677–83.
125. Santangelo G, Vitale C, Picillo M, Moccia M, Erro R, Pisano G, Pezzella D, Cuoco S, Longo K, Pellecchia MT, Amboni M, De Rosa A, De Michele G, Trojano L, Barone P. Relationship between apathy and cognitive dysfunctions in de novo, untreated Parkinson's Disease patients : a prospective longitudinal study. Eur J Neurol. 2014 May 22 [Epub ahead of print].

126. Dujardin K, Sockeel P, Delliaux M, Deste'e A, Defebvre L. Apathy may herald cognitive decline and dementia in Parkinson's disease. Mov Disord. 2009;24:2391–7.
127. Isella V, Melzi P, Grimaldi M, Iurlaro S, Piolti R, Ferrarese C, Frattola L, Appollonio I. Clinical, neuropsychological, and morphometric correlates of apathy in Parkinson's disease. Mov Disord. 2002;17:366–71.
128. Zgaljardic DJ, Borod JC, Foldi NS, Rocco M, Mattis PJ, Gordon MF, Feigin AS, Eidelberg D. Relationship between self- reported apathy and executive dysfunction in nondemented patients with Parkinson disease. Cogn Behav Neurol. 2007;20:184–92.
129. Grossi D, Santangelo G, Barbarulo AM, Vitale C, Castaldo G, Proto MG, Siano P, Barone P, Trojano L. Apathy and related executive syndromes in dementia associated with Parkinson's disease and in Alzheimer's disease. Behav Neurol. 2013;27:515–22.
130. Santangelo G, Vitale C, Trojano L, Errico D, Amboni M, Barbarulo AM, Grossi D, Barone P. Neuropsychological correlates of theory of mind in patients with early Parkinson's disease. Mov Disord. 2012;27:98–105.
131. Czernecki V, Pillon B, Houeto JL, Pochon JB, Levy R, Dubois B. Motivation, reward, and Parkinson's disease: influence of dopa therapy. Neuropsychologia. 2002;40:2257–67.
132. Czernecki V, Schipbach M, Yaici S, Levy R, Bardinet E, Yelnik J, Dubois B, Agid Y. Apathy following subthalamic stimulation in Parkinson disease: a dopamine responsive symptom. Mov Disord. 2008;23:964–9.
133. Leentjens AF, Koester J, Fruh B, Shephard DT, Barone P, Houben JJ. The effect of pramipexole on mood and motivational symptoms in Parkinson's disease: a meta-analysis of placebo-controlled studies. Clin Ther. 2009;31:89–98.
134. Chaudhuri RK, Martinez-Martin P, Antonini A, Brown RG, Friedman JH, Onofrj M, Surmann E, Ghys L, Trenkwalder C. Rotigotine and specific non-motor symptoms of Parkinson's disease: post hoc analysis of RECOVER. Parkinsonism Relat Disord. 2013;19:660–5.
135. Thobois S, Lhommée E, Klinger H, Ardouin C, Schmitt E, Bichon A, Kistner A, Castrioto A, Xie J, Fraix V, Pelissier P, Chabardes S, Mertens P, Quesada JL, Bosson JL, Pollak P, Broussolle E, Krack P. Parkinsonian apathy responds to dopaminergic stimulation of D2/D3 receptors with piribedil. Brain. 2013;136(Pt 5):1568–77.
136. Litvinenko IV, Odinak MM, Mogil'naya VI, Emelin AY. Efficacy and safety of galantamine (reminyl) for dementia in patients with Parkinson's disease (an open controlled trial). Neurosci Behav Physiol. 2008;38:937–45.
137. Grace J, Amick MM, Friedman JH. A double-blind comparison of galantamine hydrobromide ER and placebo in Parkinson disease. J Neurol Neurosurg Psychiatry. 2009;80:18–23.
138. Stevens A, Peschk I, Schwarz J. Implicit learning, executive function and hedonic activity in chronic polydrug abusers, currently abstinent polydrug abusers and controls. Addiction. 2007;102:937–46.
139. Gard DE, Kring AM, Gard MG, Horan WP, Green MF. Anhedonia in schizophrenia: distinctions between anticipatory and consummatory pleasure. Schizophr Res. 2007;93:253–60.
140. Gard D, Germans Gard M, Kring A, John O. Anticipatory and consummatory components of the experience of pleasure: a scale development study. J Res Pers. 2006;40:1086–102.
141. Assogna F, Cravello L, Caltagirone C, Spalletta G. Anhedonia in Parkinson's disease: a systematic review of the literature. Mov Disord. 2011;26:1825–34.
142. Weintraub D, Cary M, Stern M, et al. Daily affect in Parkinson disease is responsive to life events and motor symptoms. Am J Geriatr Psychiatry. 2006;14:161–8.
143. Jordan LL, Zahodne LB, Okun MS, Bowers D. Hedonic and behavioral deficits associated with apathy in Parkinson's disease: potential treatment implications. Mov Disord. 2013;28:1301–4.
144. Santangelo G, Morgante L, Savica R, et al. Anhedonia and cognitive impairment in Parkinson's disease: Italian validation of the Snaith-Hamilton Pleasure Scale and its application in the clinical routine practice during the PRIAMO study. Parkinsonism Relat Disord. 2009;15:576–81.
145. Reichmann H, Brecht MH, Koster J, Kraus PH, Lemke MR. Pramipexole in routine clinical practice: a prospective observational trial in Parkinson's disease. CNS Drugs. 2003;17:965–73.

146. Isella V, Iurlaro S, Piolti R, Ferrarese C, Frattola L, Appollonio I, et al. Physical anhedonia in Parkinson's disease. J Neurol Neurosurg Psychiatry. 2003;74:1308–11.
147. Lemke MR, Brecht HM, Koester J, Reichmann H. Effects of the dopamine agonist pramipexole on depression, anhedonia and motor functioning in Parkinson's disease. J Neurol Sci. 2006;248:266–70.
148. Matsui K, Tachibana H, Yamanishi T, Oguru M, Toda K, Okuda B, Oka N. Clinical correlates of anhedonia in patients with Parkinson's disease. Clin Neurol Neurosurg. 2013;115:2524–7.
149. Nagayama H, Kubo S, Hatano T, Hamada S, Maeda T, Hasegawa T, Kadowaki T, et al. Validity and reliability assessment of a Japanese version of the Snaith-Hamilton pleasure scale. Intern Med. 2012;51:865–9.
150. Reichmann H, Odin P, Brecht HM, Koster J, Kraus PH. Changing dopamine agonist treatment in Parkinson's disease: experiences with switching to pramipexole. J Neural Transm Suppl. 2006;71:17–25.
151. Kluger BM, Krupp LB, Enoka RM. Fatigue and fatigability in neurologic illnesses: proposal for a unified taxonomy. Neurology. 2013;80:409–16.
152. Fabbrini G, Latorre A, Suppa A, Bloise M, Frontoni M, Berardelli A. Fatigue in Parkinson's disease: motor or non-motor symptom? Parkinsonism Relat Disord. 2013;19:148–52.
153. Brown RG, Dittner A, Findley L, Wessely SC. The Parkinson fatigue scale. Parkinsonism Relat Disord. 2005;11:49–55.
154. Berardelli A, Conte A, Fabbrini G, Bologna M, Latorre A, Rocchi L, Suppa A. Pathophysiology of pain and fatigue in Parkinson's disease. Parkinsonism Relat Disord. 2012;18(S1):226–8.
155. Abe K, Takanashi M, Yanagihara T. Fatigue in patients with Parkinson's disease. Behav Neurol. 2000;2:103–6.
156. Pavese N, Metta V, Bose SK, Chaudhuri KR, Brooks DJ. Fatigue in Parkinson's disease is linked to striatal and limbic serotonergic dysfunction. Brain. 2010;133:3434–43.
157. Lou JS, Benice T, Kearns G, Sexton G, Nutt J. Levodopa normalizes exercise related cortico-motoneuron excitability abnormalities in Parkinson's disease. Clin Neurophysiol. 2003;114:930–7.
158. Friedman J, Friedman H. Fatigue in Parkinson's disease. Neurology. 1993;43:2016–8.
159. Karlsen K, Larsen JP, Tandberg E, Jørgensen K. Fatigue in patients with Parkinson's disease. Mov Disord. 1999;14:237–41.
160. Herlofson K, Larsen JP. The influence of fatigue on health-related quality of life in patients with Parkinson's disease. Acta Neurol Scand. 2003;107:1–6.
161. Alves G, Wentzel-Larsen T, Larsen JP. Is fatigue an independent and persistent symptom in patients with Parkinson disease? Neurology. 2004;63:1908–11.
162. Skorvanek M, Nagyova I, Rosenberger J, Krokavcova M, Ghorbani Saeedian R, Groothoff JW, Gdovinova Z, van Dijk JP. Clinical determinants of primary and secondary fatigue in patients with Parkinson's disease. J Neurol. 2013;260:1554–61.
163. Beiske AG, Loge JH, Hjermstad MJ, Svensson E. Fatigue in Parkinson's disease: prevalence and associated factors. Mov Disord. 2010;25:2456–60.
164. Hagell P, Brundin L. Towards an understanding of fatigue in Parkinson disease. J Neurol Neurosurg Psychiatr. 2009;80:489–92.
165. Barone P, Antonini A, Colosimo C, Marconi R, Morgante L, Avarello TP, PRIAMO Study Group, et al. The PRIAMO study: a multicenter assessment of nonmotor symptoms and their impact on quality of life in Parkinson's disease. Mov Disord. 2009;24:1641–9.
166. Elbers R, van Wegen EE, Rochester L, Hetherington V, Nieuwboer A, Willems AM, et al. Is impact of fatigue an independent factor associated with physical activity in patients with idiopathic Parkinson's disease? Mov Disord. 2009;24:1512–8.
167. Friedman J, Brown R, Comella C, Garber C, Krupp L, Lou J, et al. Fatigue in Parkinson's disease: a review. Mov Disord. 2007;22:297–308.
168. Falup-Pecurariu C. Fatigue assessment of Parkinson's disease patient in clinic: specific versus holistic. J Neural Transm. 2013;120:577–81.

169. Friedman JH, Alves G, Hagell P, Marinus J, Marsh L, Martinez-Martin P, Goetz CG, Poewe W, Rascol O, Sampaio C, Stebbins G, Schrag A. Fatigue rating scales critique and recommendations by the Movement Disorders Society task force on rating scales for Parkinson's disease. Mov Disord. 2010;25:805–22.
170. Krupp LB, La Rocca NG, Muir-Nash J, Steinberg AD. The fatigue severity scale. Application to patients with multiple sclerosis and systemic lupus erythematosus. Arch Neurol. 1989;46:1121–3.
171. Yellen SB, Cella DF, Webster K, Blendowski C, Kaplan E. Measuring fatigue and other anemia-related symptoms with the functional assessment of cancer therapy (FACT) measurement system. J Pain Symptom Manage. 1997;13:63–74.
172. Smets EMA, Garseen B, Bonke B, Dehaes JCJM. The multidimensional fatigue inventory (MFI). Psychometric properties of an instrument to assess fatigue. J Psychosom Res. 1995;39:315–25.
173. Hagell P, Ho¨glund A, Reimer J, Eriksson B, Knutsson I, Widner H, Cella D. Measuring fatigue in Parkinson's disease: a psychometric study of two brief generic fatigue questionnaires. J Pain Symptom Manage. 2006;32:420–32.
174. Grace J, Mendelsohn A, Friedman JH. A comparison of fatigue measures in Parkinson's disease. Parkinsonism Relat Disord. 2007;13:443–5.
175. Elbers RG, Rietberg MB, van Wegen EE, Verhoef J, Kramer SF, Terwee CB, Kwakkel G. Self-report fatigue questionnaires in multiple sclerosis, Parkinson's disease and stroke: a systematic review of measurement properties. Qual Life Res. 2012;21:925–44.
176. Elbers RG, van Wegen EE, Verhoef J, Kwakkel G. Reliability and structural validity of the Multidimensional Fatigue Inventory (MFI) in patients with idiopathic Parkinson's disease. Parkinsonism Relat Disord. 2012;18:532–6.
177. Fisk JD, Doble SE. Construction and validation of a fatigue impact scale for daily administration (D-FIS). Qual Life Res. 2002;11:263–72.
178. Martinez-Martin P, Catalan MJ, Benito-Leon J, Moreno AO, Zamarbide I, Cubo E, van Blercon N, Arillo VC, Pondal M, Linazasoro G, Alonso F, Ruiz PG, Frades B. Impact of fatigue in Parkinson's Disease: the fatigue impact scale for daily use (D-FIS). QualLife Res. 2006;15:597–606.
179. Schiehser DM, Ayers CR, Liu L, Lessig S, Song DS, Filoteo JV. Validation of the modified fatigue impact scale in Parkinson's disease. Parkinsonism Relat Disord. 2013;19:335–8.
180. Dooneief G, Mirabello E, Bell K, Marder K, Stern Y, Mayeux R. An estimate of the incidence of depression in idiopathic Parkinson's disease. Arch Neurol. 1992;49:305–7.
181. Havlikova E, Rosenberger J, Nagyova I, Middel B, Dubayova T, Gdovinova Z, et al. Clinical and psychosocial factors associated with fatigue in patients with Parkinson's disease. Parkinsonism Relat Disord. 2008;14:187–92.
182. Miwa H, Miwa T. Fatigue in patients with Parkinson's disease: impact on quality of life. Intern Med. 2011;50:1553–8.
183. Shulman LM, Taback RL, Bean J, Weiner WJ. Comorbidity of the nonmotor symptoms of Parkinson's disease. Mov Disord. 2001;16:507–10.
184. Friedman JH, Fernandez HH. The nonmotor problems of Parkinson's disease. Neurologist. 2000;6:8–27.
185. Nakamura T, Hirayama M, Hara T, Hama T, Watanabe H, Sobue G. Does cardiovascular autonomic dysfunction contribute to fatigue in Parkinson's disease? Mov Disord. 2011;26:1869–74.
186. Sáez-Francàs N, Hernández-Vara J, Corominas-Roso M, Alegre J, Jacas C, Casas M. Relationship between poor decision-making process and fatigue perception in Parkinson's disease patients. J Neurol Sci. 2014;337(1–2):167–72.
187. Sáez-Francàs N, Hernández-Vara J, Corominas Roso M, AlegreMartín J, CasasBrugué M. The association of apathy with central fatigue perception in patients with Parkinson's disease. Behav Neurosci. 2013;127:237–44.

188. Havlikova E, Rosenberger J, Nagyova I, Middel B, Dubayova T, Gdovinova Z, et al. Impact of fatigue on quality of life in patients with Parkinson's disease. Eur J Neurol. 2008;15:475–80.
189. Kang SY, Ma HI, Lim YM, Hwang SH, Kim YJ. Fatigue in drug-naïve Parkinson's disease. Eur Neurol. 2013;70:59–64.
190. Lou JS, Kearns G, Benice T, Oken B, Sexton G, Nutt J. Levodopa improves physical fatigue in Parkinson's disease: a double-blind, placebo-controlled, crossover study. Mov Disord. 2003;18:1108–14.
191. Abe K, Takanashi M, Yanagihara T, Sakoda S. Pergolide mesylate may improve fatigue in patients with Parkinson's disease. Behav Neurol. 2001–2002;13:117–21.
192. Mendonça DA, Menezes K, Jog MS. Methylphenidate improves fatigue scores in Parkinson disease: a randomized controlled trial. Mov Disord. 2007;22:2070–6.
193. Stocchi F, The ADAGIO Investigators. Benefits of treatment with rasagiline for fatigue symptoms in patients with early Parkinson's disease. Eur J Neurol. 2014;21(2):357–60.

Chapter 2
Mild Cognitive Impairment in Parkinson's Disease

Saul Martínez-Horta and Jaime Kulisevsky

Abbreviations

AD	Alzheimer's disease
DLPFC	Dorsal lateral prefrontal cortex
MCI	Mild cognitive impairment
OFC	Orbitofrontal cortex
PD	Parkinson's disease
PFC	Prefrontal cortex

S. Martínez-Horta, PhD
Movement Disorders Unit, Department of Neurology, Hospital de la Santa Creu i Sant Pau, Universitat Autònoma de Barcelona, Barcelona, Spain

Sant Pau Institute of Biomedical Research (IIB-Sant Pau), Barcelona, Spain

Centro Investigación Biomedica en Red-Enfermedades Neurodegenerativas (CIBERNED), Sant Antoni Maria Claret 167, Barcelona 08025, Spain
e-mail: smartinezho@santpau.cat

J. Kulisevsky, MD, PhD (✉)
Movement Disorders Unit, Department of Neurology, Hospital de la Santa Creu i Sant Pau, Universitat Autònoma de Barcelona, Barcelona, Spain

Sant Pau Institute of Biomedical Research (IIB-Sant Pau), Barcelona, Spain

Centro Investigación Biomedica en Red-Enfermedades Neurodegenerativas (CIBERNED), Sant Antoni Maria Claret 167, Barcelona 08025, Spain

Universitat Oberta de Catalunya (UOC), Barcelona, Spain
e-mail: jkulisevsky@santpau.cat

H. Reichmann (ed.), *Neuropsychiatric Symptoms of Movement Disorders*,
Neuropsychiatric Symptoms of Neurological Disease,
DOI 10.1007/978-3-319-09537-0_2

Introduction

Motor features such as resting tremor, bradykinesia, or postural instability historically characterized Parkinson's disease (PD). However, compelling evidence proved that cognitive impairment is also pervasive in PD, constituting a clinical characteristic of the disease [1]. Cognitive impairment in PD can be identified as both minor cognitive defects—present in up to 30 % of patients at time of diagnosis—and up to dementia [2]. In fact, in cross-sectional studies dementia is seen in more than 20 % of PD patients [3] and shows a cumulative prevalence up to 80 % after 20 years of follow-up [4–8].

Although the trajectory of cognitive impairment is variable along the course of the disease, these alterations have a high impact on the quality of life of the patients and on caregiver distress [9–11]. While most PD subjects exhibit relatively subtle cognitive deficits when compared with controls, [2] an intermediate transitional state of mild cognitive impairment (MCI) has been defined and suggested to be a predictor of further development of PD dementia (PDD) [3, 12, 13]. Given that PD supposes a four to six times greater risk of developing dementia, the definition and identification of neurocognitive predictors of PDD currently constitutes one of the major topics of interest in PD research. Henceforth, whether different profiles of early cognitive alterations in non-demented patients have different prognostic implications still remains to be determined [13, 14].

Unlike the construct of MCI in the general population considered as prodromic of Alzheimer's disease (AD) [15], MCI in PD (PD-MCI) must not necessarily announce short-term dementia [6, 16]. With a relative independence on the degree of early cognitive alterations seen in most of the patients from the beginning of the disease, some patients rapidly convert to dementia, while others remain stable for years [17].

This emphasized the need: (a) for a better understanding of the underlying mechanisms of early cognitive alterations in PD, (b) to define standardized methods for cognitive assessment, and (c) to determine the prognostic implications of specific cognitive profiles [13, 16].

Along this chapter we will describe the concept and underlying mechanisms of PD-MCI, the recommended evidence-based methods to assess early cognitive alterations and the clinical and prognostic implications of the different cognitive profiles that can be recognized as PD-MCI. Thus, we will review current and validated measures for cognitive assessment in PD, the methods to determine whether a cognitive performance pattern represents a decline from the previous level or current expected level, and the methods to assess the impact of cognitive abilities over activities of daily living.

Cognition in Parkinson's Disease

Cognitive impairment is intrinsic to PD [2]. From the earliest stages of the disease, patients suffering from PD may exhibit some degree of cognitive alterations [4, 18]. These early cognitive alterations seen in up to 80 % of PD patients at time of diagnosis resemble those observed in patients with lesions involving the prefrontal cortex

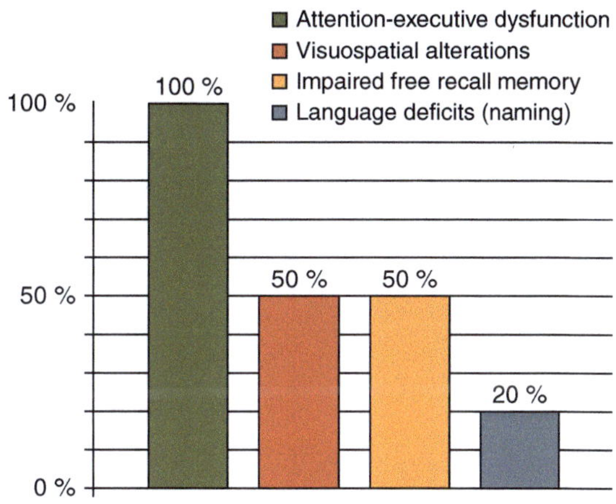

Fig. 2.1 Cognitive profile of patients with newly diagnosed PD [2]

(PFC) [19, 20] (Fig. 2.1). Thus, cognitive impairment in PD is mainly characterized by defects on executive functions such as alterations in working memory, cognitive flexibility, planning, and attention [2, 16, 19]. However, when cognition is adequately explored, alterations involving other cognitive domains—such as memory and visuospatial/visuoconstructive functions—can be seen accompanying executive dysfunction in up to 50 % of the patients [2, 3].

Cognitive changes seen in PD probably have a multifactorial causality with the pattern of observed deficits varying in accordance to the progressive course of the pathologic and neurochemical changes of the disease [21]. Most of the frontal-executive deficits seen in PD are closely related to the progressive dopaminergic depletion that occurs in the early stages of the disease [22–24]. Accordingly, the main neuropsychological profile of PD has been classically defined as a predominant "frontal-subcortical" syndrome with preserved performance on instrumental tasks, the latter considered to be specific to neurodegenerative diseases with a cortical involvement such as AD [19, 20]. Nevertheless, it is currently known that up to 20 % of non-demented PD patients can also exhibit alterations in tasks mainly involving posterior-cortical functions such as encoding information, confrontation naming, or picture copying [2, 21, 25, 26]. Thus, it was proposed that the transition from PD-MCI to PDD appears characterized by a pattern of significant addition of this kind of AD-like cognitive alterations [6, 12, 25, 26]. This emphasized the need for accurate and standardized methods for cognitive assessment in PD to better clarify whether cognitive alterations evidenced at a given time point of the disease might be taken as consistent markers of conversion to dementia [27].

The Role of Dopamine in Cognitive Impairment in PD

The involvement of dopamine in high-order cognition has been largely supported by numerous studies [24]. The massive number of dopaminergic projections emerging from the PFC to the caudate nucleus and the reciprocal

Table 2.1 Effects of dopaminergic replacement therapy over cognitive functions in PD [42]

Cognitive benefit
Set shifting
Working memory
Spatial working memory
Cognitive deterioration
Concurrent learning
Probabilistic reversal learning
Decision making
Visual hallucinations
No effect
Attentional set shifting
Task switching-abstract rules
Pattern and spatial recognition memory
Associative learning
Verbal memory

Adapted from Kehagia et al. [42], with permission

striato-pallido-thalamo-cortical projections to the PFC through the basal ganglia indicates the importance of the frontal-subcortical systems over cognition [22, 28, 29]. In humans, well-differentiated frontal-subcortical circuits emerge from different portions of the striatum establishing connections with segregated regions of the PFC [30–32]. Thus, while dorsal caudate nucleus mainly projects to dorsal lateral PFC (DLPFC), the ventral striatum projects to medial and orbital PFC (mPFC; oPFC), anterior cingulate cortex (ACC), and limbic system [22, 33, 34].

During the earliest stages of PD, massive loss of dopaminergic neurons mainly disrupts both motor putamen and dorsal caudate [22, 29, 33–35]. Lack of coactivation of the striatum with functionally related DLPFC is critical in the development of executive defects [35, 36]. These functional defects characteristic of early cognitive impairment in PD resemble those presented by patients suffering from conditions with structural involvement of the DLPFC [24, 36]. This dopaminergic dependence of frontal-executive functions in PD supports the remediation or improvement seen on the performance of some frontal-related tasks after initiation of dopaminergic replacement therapy [37–39] that partially compensate the dorsal caudate dopaminergic deficiency [35, 40].

However, a paradoxical cognitive effect also mediated by the treatment with dopaminergic drugs can be seen in PD and explains the occurrence of other cognitive alterations (Table 2.1). As indicated, dorsal caudate projections are known to be significantly impaired from the earliest stages of the disease. However, the ventral striatum and its related projections are known to remain relatively spared during the early and middle stages of the disease [33, 34]. Thus, the doses of dopaminergic drugs used to remediate the motor alterations of PD related to dopaminergic deficiency in the putamen result excessive and lead to an overdose of other unaffected or less dopamine-depleted regions [35]. Consequently, those cognitive functions more

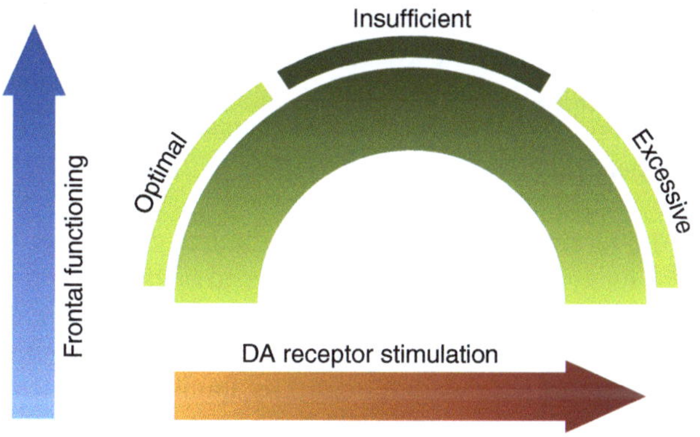

Fig 2.2 Effect of dopaminergic replacement therapy over frontal functions

dependent on ventral striatum projections to orbital and medial PFC that appeared intact before initiation of dopaminergic replacement therapy (i.e., decision making, reversal learning) tend to appear altered, while those more dependent on dorsal caudate projections to DLPFC previously altered show consistent improvement [35, 38, 40–42]. This inverted-U relationship (Fig. 2.2) has been demonstrated in numerous controlled studies, indicating that cognitive alterations seen in PD may variably depend on dopaminergic depletion and neurodegeneration, disease staging, and dopaminergic overdose over spared regions [34, 38].

The paradoxical dopamine-dependent response demonstrates the fragile relationship between optimum levels of dopamine and cognition [38, 40, 41] which should be taken into account when assessing cognitive functions in PD.

The Role of Acetylcholine in Cognitive Impairment in PD

While most of the cognitive defects initially seen in non-demented PD can be understood within the framework of frontal-executive alterations fueled by dopaminergic deficits, not all the cognitive alterations seen in early PD respond to dopaminergic replacement therapy. This suggests that other neurotransmitters are involved on the pathogenesis of cognitive impairment. Loss of cholinergic cells at the basal nucleus of Meynert (bNM) and pedunculopontine nucleus (PPN) is also known to be present in PD [43, 44]. Alterations on the cholinergic projections have been consistently related to cognitive deterioration in PD [23]. Alterations in cognitive domains such as visuospatial and visuoconstructive skills or memory, that do not significantly ameliorate after initiation of dopaminergic replacement therapy, may obey to cortical cholinergic deficit [23, 25, 45]. In this line, disregarding disease duration, cholinergic depletion in patients presenting dementia associated to PD (PDD) is comparable to that observed in patients with Lewy body dementia [46]. It was suggested that the conversion of PD-MCI to PDD, signaled by the addition of significant neuropsychological deficits related to posterior cortical dysfunction (i.e., visuospatial or language defects), is related to progressive cholinergic deficit [6, 14, 47–49]. Accordingly, PD-cholinergic alterations and related cognitive impairment seem to be more relevant than dopamine-dependent features on the definition of the prognostic implications of a given cognitive profile [13].

In line with the recent formalization of the clinical criteria for both PDD and PD-MCI [50, 51], many studies have been developed on the topic of identifying the neurobiological correlates of cognitive deterioration in PD. Severe dopamine deficits have been emphasized to follow the emergence of cognitive alterations. However, alpha-synuclein pathology followed by limbic and cortical loss of dopamine, noradrenaline, serotonin, and acetylcholine neurons has been significantly pointed as added mechanisms leading to cognitive deterioration and dementia in PD [33, 52]. In addition, genetic factors such as triplications in the alpha-synuclein gene or MAP-t haplotypes have been also linked to cognitive decline [53, 54].

Parkinson's Disease Mild Cognitive Impairment: Definition and Clinical Implications

The concept of mild cognitive impairment (MCI) was defined in the field of AD indicating the transitional stage between normal cognition and dementia [55]. Thus, mild cognitive impairment (MCI) refers to the stage between normal aging and dementia [56] and was originally used to describe prodromal AD. More recently, MCI has become important in studies on PD, [57] where it is called MCI in PD (PD-MCI) [50]. Whereas MCI due to AD is primarily characterized by memory impairment, cognitive deficits of PD-MCI in newly diagnosed patients more often concern a range of cognitive domains, including memory, visual-spatial, and attention/executive abilities [2, 4].

AD-MCI occurs when, in the presence of significant and measurable cognitive alterations in one or more cognitive domains, independent activities of daily living (IADL) are preserved. In the field of AD, diagnosis of MCI should be unequivocally linked to a progressive linear worsening leading to dementia [15]. More specifically, it is known to occur in those patients presenting an amnesic type of MCI. However, this concept pointing for a transitional stage towards dementia results more complex when it refers to PD [16, 58]. In the context of PD, most patients present relatively mild but significant cognitive alterations since the beginning of the disease, and there is an unclear relationship between the occurrence of these symptoms and unequivocal transition to dementia [14, 18].

Epidemiological studies have demonstrated that from the beginning of the disease to more advanced stages, the cognitive profile of PD patients is largely heterogeneous (Table 2.2) [2–4, 13, 18, 50, 59, 60]. Hence, the prospective Sydney Multicenter Study [8] identified three cognitive phenotypes in PD: (i) PD patients with early and prominent dementia clinically corresponding with dementia with

Table 2.2 Studies of prevalence and MCI subtypes in PD [2, 3, 5, 13, 18, 57, 59, 60]

Authors	Year	Sample size	Disease duration	PD-MCI (%)	PD-MCI type (%)
Muslimovic et al. [2]	2005	115	1.6	24 %	Múltiples dominios
Janvin et al. [13]	2006	72	11	52 %	44 % non-amnesic single domain
					39 % multiple domains
					15 % amnesic single domain
Caviness et al. [3]	2007	86	9.2	21 %	39 % non-amnesic single domain
					22 % non-amnesic multiple domains
					22 % nmnesic single domain
Aarsland et al. [18]	2009	196	2.4	18.9 %	62.2 % non-amnesic single domain
					2.7 % non-amnesic multiple domains
					24.3 % amnesic single domain
					10.8 % amnesic multiple domain
Aarsland et al. [5]	2010	1,346	6.1	26 %	11.3 % non-amnesic single domain
					8.9 % amnesic single domain
					4.8 % amnesic multiple domain
					1.3 % non-amnesic multiple domain
Litvan et al. [57]	2011	776	ND	26.7 %	Non-amnesic more frequent tan amnesic in 8 reviewed studies
Goldman et al. [59]	2012	125	7	ND	47.7 % non-amnesic single domain
					24.2 % amnesic single domain
					18.8 % non-amnesic multiple domain
					9.5 % no amnésico múltiples dominios
Yu et al. [60]	2012	94	4.4	46.8 %	25.5 % non-amnesic single domain
					7.4 % non-amnesic multiple domains
					7.4 % amnesic multiple domain
					6.4 % amnesic single domain

Levy bodies, (ii) older patients (>70 years old) developing dementia after 3–10 years clinically corresponding to PDD, and (iii) a younger group who may remain cognitively intact during many years and eventually develop dementia at a given point [17, 18]. As a result, main interest relates on whether it is possible to differentiate these early cognitive profiles predicting a benign or relatively slow course to those with a more malignant course to dementia [6, 12, 25, 61].

As previously stated, an estimated 15–20 % of non-demented PD patients also exhibit deficits in more cortical-dependent tasks such as confrontation naming or encoding deficits [2, 3, 13]. This pattern of added posterior-cortical alterations is commonly evidenced in patients who convert to PDD [12, 21, 27]. Notably, while the progression of frontal-executive deficits usually follows a slow and linear decline, the addition of posterior-cortical alterations occurs in an abrupt nonlinear and faster fashion [6, 27].

The importance of exploring for posterior cortical defects as possible prodromal markers of dementia is highlighted by the fact that even in drug-naïve PD patients with mild cognitive impairment (PD-MCI), decline in executive/attentional, visuospatial, and memory functions appeared directly related to cortical hypometabolism in prefrontal but also in posterior cortical networks. Such pattern is shared in advanced stages of PD-MCI and PD with dementia [62, 63].

Given the proposed heterogeneity on both clinical characteristics and prognostic implications of PD-MCI, a task force commissioned by the Movement Disorders Society (MDS) recently established the diagnostic criteria for MCI in PD (PD-MCI) [50]. These criteria (Table 2.3), based on literature review and expert consensus, presuppose that PD-MCI might also be associated with impairments in daily functioning and quality of life. The criteria are presently under validation and are open to modification when further research improves knowledge of the clinical syndrome of PD-MCI and its subtypes [4, 18, 26, 27].

Neuropsychological Assessment of Cognitive Impairment in PD

Per definition, neuropsychological assessment methods differ from other specialties—such as cognitive neurology or neuropsychiatry—by the use of standardized, quantitative, and norm-referenced procedures [64]. Clinical neuropsychology provides clinicians and researchers with a large list of standardized and normalized assessment tools able to cover for all the cognitive domains of interest when assessing cognitive status in PD. However, test selection on the setting up of comprehensive neuropsychological assessments should be always done taking into account the study population of interest (i.e., AD, PD, traumatic brain injury) and the information that will be provided by the tools employed (i.e., global cognitive status addressed through screening methods, detailed cognitive performance at different

Table 2.3 Diagnostic criteria for PD-MCI [50]

Inclusion criteria
Diagnosis of Parkinson's disease as based on the UK PD Brain Bank Criteria
Gradual decline, in the context of established PD, in cognitive ability reported by either the patient or informant, *or* observed by the clinician
Cognitive deficitcis on either formal neuropsychological testing or a scale of global cognitive abilities
Cognitive deficits are not sufficient to interfere significantly with functional independence, although subtle difficulties on complex functional tasks may be present
Exclusion criteria
Diagnosis of PD dementia based on MDS task force proposed criteria
Other primary explanations for cognitive impairment (e.g., delirium, stroke, major depression, metabolic abnormalities, adverse effects of medication, or head trauma)
Other PD-associated comorbid conditions (e.g., motor impairment or severe anxiety, depression, excessive daytime sleepiness, or psychosis) that, in the opinion of the clinician, significantly influence cognitive testing
Specific guidelines for PD-MCI level I and level II categories
A. Level I (abbreviated assessment)
Impairment on a scale of global cognitive abilities validated for use in PD *or*
Impairment on at least two tests, when a limited battery of neuropsychological tests is performed (i.e., the battery includes less than two tests within each of the five cognitive domains, or less than five cognitive domains are assessed)
B. Level II (comprehensive assessment)
Neuropsychological testing that includes two tests within each of the five cognitive domains (i.e., attention and working memory, executive, language, memory, and visuospatial)
Impairment on at least two neuropsychological tests, represented by either two impaired tests in one cognitive domain or one impaired test in two different cognitive domains
Impairment on neuropsychological tests may be demonstrated by:
Performance approximately 1–2 SDs below appropriate norms *or*
Significant decline demonstrated on serial cognitive testing *or*
Significant decline from estimated premorbid levels
Subtype classification for PD-MCI (optional, requires two tests for each of the five cognitive domains assessed and is strongly suggested for research purposes)
PD-MCI single-domain—abnormalities on two tests within a single cognitive domain (specify the domain), with other domains unimpaired *or*
PD-MCI multiple-domain—abnormalities on at least one test in two or more cognitive domains (specify the domains)

Diagnostic criteria for PD-MCI from the Movement Disorders Society Task Force guidelines [50]

cognitive domains, detailed performance in a specific subprocess involved in a given cognitive domain) [64].

In the context of PD, assessment of cognitive status can be performed with clinical and/or research interests [25]. In both contexts, accurate neuropsychological assessment must be defined based on the accomplishment of psychometric standards with a relatively independence on the effect that motor symptoms might exert over cognitive performance. However, focusing on clinical or diagnostic proposes, test selection must be done in accordance of the capacity of the tools employed to identify whether or not the patient fulfills the proposed diagnostic criteria for PD-MCI or PDD [25, 50].

On the context of screening and diagnosis of PD-MCI, the selection of the tests to be used should be made on the basis of covering for all the cognitive domains of interest [25, 50, 57, 65]. It should be also taken into account that the assignment of specific cognitive tasks to single domains is a bit arbitrary. Some tests may cover more than one domain (e.g., the Rey-Osterrieth Complex Figure Test, widely used for the evaluation of visuospatial constructional ability and visual memory and also a useful tool for measuring executive function); then the intervention of an experienced neuropsychologist is highly recommendable for the selection of the instruments to be used.

As previously pointed out, from a clinical perspective, neuropsychological assessment can be constructed on the basis of allowing clinicians to determine if a given patient is fulfilling diagnostic criteria for PD-MCI and also to identify the cognitive profile [50, 66]. Thus, based on the previous described characteristics that differentiate the prognostic implications of frontal-subcortical to posterior-cortical alterations and the need to cover a full range of possible alterations, patients should be assessed in different cognitive domains [25].

Numerous cognitive assessment approaches are currently available. As noted, the preliminary consideration on test selection refers to the psychometric properties of the test. Thus, beyond the existence of good normative data, how free of producing random and nonrandom errors is the test, how well it measures and predicts all for what it was designed and how practice modulates performance.

Once focused on clinical cognitive assessment, a first approach should be done as a preliminary screening method to generally determine whether or not some degree of cognitive impairment is significantly present. Screening methods, also known as "Level 1" tests, allow a first approach to the global cognitive status of the patient and serve for the screening of PD-MCI [50]. For research purposes and formal diagnosis of PD-MCI, it is recommended to use "Level 2" tests. These latter refer to both specific neuropsychological assessment batteries compiled in order to provide an in-depth assessment of at least five cognitive domains (attention, memory, executive functions, language, and visuoperception/visuoconstruction). Thus, comprehensive neuropsychological assessment allows (a) the formal diagnosis of a given cognitive syndrome; (b) the identification of specific cognitive profiles; and (c) the reliable measurement of follow-up changes.

Functionality and day-to-day activities are also a key feature to be assessed in the context of the neuropsychological evaluation [67]. Specifically, both motor and cognitive features can independently disrupt independence on ADL. Thus, functional scales to be used should be selected on the basis of covering for the impact of cognitive—rather than just motor—alterations over functionality that may cause a significant impact on instrumental activities of daily living (IADL).

Tools for Cognitive Assessment in PD

Level 1 Tests

The Mini-Mental State Examination (MMSE)

The MMSE [68] is a general screening instrument for cognitive impairment. It can be easily and rapidly performed by a clinician and is currently the most commonly used screening test for dementia. Dependence of the MMSE on age and educational level hinders the use of a rigid cutoff score. In elderly populations, the MMSE demonstrates floor effects in subjects with severe cognitive impairment and ceiling effects in subjects with mild cognitive impairment.

It was widely used in PD as a screening tool, despite that it was not designed nor validated to assess cognitive impairment and dementia in PD. Although widely used, the Mini-Mental State Examination (MMSE) does not capture domains germane to PD (i.e., executive dysfunction) and suffers from ceiling effects (i.e., a normal score does not rule out cognitive disturbances or dementia in PD). In conclusion, the MMSE is not a recommended instrument to be used in the screening of PD-MCI [25, 50].

The Montreal Cognitive Assessment (MoCA)

The MoCA [69] was initially developed as a brief screening assessment for MCI in AD with the intention to address the limitations of the MMSE. Interestingly, the MoCA divides subscores in visuospatial/executive, language, memory, attention, abstraction, and orientation and sums an extra point when years of education are below <12 years. However, the validity of the MoCA in PD has not been unequivocally established against formal criteria or a comprehensive neuropsychological battery used to provide a criterion standard diagnosis of MCI and dementia. In a study comparing the accuracy of MMSE versus MoCA in PD patients with MCI or dementia, a cutoff score <26 was proposed for screening of MCI. When compared with the MMSE, the MoCA appeared to be more sensitive to mild frontal-subcortical cognitive defects. However, its substandard accuracy in diagnosing PD-MCI (sensitivity = 0.83, specificity = 0.53) cast some doubts on recommending this scale in PD-MCI as a useful tool other than for screening purposes [70, 71]. A MoCA cutoff point of 26 that has been established as optimal for screening cognitive impairment in PD was mostly established on how it relates to MMSE performance. Nevertheless, a positive screen using either instrument requires additional assessment due to suboptimal specificity at the recommended screening cutoff point [71, 72]. In a more recent study, the optimal MoCA screening cutoffs differed significantly, with a proposed score of <26 for PD-MCI, with sensitivity 90 % and specificity 75 %. Although the accuracy of MoCA in this study is clearly better, a specificity <80 % for screening PD-MCI is still of doubtful usefulness in clinical practice. While the MoCA still requires further study of its diagnostic utility in PD populations, among the brief tests of level 1, it can be considered a minimum cognitive screening measure in clinical trials of PD. Its value as outcome measure was not established yet.

Mini-Mental Parkinson (MMP)

The MMP [19] is a brief screening instrument derived from the MMSE initially oriented to patients who need a more comprehensive cognitive assessment. It includes seven-ordered sections assessing orientation, visual registration, attention, verbal fluency, visual recall, set shifting, and concept processing. Limitations of the scale include heavy representation of the orientation item (10 of 32 points), which is also the item contributing least to scale variance, and a lack of cortical items. The MMP also differs significantly between different stages of the disease [73].

The MMP was not subjected to an extensive clinimetric evaluation, and data is lacking regarding internal consistency, test-retest, or inter-rater reliability. In a recent work, the psychometric and validity properties of the MMP were evaluated in 69 cognitively intact and 52 cognitively impaired PD patients, classified according to their performance at the Dementia Rating Scale. The MMP showed better metrics and convergent validity and higher screening ability. However, its performance was not fully satisfying in terms of data distribution, coefficient of variation, and specificity, and ROC curves did not show clear cut superiority of either scale at their best sensitivity-specificity trade-off. The MMP seems to be slightly preferable to the MMSE only at a cutoff that favors sensitivity with respect to specificity, for screening purposes. The test is simple and quick, but has limitations in terms of validity [73].

PDD-Short Screen

The PDD-Short Screen (PDD-SS) [74] was designed and validated as a PD-specific brief cognitive test for screening dementia in PD. Based on regression analyses, and from an initial version covering different cognitive domains, a final brief version taking from 5 to 7 min to be administered disclosed a high accuracy in screening PDD. The final version included tasks assessing verbal fluency, free-recall verbal memory, clock copying, and a questionnaire on cognitive and associated psychiatric symptoms in PD. Score ranges from 0 to 22 points. ROC curves showed that a cut-off score ≤ 11 on the PDD-SS yielded high sensitivity (89.8 %), specificity (88.5 %), and positive and negative predictive values (PPV 80.7 %, NPV 93.6 %) for screening PDD. Although the accuracy for PDD was similar to that found with the Mattis Dementia Rating Scale, no further studies were still conducted to address the question of whether or not it is a feasible method for the screening of PD-MCI.

Clinical Dementia Rating Scale (CDR)

The Clinical Dementia Rating (CDR) [75] scale was developed to distinguish between normal cognition (CDR = 0), questionable dementia (CDR = 0.5), and mild, moderate, or severe dementia (CDR = 1–3). Employing a semi-structured interview, the CDR is a global rating device for assessing stages of dementia. It measures cognitive function across six domains: memory, orientation, judgment and problem solving, community affairs, home and hobby, and personal care. Information collected by the CDR allows assessment of cognitive impairment without reference to psychometric performance. The CDR has been used in patients with PD and has been shown to be sensitive to very mild cognitive impairment [27]. Relative to healthy control subjects, subjects with PD and questionable dementia (CDR = 0.5) exhibited impairment on all psychometric measures examined, except digit span and word fluency. Quantitative impairments detected during psychometric assessment of a group of PD patients with a CDR score of 0 were not detected by the physician. This observation suggests that screening for PD-MCI using the CDR still depends on information provided by patients and caregivers and on the subjective impression of the examiner. When applied in PD, the description of progressive memory loss is ambiguous; the orientation task is not useful in differentiating between PD patients with no or very mild cognitive impairment because this cognitive function is generally not altered in PD until moderate or severe dementia appears. In addition, scoring in the items "community affairs," "home and hobbies," and "personal care" is clearly influenced by PD motor symptoms.

The Frontal Assessment Battery

The FAB [62] is a short, bedside, cognitive battery assessing frontal lobe function. It comprises six subtests mainly exploring cognitive functions mediated by the medial prefrontal cortex: conceptualization/similarities, verbal fluencies, motor programming, sensitivity to interference, inhibitory control, and environmental autonomy. It was validated in normal control subjects and in patients with frontal lobe dysfunction (PD, multiple system atrophy, corticobasal degeneration, frontotemporal dementia (FTD), and progressive supranuclear palsy (PSP)). The FAB can be considered a useful scale to capture the cognitive impairment characteristic of pathologies with predominantly medial-prefrontal dysfunction. In PD, the FAB correlates well with measures of executive functions. The FAB does not cover for the full spectrum of cognitive impairment in PD [21, 25]. No formal studies assessed the discriminative properties of the FAB in screening or diagnosing of PD-MCI.

Level 2 Tests

The Mattis Dementia Rating Scale

Compared with the Mini-Mental State Examination (MMSE), the MDRS [76] is a more sensitive tool to detect frontal lobe dysfunction in PDD. In PD, it also accounts for more variation in the level of cognitive function. The MDRS appears to be valid and reliable; however, the first reported study attempting to validate this tool as a screening test for cognitive impairment in PD only included 14 patients. Most of the sample showed no cognitive deficits, and no cutoff scores were provided to differentiate between the cognitive groups. A main limitation of the MDRS is length, as the estimated administration time in the general population is 20–45 min. Normative data indicates that performance on the MDRS is largely influenced by both age and educational level. When using standard diagnostic criteria for diagnosing PD-MCI, a recent paper found different cutoff scores on regard the purposes of the assessment. Thus, ≤140 and ≤137 appeared as the more accurate cutoff scores for screening and diagnostic purposes, respectively. However, an in-depth examination of sensitivity/specificity for the screening cutoff revealed that a ≤139 yielded a better balance between sensitivity (77 %) and specificity (65 %).

While some limitations of the MDRS are the relatively weak coverage of visuospatial function and language, these recent data suggest that this instrument can be used both, for a preliminary screening (cutoff ≤139) and classification purposes on research (cutoff ≤137) [77].

SCOPA-COG (Scales for Outcomes of Parkinson's Disease-Cognition)

The SCOPA-COG was developed to specifically assess cognitive defects in PD [78]. Administration takes 10–15 min and the scale demonstrated good clinimetric properties. The main known limitation of the scale is that it mostly includes items assessing frontal-subcortical functioning (orientation, attention, memory/learning, executive functions, visuospatial functions, thinking, and reasoning), but there are no items assessing instrumental-cortical functions. Accordingly, the exclusive use of this scale for the assessment of longitudinal changes in PD might be inappropriate by an insufficient identification of subgroups of non-demented PD patients with posterior-cortical patterns of cognitive impairment suggesting an increased risk of dementia [25]. Accounting for these limitations, it is a good instrument to be used in both clinical and research settings.

PANDA (Parkinson Neuropsychometric Dementia Assessment)

The PANDA [79] is a short test (8–10 min) designed to screen for cognitive impairment in PD. It includes items covering distinct cognitive domains (immediate and delayed recall memory, verbal fluency, visuospatial skills, attentions, and working memory). Despite the validation study showed appropriate discriminative properties between controls, PD, PD-MCI, and PDD patients, it was not subjected to an extensive clinimetric evaluation. As it occurs with other tools developed following the concept of cognitive impairment in PD as a predominant dysexecutive syndrome, it was eminently addressed to assess frontal-subcortical functions but does not include any item assessing instrumental-cortical functions. Nevertheless, PANDA shows superiority against the MMSE on detecting cognitive impairment in PD.

PD-CRS (Parkinson's Disease-Cognitive Rating Scale)

The PD-CRS [27] is a new instrument specifically designed to capture from subtle, mild, to major cognitive defects appearing along the course of PD. The PD-CRS displayed very good clinimetric properties, and its time of application is relatively short (ranging from 15 min in non-demented to 26 min in PDD). The PD-CRS consists of nine tasks differentially assessing frontal-subcortical and instrumental-cortical functions. The seven frontal-subcortical tasks include sustained attention, working memory, alternating and action verbal fluency, clock drawing, and immediate and delayed free-recall verbal memory. The two instrumental posterior cortical items include confrontation naming and copying a clock. In the validation study, it showed a very good power differentiating cognitively intact PD patients from both PD-MCI and PDD. As expected, instrumental-cortical items selectively differentiated PDD from non-demented PD patients. A total score of ≤64 yielded high sensitivity (94 %), specificity (94 %), positive predictive value (PPV) (91 %), and negative predictive value (NPV) (96 %) for screening PDD. These data were confirmed by an independent evaluation of the psychometric attributes of the PD-CRS that found that the scale displayed satisfactory levels of acceptability, internal consistence, construct validity, and precision [69]. The PD-CRS is a recommended instrument by the MDS task force on MCI for the evaluation of PD-MCI. Recent findings highlighting the early involvement of posterior cortical regions in PD patients with cognitive deficits and the probable relevance of this pattern in predicting prodromal dementia [21, 26] stress the additional advantage of the PD-CRS relative to other instruments in distinguishing frontal-striatal and posterior cortical patterns of cognitive impairment. A recent validation study indicated that a score ≤81 of 134 was the optimal cutoff point on the total score for the PD-CRS (sensitivity, 79 %; specificity, 80 %; positive predictive value, 59 %; negative predictive value, 91 %). In addition, a range of change from 10 to 13 points on the PD-CRS total score appeared indicative of clinically significant change [69].

Cambridge Cognitive Assessment (CAMCOG)

This is the cognitive section of the Cambridge Examination of Mental Disorders. Validation studies showed the CAMCOG as a valid and reliable scale for assessing cognitive function and screening for dementia in elderly populations [80]. It includes eight subscales: orientation, language, recall and recognition memory, attention, calculation, praxis, and perception. While the CAMCOG showed extremely good clinimetric properties for the diagnosis of PDD, no validation studies were done on the context of usefulness of CAMCOG for the screening and diagnosis of PD-MCI. In addition, disadvantages of the CAMCOG are lengthy administration time (25–30 min), and aging associated with significantly poorer scores.

Recommendations for the Interpretation of Test Results

Measurement of whether or not a given cognitive performance pattern represents a significant decline on premorbid competences or expected age-referred level is crucial for the diagnosis of any cognitive syndrome. In an ideal context, premorbid cognitive evaluation will allow clinicians to compare current and further evaluations to determine if a rate of significant decline is present. However, in most cases, cognitive assessment is done once some degree of subjective cognitive complains are indicated by the patient. Thus, no clear premorbid cognitive status uses to be available. Estimating premorbid IQ represents a standardized approach to address this question that can be done using instruments such the Wechsler Test of Adult Reading or the National Adult Reading Test. Accordingly, current cognitive status can be then compared to premorbid IQ. The follow-up routine along these time points where minimum clinical change is expected to be significantly measured represents a core method [64].

Tests results falling between −1 and −2 SD from the expected or premorbid level can be considered as characteristic of MCI, while larger deviations of more than −2 SD are more typical for patients who crossed the threshold of dementia. As mentioned before, the construct of PD-MCI is still waiting for a validation consensus, and their diagnostic criteria have been recently defined in consensus by the MDS task force on PD-MCI to avoid potential confusion arising from different definitions that may hamper targeted intervention. These criteria require validation with further research using comprehensive neuropsychological assessment and comparison with commonly used standardized rating scales. When using ad hoc comprehensive neuropsychological batteries for research, the definition of PD-MCI can be based on patient's performance in different cognitive domains (including attention, execution, memory, visuospatial, and language). For each cognitive domain, averaged z scores of tests included in that domain can be calculated and compared with normalized data for each test or using a control group of healthy subjects without dementia and performing multiple regression analysis adjusting for age, education, and sex. Using this method, PD patients can be diagnosed with PD-MCI when the difference between the actual cognitive domain z score and the expected z score is below −1.5 or 2 on at least one out of the five cognitive domains. It is not recommendable using more than two tests for domain to avoid increasing the probabilities of statistical bias towards overdiagnosing cognitive impairment.

Tools for Functional Assessment in PD

Functional assessment results crucial in front of the need to delimitate the cognitive status of the patient [67]. Given the course of PD-MCI, functional assessment should be done to delineate whether or not cognitive alterations have an impact over

IADL. Functional assessment instruments should be selected based on the avoidance of confounders such as motor impairment.

The Parkinson's Disease: Cognitive Functional Rating Scale (PD-CFRS)

The PD-CFRS was developed based on the lack of specific instruments of functional assessment controlling for motor aspects. The PD-CFRS is a brief questionnaire addressed to explore a wide range of functional aspects suspected to be sensible to CI in PD, minimizing the motor impact of the disease. The scale is administered to a knowledgeable informant in an interview form by 12 items selected to cover the spectrum of instrumental cognitive changes seen in PD over the last 2 weeks before the evaluation. Cutoff score ≥3 points demonstrated good clinimetric properties (sensitivity: 0.84; NPV: 0.83) recognizing patients presenting PD-MCI and some degree of functional impairment. Moreover, an increase of 2 points after 6-month follow-up was associated with a clinically significant worsening of the cognitive functional status.

The Brief Penn Daily Activities Questionnaire (PDAQ)

The PDAQ is a 15-item functional scale focused on specific issues regarding cognitive impairment in PD. Preliminary results showed that the PDAQ presents good discriminant validity across stages of cognitive impairment in PD and correlates highly with global cognitive performance.

Management of Cognitive Impairment in PD

Effects of Dopaminergic Stimulation on Cognition

Mild cognitive impairment in PD is mainly characterized by dopaminergic-related dysfunctions, such as defects in verbal fluencies, working-memory, sustained attention, visuospatial disturbances, and free-recall verbal memory. As stated before, in the early to mid PD stages, in which patients still have a stable motor response to dopaminergic agents, several studies have demonstrated an improvement of all these domains, either on dopamine agonists or levodopa, that is maintained 12–18 months after treatment onset. Compared to levodopa, pramipexole exhibited lower benefits in verbal fluency and Luria's palm-edge-fist test [39]. Recently, in a double-blind, placebo-controlled, multicenter study, patients receiving rasagiline, a selective monoamine oxidase type-B inhibitor that enhances central dopaminergic transmission, attentional and executive tasks improved, with no changes in other cognitive domains [81].

All these benefits, however, are not usually sufficient so as to compensate for all deficits, and tend to deteriorate at 18–24 months of follow-up, despite optimal control of motor parkinsonian signs. In advanced patients with motor complications, levodopa may even induce impairment in frontal-executive tasks (i.e., Wisconsin card sorting test) 1–4 h after each levodopa dose [37, 39].

As a whole, it seems that dopaminergic replacement does not recover cognition efficiently and has a limited effect in time, with very modest or even transient deleterious effects on cognition from mid to advanced stages of the disease [39, 40, 82].

Effects of Cholinergic Stimulation on Cognition

Despite the long-standing evidence supporting the role of cholinergic deficits for the development and progression of cognitive deterioration in PD, few studies have accomplished to demonstrate a benefit in cognition through cholinergic stimulation.

Initial open-label studies with different cholinesterase inhibitors (donepezil, rivastigmine, galantamine) observed significant improvement in attention, memory, and visuoperceptive tasks in PDD. Regarding PD-MCI, there is a lack of clinical trials focusing on the potential therapeutic and/or neuroprotective effects that cholinergic stimulation should exert on transition to PDD.

Conclusion

Cognitive impairment is a key feature of PD that can be recognized in most of the patients from the earliest stages and at any time along the course of the disease [2]. Cognitive impairment has important clinical implications since it can indicate an aggregated risk for further development of dementia [7, 12, 25]. However, dissimilarly than the observed in the field of AD, in PD the presence of cognitive alterations that can be labeled, MCI does not always indicate progression to dementia in a short period of time [14, 26].

In PD, different cognitive profiles have been linked to major or minor risk for developing dementia [13, 16, 26, 27]. Thus, common frontal-subcortical cognitive alterations seen in most of the patients and mainly attributable to the concurrent dopaminergic deficiency can result in a relatively benign course remaining stable a long time [26]. In contrast, with independence on the degree of frontal-subcortical alterations, the addition of AD-like or more posterior cortical defects appears to herald higher risk for developing dementia.

PD-MCI can be characterized as the presence of a sum of measurable cognitive alterations fulfilling with the standards proposed by the MDS [50]. These alterations can affect single or multiple domains despite that the more common early findings are alteration on executive functions. While dysexecutive alterations may follow a linear pattern of decline, cortical alterations can appear at any time along the course of the disease added to frontal-subcortical alterations. These posterior cortical alterations seem to define a more aggressive pattern of cognitive impairment [26, 27]. Thus, cognitive assessment in PD must be done focusing on the whole spectrum of PD-associated cognitive impairment. As there is considerable heterogeneity within PD-MCI, further stratification of different subtypes may be necessary when selecting patients for clinical trials if certain subtypes or cognitive domains are shown to be more relevant than others for predicting dementia. To properly characterize PD-MCI, accurate neuropsychological assessment is needed. Different tools have been tested in the field of cognitive assessment in PD. However, a first approach should be done through screening methods [25].

Mild cognitive impairment can have some degree of impact over ADL [67]. Based on the interference that motor alteration should exert over IADL, the impact of cognition over functionality should be addressed through specific instruments that control for this confounding variable [67].

References

1. Janvin C, Aarsland D, Larsen JP, Hugdahl K. Neuropsychological profile of patients with Parkinson's disease without dementia. Dement Geriatr Cogn Disord. 2003;15(3):126–31. Epub 2003/02/14.
2. Muslimovic D, Post B, Speelman JD, Schmand B. Cognitive profile of patients with newly diagnosed Parkinson disease. Neurology. 2005;65(8):1239–45. Epub 2005/10/26.
3. Caviness JN, Driver-Dunckley E, Connor DJ, Sabbagh MN, Hentz JG, Noble B, et al. Defining mild cognitive impairment in Parkinson's disease. Mov Disord. 2007;22(9):1272–7. Epub 2007/04/07.
4. Aarsland D, Bronnick K, Williams-Gray C, Weintraub D, Marder K, Kulisevsky J, et al. Mild cognitive impairment in Parkinson disease: a multicenter pooled analysis. Neurology. 2010;75(12):1062–9. Epub 2010/09/22.
5. Aarsland D, Kurz MW. The epidemiology of dementia associated with Parkinson's disease. Brain Pathol. 2010;20(3):633–9. Epub 2010/06/05.
6. Aarsland D, Muniz G, Matthews F. Nonlinear decline of mini-mental state examination in Parkinson's disease. Mov Disord. 2011;26(2):334–7. Epub 2010/10/21.
7. Buter TC, van den Hout A, Matthews FE, Larsen JP, Brayne C, Aarsland D. Dementia and survival in Parkinson disease: a 12-year population study. Neurology. 2008;70(13):1017–22. Epub 2008/03/26.
8. Clarimon J, Kulisevsky J. Parkinson's disease: from genetics to clinical practice. Curr Genomics. 2013;14(8):560–7. Epub 2014/02/18.
9. Committee GPsDSS. Factors impacting on quality of life in Parkinson's disease: results from an international survey. Mov Disord. 2002;17(1):60–7. Epub 2002/02/09.
10. Aarsland D, Bronnick K, Ehrt U, De Deyn PP, Tekin S, Emre M, et al. Neuropsychiatric symptoms in patients with Parkinson's disease and dementia: frequency, profile and associated care giver stress. J Neurol Neurosurg Psychiatry. 2007;78(1):36–42. Epub 2006/07/06.
11. Muslimovic D, Post B, Speelman JD, Schmand B, de Haan RJ. Determinants of disability and quality of life in mild to moderate Parkinson disease. Neurology. 2008;70(23):2241–7. Epub 2008/06/04.

12. Aarsland D, Andersen K, Larsen JP, Lolk A, Kragh-Sorensen P. Prevalence and characteristics of dementia in Parkinson disease: an 8-year prospective study. Arch Neurol. 2003;60(3):387–92. Epub 2003/03/14.
13. Janvin CC, Larsen JP, Aarsland D, Hugdahl K. Subtypes of mild cognitive impairment in Parkinson's disease: progression to dementia. Mov Disord. 2006;21(9):1343–9. Epub 2006/05/25.
14. Williams-Gray CH, Foltynie T, Brayne CE, Robbins TW, Barker RA. Evolution of cognitive dysfunction in an incident Parkinson's disease cohort. Brain. 2007;130(Pt 7):1787–98. Epub 2007/05/31.
15. Petersen RC, Smith GE, Waring SC, Ivnik RJ, Tangalos EG, Kokmen E. Mild cognitive impairment: clinical characterization and outcome. Arch Neurol. 1999;56(3):303–8. Epub 1999/04/06.
16. Martinez-Horta S, Kulisevsky J. Is all cognitive impairment in Parkinson's disease "mild cognitive impairment"? J Neural Transm. 2011;118(8):1185–90. Epub 2011/06/23.
17. Hely MA, Reid WG, Adena MA, Halliday GM, Morris JG. The Sydney multicenter study of Parkinson's disease: the inevitability of dementia at 20 years. Mov Disord. 2008;23(6):837–44. Epub 2008/03/01.
18. Aarsland D, Bronnick K, Larsen JP, Tysnes OB, Alves G. Cognitive impairment in incident, untreated Parkinson disease: the Norwegian ParkWest study. Neurology. 2009;72(13):1121–6. Epub 2008/11/21.
19. Pagonabarraga J, Corcuera-Solano I, Vives-Gilabert Y, Llebaria G, Garcia-Sanchez C, Pascual-Sedano B, et al. Pattern of regional cortical thinning associated with cognitive deterioration in Parkinson's disease. PLoS One. 2013;8(1):e54980. Epub 2013/01/30.
20. Martinez-Horta S, Pagonabarraga J, Fernandez de Bobadilla R, Garcia-Sanchez C, Kulisevsky J. Apathy in Parkinson's disease: more than just executive dysfunction. J Int Neuropsychol Soc. 2013;19(5):571–82. Epub 2013/02/22.
21. Pagonabarraga J, Kulisevsky J. Cognitive impairment and dementia in Parkinson's disease. Neurobiol Dis. 2012;46(3):590–6. Epub 2012/04/10.
22. Nandhagopal R, Kuramoto L, Schulzer M, Mak E, Cragg J, McKenzie J, et al. Longitudinal evolution of compensatory changes in striatal dopamine processing in Parkinson's disease. Brain. 2011;134(Pt 11):3290–8. Epub 2011/11/15.
23. Pillon B, Dubois B, Cusimano G, Bonnet AM, Lhermitte F, Agid Y. Does cognitive impairment in Parkinson's disease result from non-dopaminergic lesions? J Neurol Neurosurg Psychiatry. 1989;52(2):201–6. Epub 1989/02/01.
24. Monchi O, Petrides M, Doyon J, Postuma RB, Worsley K, Dagher A. Neural bases of set-shifting deficits in Parkinson's disease. J Neurosci. 2004;24(3):702–10. Epub 2004/01/23.
25. Kulisevsky J, Pagonabarraga J. Cognitive impairment in Parkinson's disease: tools for diagnosis and assessment. Mov Disord. 2009;24(8):1103–10. Epub 2009/04/09.
26. Williams-Gray CH, Evans JR, Goris A, Foltynie T, Ban M, Robbins TW, et al. The distinct cognitive syndromes of Parkinson's disease: 5 year follow-up of the CamPaIGN cohort. Brain. 2009;132(Pt 11):2958–69. Epub 2009/10/09.
27. Pagonabarraga J, Kulisevsky J, Llebaria G, Garcia-Sanchez C, Pascual-Sedano B, Gironell A. Parkinson's disease-cognitive rating scale: a new cognitive scale specific for Parkinson's disease. Mov Disord. 2008;23(7):998–1005. Epub 2008/04/03.
28. Scatton B, Rouquier L, Javoy-Agid F, Agid Y. Dopamine deficiency in the cerebral cortex in Parkinson disease. Neurology. 1982;32(9):1039–40. Epub 1982/09/01.
29. Halliday GM, McCann H. The progression of pathology in Parkinson's disease. Ann N Y Acad Sci. 2010;1184:188–95. Epub 2010/02/12.
30. Yeterian EH, Pandya DN. Prefrontostriatal connections in relation to cortical architectonic organization in rhesus monkeys. J Comp Neurol. 1991;312(1):43–67. Epub 1991/10/01.
31. Yeterian EH, Pandya DN. Corticothalamic connections of the superior temporal sulcus in rhesus monkeys. Exp Brain Res. 1991;83(2):268–84. Epub 1991/01/01.
32. Pagonabarraga J, Soriano-Mas C, Llebaria G, Lopez-Sola M, Pujol J, Kulisevsky J. Neural correlates of minor hallucinations in non-demented patients with Parkinson's disease. Parkinsonism Relat Disord. 2014;20(3):290–6. Epub 2014/01/01.

33. Braak H, Ghebremedhin E, Rub U, Bratzke H, Del Tredici K. Stages in the development of Parkinson's disease-related pathology. Cell Tissue Res. 2004;318(1):121–34. Epub 2004/09/01.
34. MacDonald AA, Monchi O, Seergobin KN, Ganjavi H, Tamjeedi R, MacDonald PA. Parkinson's disease duration determines effect of dopaminergic therapy on ventral striatum function. Mov Disord. 2013;28(2):153–60. Epub 2012/11/21.
35. Gotham AM, Brown RG, Marsden CD. 'Frontal' cognitive function in patients with Parkinson's disease 'on' and 'off' levodopa. Brain. 1988;111(Pt 2):299–321. Epub 1988/04/01.
36. Monchi O, Petrides M, Mejia-Constain B, Strafella AP. Cortical activity in Parkinson's disease during executive processing depends on striatal involvement. Brain. 2007;130(Pt 1):233–44. Epub 2006/11/24.
37. Kulisevsky J. Role of dopamine in learning and memory: implications for the treatment of cognitive dysfunction in patients with Parkinson's disease. Drugs Aging. 2000;16(5):365–79. Epub 2000/08/05.
38. Kulisevsky J, Avila A, Barbanoj M, Antonijoan R, Berthier ML, Gironell A. Acute effects of levodopa on neuropsychological performance in stable and fluctuating Parkinson's disease patients at different levodopa plasma levels. Brain. 1996;119(Pt 6):2121–32. Epub 1996/12/01.
39. Kulisevsky J, Garcia-Sanchez C, Berthier ML, Barbanoj M, Pascual-Sedano B, Gironell A, et al. Chronic effects of dopaminergic replacement on cognitive function in Parkinson's disease: a 2-year follow-up study of previously untreated patients. Mov Disord. 2000;15(4):613–26. Epub 2000/08/06.
40. Cools R, Stefanova E, Barker RA, Robbins TW, Owen AM. Dopaminergic modulation of high-level cognition in Parkinson's disease: the role of the prefrontal cortex revealed by PET. Brain. 2002;125(Pt 3):584–94. Epub 2002/03/02.
41. Cools R, Lewis SJ, Clark L, Barker RA, Robbins TW. L-DOPA disrupts activity in the nucleus accumbens during reversal learning in Parkinson's disease. Neuropsychopharmacology. 2007;32(1):180–9. Epub 2006/07/15.
42. Kehagia AA, Barker RA, Robbins TW. Neuropsychological and clinical heterogeneity of cognitive impairment and dementia in patients with Parkinson's disease. Lancet Neurol. 2010;9(12):1200–13. Epub 2010/10/01.
43. Nakano I, Hirano A. Parkinson's disease: neuron loss in the nucleus basalis without concomitant Alzheimer's disease. Ann Neurol. 1984;15(5):415–8. Epub 1984/05/01.
44. Dubois B, Pilon B, Lhermitte F, Agid Y. Cholinergic deficiency and frontal dysfunction in Parkinson's disease. Ann Neurol. 1990;28(2):117–21. Epub 1990/08/01.
45. Pillon B, Dubois B, Bonnet AM, Esteguy M, Guimaraes J, Vigouret JM, et al. Cognitive slowing in Parkinson's disease fails to respond to levodopa treatment: the 15-objects test. Neurology. 1989;39(6):762–8. Epub 1989/06/01.
46. Shimada H, Hirano S, Shinotoh H, Aotsuka A, Sato K, Tanaka N, et al. Mapping of brain acetylcholinesterase alterations in Lewy body disease by PET. Neurology. 2009;73(4):273–8. Epub 2009/05/29.
47. Galvin JE. Cognitive change in Parkinson disease. Alzheimer Dis Assoc Disord. 2006;20(4):302–10. Epub 2006/11/30.
48. Klein JC, Eggers C, Kalbe E, Weisenbach S, Hohmann C, Vollmar S, et al. Neurotransmitter changes in dementia with Lewy bodies and Parkinson disease dementia in vivo. Neurology. 2010;74(11):885–92. Epub 2010/02/26.
49. Hilker R, Thomas AV, Klein JC, Weisenbach S, Kalbe E, Burghaus L, et al. Dementia in Parkinson disease: functional imaging of cholinergic and dopaminergic pathways. Neurology. 2005;65(11):1716–22. Epub 2005/12/14.
50. Litvan I, Goldman JG, Troster AI, Schmand BA, Weintraub D, Petersen RC, et al. Diagnostic criteria for mild cognitive impairment in Parkinson's disease: movement disorder society task force guidelines. Mov Disord. 2012;27(3):349–56. Epub 2012/01/26.
51. Emre M, Aarsland D, Brown R, Burn DJ, Duyckaerts C, Mizuno Y, et al. Clinical diagnostic criteria for dementia associated with Parkinson's disease. Mov Disord. 2007;22(12):1689–707; quiz 837; Epub 2007/06/02.
52. Jellinger KA. Neurobiology of cognitive impairment in Parkinson's disease. Expert Rev Neurother. 2012;12(12):1451–66. Epub 2012/12/15.

53. Seto-Salvia N, Clarimon J, Pagonabarraga J, Pascual-Sedano B, Campolongo A, Combarros O, et al. Dementia risk in Parkinson disease: disentangling the role of MAPT haplotypes. Arch Neurol. 2011;68(3):359–64. Epub 2011/03/16.
54. Seto-Salvia N, Pagonabarraga J, Houlden H, Pascual-Sedano B, Dols-Icardo O, Tucci A, et al. Glucocerebrosidase mutations confer a greater risk of dementia during Parkinson's disease course. Mov Disord. 2012;27(3):393–9. Epub 2011/12/17.
55. Petersen RC. Mild cognitive impairment as a diagnostic entity. J Intern Med. 2004;256(3):183–94. Epub 2004/08/25.
56. Petersen RC, Doody R, Kurz A, Mohs RC, Morris JC, Rabins PV, et al. Current concepts in mild cognitive impairment. Arch Neurol. 2001;58(12):1985–92. Epub 2001/12/26.
57. Litvan I, Aarsland D, Adler CH, Goldman JG, Kulisevsky J, Mollenhauer B, et al. MDS Task Force on mild cognitive impairment in Parkinson's disease: critical review of PD-MCI. Mov Disord. 2011;26(10):1814–24. Epub 2011/06/11.
58. Dubois B. Is PD-MCI a useful concept? Mov Disord. 2007;22(9):1215–6. Epub 2007/06/09.
59. Goldman JG, Weis H, Stebbins G, Bernard B, Goetz CG. Clinical differences among mild cognitive impairment subtypes in Parkinson's disease. Mov Disord. 2012;27(9):1129–36. Epub 2012/07/11.
60. Yu RL, Wu RM, Tai CH, Lin CH, Cheng TW, Hua MS. Neuropsychological profile in patients with early stage of Parkinson's disease in Taiwan. Parkinsonism Relat Disord. 2012;18(10):1067–72. Epub 2012/07/04.
61. Foltynie T, Brayne CE, Robbins TW, Barker RA. The cognitive ability of an incident cohort of Parkinson's patients in the UK. The CamPaIGN study. Brain. 2004;127(Pt 3):550–60. Epub 2003/12/24.
62. Villa-Bonomo C, Pagonabarraga J, Martinez-Horta S, Fernandez de Bobadilla R, Garcia-Sanchez C, Campolongo A, et al. Short-lasting episodes of prosopagnosia in Parkinson's disease. Parkinsonism Relat Disord. 2013;19(3):375–7. Epub 2012/12/15.
63. Hosokai Y, Nishio Y, Hirayama K, Takeda A, Ishioka T, Sawada Y, et al. Distinct patterns of regional cerebral glucose metabolism in Parkinson's disease with and without mild cognitive impairment. Mov Disord. 2009;24(6):854–62. Epub 2009/02/10.
64. Marras C, Troster AI, Kulisevsky J, Stebbins GT. The tools of the trade: a state of the art "How to Assess Cognition" in the patient with Parkinson's disease. Mov Disord. 2014;29(5):584–96. Epub 2014/04/24.
65. Troster AI. A precis of recent advances in the neuropsychology of mild cognitive impairment(s) in Parkinson's Disease and a proposal of preliminary research criteria. J Int Neuropsychol Soc. 2011;3:393–406. Epub 2011/04/09.
66. Dubois B, Burn D, Goetz C, Aarsland D, Brown RG, Broe GA, et al. Diagnostic procedures for Parkinson's disease dementia: recommendations from the movement disorder society task force. Mov Disord. 2007;22(16):2314–24. Epub 2007/12/22.
67. Kulisevsky J, Fernandez de Bobadilla R, Pagonabarraga J, Martinez-Horta S, Campolongo A, Garcia-Sanchez C, et al. Measuring functional impact of cognitive impairment: validation of the Parkinson's disease cognitive functional rating scale. Parkinsonism Relat Disord. 2013;19(9):812–7. Epub 2013/06/19.
68. Marti MJ, Kulisevsky J. Candidate patient for treatment with continuous apomorphine infusion. Rev Neurol. 2012;55 Suppl 1:S15–9. Epub 2012/10/20. Paciente candidato a tratamiento con apomorfina en infusion continua.
69. Fernandez de Bobadilla R, Pagonabarraga J, Martinez-Horta S, Pascual-Sedano B, Campolongo A, Kulisevsky J. Parkinson's disease-cognitive rating scale: psychometrics for mild cognitive impairment. Mov Disord. 2013;28(10):1376–83. Epub 2013/07/23.
70. Kasten M, Bruggemann N, Schmidt A, Klein C. Validity of the MoCA and MMSE in the detection of MCI and dementia in Parkinson disease. Neurology. 2010;75(5):478; author reply -9. Epub 2010/08/04.
71. Hoops S, Nazem S, Siderowf AD, Duda JE, Xie SX, Stern MB, et al. Validity of the MoCA and MMSE in the detection of MCI and dementia in Parkinson disease. Neurology. 2009;73(21):1738–45. Epub 2009/11/26.

72. Dalrymple-Alford JC, MacAskill MR, Nakas CT, Livingston L, Graham C, Crucian GP, et al. The MoCA: well-suited screen for cognitive impairment in Parkinson disease. Neurology. 2010;75(19):1717–25. Epub 2010/11/10.
73. Isella V, Mapelli C, Morielli N, De Gaspari D, Siri C, Pezzoli G, et al. Validity and metric of MiniMental Parkinson and MiniMental State Examination in Parkinson's disease. Neurol Sci. 2013;34(10):1751–8. Epub 2013/02/21.
74. Volkmann J, Albanese A, Antonini A, Chaudhuri KR, Clarke CE, de Bie RM, et al. Selecting deep brain stimulation or infusion therapies in advanced Parkinson's disease: an evidence-based review. J Neurol. 2013;260(11):2701–14. Epub 2013/01/05.
75. Berardelli A, Wenning GK, Antonini A, Berg D, Bloem BR, Bonifati V, et al. EFNS/MDS-ES/ENS [corrected] recommendations for the diagnosis of Parkinson's disease. Eur J Neurol. 2013;20(1):16–34. Epub 2013/01/03.
76. Llebaria G, Pagonabarraga J, Kulisevsky J, Garcia-Sanchez C, Pascual-Sedano B, Gironell A, et al. Cut-off score of the Mattis Dementia Rating Scale for screening dementia in Parkinson's disease. Mov Disord. 2008;23(11):1546–50. Epub 2008/06/12.
77. Pirogovsky E, Schiehser DM, Litvan I, Obtera KM, Burke MM, Lessig SL, et al. The utility of the Mattis Dementia Rating Scale in Parkinson's disease mild cognitive impairment. Parkinsonism Relat Disord. 2014;20(6):627–31. Epub 2014/04/09.
78. Moro E, Lozano AM, Pollak P, Agid Y, Rehncrona S, Volkmann J, et al. Long-term results of a multicenter study on subthalamic and pallidal stimulation in Parkinson's disease. Mov Disord. 2010;25(5):578–86. Epub 2010/03/10.
79. Davila G, Berthier ML, Kulisevsky J, Asenjo B, Gomez J, Lara JP, et al. Structural abnormalities in the substantia nigra and neighbouring nuclei in Tourette's syndrome. J Neural Transm. 2010;117(4):481–8. Epub 2010/02/05.
80. Kulisevsky J, Pagonabarraga J. Tolerability and safety of ropinirole versus other dopamine agonists and levodopa in the treatment of Parkinson's disease: meta-analysis of randomized controlled trials. Drug Saf. 2010;33(2):147–61. Epub 2010/01/20.
81. Emre M, Poewe W, De Deyn PP, Barone P, Kulisevsky J, Pourcher E, et al. Long-term safety of rivastigmine in parkinson disease dementia: an open-label, randomized study. Clin Neuropharmacol. 2014;37(1):9–16. Epub 2014/01/18.
82. Cooper JA, Sagar HJ, Doherty SM, Jordan N, Tidswell P, Sullivan EV. Different effects of dopaminergic and anticholinergic therapies on cognitive and motor function in Parkinson's disease. A follow-up study of untreated patients. Brain. 1992;115(Pt 6):1701–25. Epub 1992/12/01.

Chapter 3
Parkinson's Disease Dementia

Başar Bilgiç, Haşmet A. Hanağası, and Murat Emre

Introduction

Parkinson's disease (PD) is a neurodegenerative disorder commonly presenting with motor symptoms. Current diagnostic criteria are based on motor symptoms and signs. Although the dominant features consist of motor symptoms, neuropathological changes in the nervous system are not confined to motor related areas, but more widespread. As a consequence, nonmotor symptoms are common in the course of the disease. Sleep disturbances, cognitive and behavioral changes, and autonomic dysfunction occur in the majority of the patients.

In early descriptions of the condition, cognitive changes and dementia had been largely under-recognized. Due to the advances in the treatment of motor symptoms and the subsequent increase in life expectancy, cognitive impairment and dementia in PD have become increasingly more recognized with substantially increased amount of research in this field. In the last 5 years operational diagnostic criteria have been published for both mild cognitive impairment (PD-MCI) and dementia in PD (PD-D), and more has been understood about the pathological and biochemical changes underlying cognitive changes and first specific treatment for PD-D became available.

In this chapter we will describe the epidemiological features, clinical characteristics, pathology, genetic background, diagnosis, and treatment of PD-D.

B. Bilgiç, MD (✉) • H.A. Hanağası, MD • M. Emre, MD
Behavioral Neurology and Movement Disorders Unit,
Department of Neurology, Istanbul Faculty of Medicine,
Istanbul University, Millet cad., Capa, Istanbul 34093, Turkey
e-mail: bilgicb@gmail.com; hasmet@yahoo.com; muratemre@superonline.com

H. Reichmann (ed.), *Neuropsychiatric Symptoms of Movement Disorders*,
Neuropsychiatric Symptoms of Neurological Disease,
DOI 10.1007/978-3-319-09537-0_3

Epidemiology and Risk Factors

Both the prevalence and the incidence of cognitive impairment and dementia are substantially higher in patients with PD compared to age-matched controls. In a study in 115 newly diagnosed PD patients, 24 % displayed impaired performance on at least three neuropsychological tests and were classified as cognitively impaired [1]. A pooled analysis of data from eight centers using a standardized evaluation and comprising 1,346 non-demented PD patients showed that 25.8 % of patients had mild cognitive impairment according to the definition used [2]. In a community-based study in the UK, 36 % of newly diagnosed patients were found to have some degree of cognitive impairment at the time of diagnosis, while 57 % of this cohort developed cognitive deficits within 3.5 (±0.7) years. In the same cohort twenty-one incident dementia cases were identified over 5.2 years of follow-up, corresponding to a dementia incidence estimate of 38.7 per 1,000 person-years of observation [3]. At 10 years, cumulative probability of dementia increased to 46 %, and estimated dementia incidence was 54.7 per 1,000 person-years [4].

A systematic review of 12 selected studies on prevalence of PD-D revealed a point prevalence of 24–31 %. The prevalence of PD-D in the general population aged 65 years and over was calculated to be 0.3–0.5 %; 3–4 % of patients with dementia in the general population were estimated to be due to PD-D [5].

Incidence rates are more reliable than the prevalence rates to estimate the risk of dementia in PD, as demented patients are less likely to survive as compared to non-demented patients. The risk of dementia in PD was reported to vary between 1.7 and 5.9 compared to controls [6, 7]. In the longitudinally followed-up Sydney cohort, 48 % of surviving patients had developed dementia 15 years after the diagnosis [8], and the cumulative incidence had risen to 83 % 20 years after the diagnosis [9]. In another longitudinal study, 8-year cumulative prevalence of dementia was 78.2 %, with 26 % of cases being demented already at baseline [10]. The 12-year cumulative probability of dementia in this cohort was 60 % at the end of the follow-up period [11]. In the Rotterdam study, which employed a door-to-door survey, 15 % of the PD patients developed dementia compared to the 4.9 % of the control group, during a mean follow-up time of 4.3 years for the incident and 6.9 years for the prevalent PD group [7]. A recent study conducted in Olmsted County revealed that the incidence of PD-D was 2.5 per 100,000 person-years overall [12].

A number of risk factors have been associated with PD-D, as associated features in cross-sectional studies and as baseline characteristics predictive of dementia in prospective studies. Most consistent risk factors are old age at disease onset or at the time of evaluation, severe motor disability, presence of mild cognitive impairment at the time of diagnosis, and atypical neurological features such as early autonomic symptoms, symmetrical disease at presentation, and poor response to dopaminergic treatment including early development of confusion, hallucinations, or psychosis.

Both cross-sectional and prospective studies indicate advanced age as a prominent risk factor. In the Olmsted County study, the incidence of PD-D increased consistently with age, ranging from 0.6 in persons aged 50–59 years to 47.0 in persons aged 80–99 years [12]. Along with severe disease, patients with old age had a 12-fold increased dementia risk compared to young patients with mild disease demonstrating the combined effect of these risk factors [13].

Presence of mild cognitive impairment at the time of diagnosis appears to be a significant risk factor for dementia. In a community-based study in 182 incident PD patients monitored for 3 years, significantly more patients with MCI at baseline progressed to dementia compared to patients without cognitive impairment [14]. Neuropsychological features such as poor verbal fluency, poor performance on verbal memory, and impairment in executive functions at baseline were significantly associated with incident dementia [15]. In another study, however, impairment in cognitive tests relying on frontal executive functions was associated with a lower risk of dementia, whereas impairment in those tests tapping more posterior cortical functions was associated with a higher risk [3].

Dementia seems to be associated with postural instability and gait disorder phenotype (PIGD type). Tremor-dominant patients seem to have lower risk of developing dementia, unless they convert to PIGD form in their disease course [16]. Similar to constituting risk factors for dementia, PIGD phenotype and longer disease duration were also found to be risk factors for mild cognitive impairment [17].

Sleep-wake cycle disturbances such as excessive daytime sleepiness and rapid eye movement (REM) sleep behavior disorder (RBD) may also be associated with increased risk of dementia. RBD is frequently seen in PD and may be more frequent in patients who eventually develop dementia. In one study, PD patients with RBD had a sixfold higher occurrence of dementia than those without [18]. Similarly RBD was associated with a 2.2-fold increased risk of developing mild cognitive impairment over 4 years [19].

In terms of potential biomarkers, reduced CSF β-amyloid levels, an established CSF biomarker in Alzheimer's disease (AD), were found to be related with cognitive decline in PD patients [20, 21]. In neuroimaging studies, white matter hyperintensities were associated with cognitive decline in PD patients, regardless of age, sex, education status, duration or severity of PD symptoms, and vascular risk factors [22]; the load of vascular lesions was found to be correlated with impairment in executive functions, memory, and language [23].

Although several environmental factors have been associated with PD, less is known about their role in PD-D. Smoking was associated with a fourfold higher risk for dementia in PD [24]. Another study with a mean follow-up of 3.6 ± 2.2 years found a twofold increase in the risk of dementia in PD patients with a history of smoking. In the same study there was no significant association with head injury, diabetes mellitus, and incident dementia [25]. Risk factors associated with PD-D are summarized in Table 3.1.

Clinical Features

Clinical features of PD-D include cognitive and behavioral changes as well as frequently associated autonomic symptoms and disturbances of sleep-wake cycle. In typical cases, the profile of dementia can be described as a dysexecutive syndrome

Table 3.1 Risk factors associated with PD-D

Clinical	Genetic associations and biomarkers
Presence of mild cognitive impairment	Tau gene MAPT H1/H1 haplotype
Advanced age	Glucocerebrosidase gene mutations
Symmetrical disease at presentation	Alpha-synuclein gene duplication or triplication
Severe motor disability	Apo E4? Apo E2?
Axial symptoms such as speech impairment and postural imbalance	White matter hyperintensities in MRI
Early autonomic symptoms	Reduced CSF β-amyloid levels
Early development of confusion, hallucinations, or psychosis on dopaminergic medication	
Excessive daytime sleepiness	
REM sleep behavior disorder	

with prominent impairment of attention, executive and visuospatial functions, moderately impaired memory, and behavioral symptoms including apathy and psychosis (Table 3.2).

Cognitive Features

PD patients may show some degree of cognitive impairment already at the time of diagnosis. Cognitive impairment without dementia is designated as mild cognitive impairment of PD (PD-MCI), where the activities of daily living are largely preserved. Diagnostic criteria for PD-MCI have been recently described by a Movement Disorder Society Task Force [26]. Cognitive deficits in PD-MCI may vary; the most common deficits are in executive functions, visuospatial functions, memory, and attention. Transition from MCI to dementia is gradual, both in terms of symptom severity as well as temporal course.

In PD-D impairment of attentional functions and working memory is an early and prominent feature. Vigilance and reaction time impaired, attention frequently fluctuates similar to what is seen in patients with dementia with Lewy bodies (DLB). Impaired attention is an important determinant of activities of daily living (ADL) in PD-D: the measure of vigilance and focused attention was the strongest cognitive predictor of ADL status, matching the strength of the effect of motor function on ADL [27].

The term executive function designates a set of cognitive skills including the ability to plan, organize, and perform goal-directed behavior (the central executive), as well as higher intellectual skills such as insight and foresight. Impairment in executive functions is one of the core features of PD-D. In the Mattis Dementia Rating scale, PD-D patients were found to have lower initiation, perseverance, and construction, but higher memory subscores [28]. Insight to impaired function,

Table 3.2 Clinical features of dementia associated with PD

I. Core features
1. Diagnosis of Parkinson's disease according to Queen Square Brain Bank criteria
2. A dementia syndrome with insidious onset and slow progression, developing within the context of established Parkinson's disease and diagnosed by history, clinical, and mental examination, defined as:
Impairment in more than one cognitive domain
Representing a decline from premorbid level
Deficits severe enough to impair daily life (social, occupational, or personal care), independent of the impairment ascribable to motor or autonomic symptoms
II. Associated clinical features
1. Cognitive features:
Attention: impaired. Impairment in spontaneous and focused attention, poor performance in attentional tasks; performance may fluctuate during the day and from day to day
Executive functions: impaired. Impairment in tasks requiring initiation, planning, concept formation, rule finding, set shifting or set maintenance; impaired mental speed (bradyphrenia)
Visuospatial functions: Impaired. Impairment in tasks requiring visual-spatial orientation, perception, or construction
Memory: impaired. Impairment in free recall of recent events or in tasks requiring learning new material, memory usually improves with cueing; recognition is usually better than free recall
Language: core functions largely preserved. Word finding difficulties and impaired comprehension of complex sentences may be present
2. Behavioral features:
Apathy: decreased spontaneity; loss of motivation, interest, and effortful behavior
Changes in personality and mood including depressive features and anxiety
Hallucinations: mostly visual, usually complex, formed visions of people, animals, or objects
Delusions: usually paranoid, such as infidelity, or phantom boarder (unwelcome guests living in the home) delusions
Excessive daytime sleepiness
III. Features which do not exclude PD-D, but make the diagnosis uncertain
Coexistence of any other abnormality which may by itself cause cognitive impairment, but judged not to be the cause of dementia, e.g., presence of relevant vascular disease in imaging
Time interval between the development of motor and cognitive symptoms not known
IV. Features suggesting other conditions or diseases as cause of mental impairment, which, when present, make it impossible to reliably diagnose PD-D
Cognitive and behavioral symptoms appearing solely in the context of other conditions such as:
Acute confusion due to
(a) Systemic diseases or abnormalities
(b) Drug intoxication
Major depression according to DSM-IV
Features compatible with probable vascular dementia criteria according to NINDS-AIREN (dementia in the context of cerebrovascular disease as indicated by focal signs in neurological exam such as hemiparesis, sensory deficits, and evidence of relevant cerebrovascular disease by brain imaging and a relationship between the two as indicated by the presence of one or more of the following: onset of dementia within 3 months after a recognized stroke, abrupt deterioration in cognitive functions, and fluctuating, stepwise progression of cognitive deficits)

Reprinted with permission from Wiley, Emre et al. [86])

however, is usually preserved in PD-D, in contrast to patients with AD, where cognitive impairment is usually denied.

All types of memory functions such as working memory, explicit (declarative) memory (both verbal and visual modalities), and implicit memory such as procedural learning can be impaired in PD-D. Deficits in working memory are found early on. The relative severity of declarative memory impairment and its profile usually differ from that seen in AD, in general being less severe. In typical cases the memory impairment is characterized by a deficit in free recall with relatively preserved recognition, indicating that information is stored, but not readily accessed; when structured cues or multiple choices are provided, retrieval usually improves. Same pattern of memory impairment is also seen in mild cognitive impairment associated with PD [29]. Memory scores in patients with PD-D were found to correlate with performance in executive function tests. Based on this observation, it was suggested that impairment of memory in PD-D may be partly due to difficulties in developing internally cued search strategies, although this view has been recently challenged [30]. Memory impairment of limbic type, similar to that seen in AD, can also be seen in a subpopulation of PD-D patients [31].

Another early impairment in PD-D is seen in visuospatial functions. Impairment, especially in visual-perceptual abilities, is more severe compared to AD patients with similar dementia severity. Visuospatial abilities such as object assembly are more impaired in PD-D, whereas visuospatial memory tasks are worse in AD. Deficits in visuospatial functions become more evident in more complex tasks, which require planning and sequencing of response or generation of strategies. These deficits may thus be partly due to problems in sequential organization of response, i.e., executive functions.

Core language functions are largely preserved in PD-D, deficits usually consist of word-finding difficulties resulting in pauses in spontaneous speech, and understanding of complex sentences may be difficult, probably due to attentional deficits.

Behavioral Features

A wide range of behavioral symptoms can be seen in PD-D. The most common symptoms include depression, apathy, anxiety, hallucinations, and insomnia, and at least one neuropsychiatric symptom is present in more than 90 % of the patients [32]. Hallucinations are mostly visual, usually well-formed figures of humans or animals; insight is usually preserved, but may become lost causing agitation, especially in more advanced stages. Auditory hallucinations may occur, but are less common. Hallucinations and delusions may emerge following treatment with dopaminergic agents. When minor forms such as feeling of presence are included, hallucinations occur in 70 % of patients with PD-D, as compared to 25 % of those with AD [33]. Delusional misidentification syndromes are found in 17 % of PD-D patients and are associated with hallucinations and more severe memory and language deficits [34]. Apathy is common in the earlier stages, while delusions increase with more severe cognitive dysfunction. In a longitudinal study, patients with PD-D were discriminated by the presence of cognitive fluctuations, visual and auditory hallucinations, depression, and sleep disturbance from patients with AD, whereas these features were identical to those observed in DLB [35].

Motor, Autonomic, and Other Associated Features

In PD-D patients motor symptoms are usually more symmetrical with predominance of bradykinesia, rigidity, and postural instability; tremor is usually a less prominent feature or may disappear all together. These features are also correlated with more rapid cognitive decline. In a cross-sectional study, PIGD subtype was found in 88 % of patients with PD-D in contrast to 38 % in non-demented patients [36]. In another study it was found that in nearly all cases, dementia was preceded by PIGD phenotype or by a transition from tremor dominant to PIGD phenotype [16]. In the CamPaign study, severity of akinetic-rigid syndrome was associated with a higher risk for dementia independent of age [37]. PD patients with falls are more likely to have lower MMSE scores than those without falls and also more likely to have overt dementia.

L-dopa responsiveness of motor symptoms may diminish as cognitive impairment emerges, although this assumption is largely based on retrospective clinical data. Mechanisms underlying relative loss of l-dopa response may include development of alpha-synuclein pathology in striatum and loss of striatal dopamine D2 and D3 receptors. On the other hand, it may also reflect the development or predominance of non-dopaminergic symptoms such as postural instability and dysarthria.

Autonomic symptoms include constipation, urinary incontinence or frequency, orthostatic or postprandial hypotension resulting in syncope and falls, reduced heart rate variability predisposing to ventricular arrhythmias, and sexual dysfunction. In a comparative study, cardiovascular autonomic dysfunction was more frequent in patients with PD-D as compared to those with DLB, vascular dementia, and AD; PD-D patients demonstrated impairment in both parasympathetic and sympathetic function tests as compared to controls [38].

Sleep and sleep-wake cycle disturbances are common in PD-D including insomnia, sleep disruption, and REM sleep behavior disorder (RBD). The latter can also occur in non-demented patients, but is probably more common in demented patients, and in some it can be an early indicator of incipient dementia. Excessive daytime sleepiness (EDS) and poor sleep quality are more common in patients with PD, PD-D, and DLB as compared to AD [39]. A PIGD phenotype predicts more frequent and severe EDS in PD-D patients, although this association may be lost during the course of the disease [39].

Genetic Factors

Genetic factors related to PD-D include susceptibility genes and increased occurrence of dementia in some monogenic forms of PD. Apolipoprotein epsilon4 (ApoE4) has been strongly linked with Alzheimer's disease and is the most frequent genetic risk factor for AD. The data on the association of ApoE4 with PD-D have been inconsistent: in one study along with ApoE4, ApoE2 was also suggested to be associated with PD-D [40]. A large meta-analysis failed to show an association between ApoE4 and risk for PD-D [41], and a large case-control study which included autopsy-proven patients revealed that ApoE4 increases the likelihood of presenting with dementia in the context of a pure synucleinopathy [42].

In the CamPaIGN cohort the H1/H1 haplotype of the tau (*MAPT*) gene has been associated with a greater rate of cognitive decline and dementia in PD patients [43, 44], and with a 12.1 odds ratio to predict dementia, it has not been associated with other neurodegenerative diseases such as DLB and AD [45].

A significantly higher frequency of heterozygote mutations in the glucocerebrosidase gene (GBA) is found in patients with PD or DLB compared with control subjects. GBA mutations may exert a large effect on susceptibility for Lewy body disorders at the individual level, but they are associated with a modest (approximately 3 %) population-attributable risk in individuals of European ancestry [46]. In one cohort up to half of the PD patients heterozygous for GBA mutations developed cognitive impairment later in their disease [47]. PD patients with GBA mutations were more likely to demonstrate cognitive dysfunction compared to patients without [48], and in another study hazard ratio for progression to dementia was found to be significantly higher in GBA mutation carriers [49].

Altered expression of or missense mutations in the alpha-synuclein gene have been linked to early-onset familial PD, sometimes associated with dementia. There is an association with cognitive decline and duplication and more so with the triplication of the alpha-synuclein gene [50, 51].

Dementia rates seem to be lower in patients with *Parkin, PINK1*, and *LRRK2* mutations. Frequency of dementia in monogenic forms of PD does not appear to be higher and may be lower than in sporadic PD [52].

Neuropathological and Biochemical Correlates of PD-D

There is a lack of unanimous agreement with regard to the main neuropathological correlate of PD-D. This may be partly due to variation in clinical diagnosis in different cohorts and partly due to methodological differences in assessing pathology. In general PD-D is characterized by variable combination of the three types of pathological changes: degeneration in subcortical nuclei, cortical cell loss combined with AD-type pathology, and Lewy body (LB)-type degeneration [53]. It is probably the topographical and temporal sequence of neuronal loss rather than the type of protein aggregation which ultimately determines the clinical phenotype. In addition, AD-type and LB pathologies do not need to be mutually exclusive; they frequently coexist; there are interactions between different protein aggregations (i.e., accumulation of alpha-synuclein, tau, and beta-amyloid). Beta-amyloid deposits in the cerebral cortex enhance alpha-synuclein-induced damage; beta-amyloid may promote the aggregation of alpha-synuclein [54]. Hence protein aggregation may be synergistic, with one protein promoting the aggregation of the other, although the consequences of these protein aggregations in terms of cellular function are uncertain.

As opposed to earlier studies which utilized ubiquitin staining, more recent studies performed using alpha-synuclein immunohistochemistry (which is more sensitive to detect cortical Lewy bodies) revealed that dementia better correlates with LB pathology. The fact that families with alpha-synuclein gene duplications and more so those with triplications develop dementia more often also supports a primary and possibly a "dose-dependent" role for synuclein-based pathology in development of PD-D. In a clinicopathological study, however, approximately 55 % of subjects with widespread alpha-synuclein pathology lacked clinical signs of dementia or extrapyramidal signs before their demise [55].

AD-type pathology of variable extent (more plaques than tangles) usually coexists in PD-D [56]. In a recent study, combination of LB-type and AD-type pathologies was found to be a better predictor of dementia than the severity of a single pathology [57].

Dementia in PD usually develops later in the disease course and may be related to an ascending order of pathological changes, as suggested by Braak et al. [58], involving the limbic and cortical structures later in the disease course. Some support for this "bottom-up" hypothesis is also provided by other studies [59]: PD patients with relatively longer disease duration prior to dementia onset had lower levels of cortical choline acetyltransferase than those with a shorter disease duration, implying greater loss of ascending cholinergic projections before dementia developed. In contrast, a more "top-down" pathological process, with greater burden of cortical pathology in PD patients with a more malignant disease course and short time before dementia onset, has also been suggested [60]. This clinicopathological study arising from the Sydney cohort suggested that there may be three types of pathological constellations associated with three different clinical phenotypes, in particular with regard to the temporal course of dementia. Younger patients who developed dementia late in the disease seem to have a predominance of alpha-synuclein pathology with little amyloid, whereas those with a later age of onset and rapid progression to dementia seem to have mixed alpha-synuclein and amyloid pathology: these patients constituting 25 % of the sample had severe neocortical LB pathology, more consistent with a "DLB-like" phenotype, but also with a high amyloid burden [60]. It is not known which factors determine this clinical and pathological variability, and age of onset is probably one of them.

Biochemically, degeneration of the subcortical nuclei results in various neurochemical changes including cholinergic, dopaminergic, serotoninergic, and noradrenergic deficits. The most profound is the cholinergic deficit although the others may also contribute to some aspects of mental dysfunction. In PD-D loss of cholinergic cells in the nucleus basalis of Meynert (nbM) is observed, which is greater than that seen in AD, and LBs are also frequently found in nbM cells. Choline acetyltransferase (ChAT) activity is markedly decreased in the frontal cortex of PD and DLB when compared to normal controls and AD [61, 62]. In contrast to AD, PD is also associated with neuronal loss in the pedunculopontine cholinergic nuclei which project to structures such as the thalamus [63]. Using SPECT and vesicular acetylcholine transporter ([^{123}I] iodobenzovesamicol (IBVM)) as a marker of cholinergic innervation, reduction in IBVM binding in parietal and occipital cortices was shown in non-demented PD patients, while demented PD cases had a more extensive decrease in cortical binding [64]. Functional imaging studies with PET demonstrated that compared with controls mean cortical AChE activity was lowest in patients with PD-D, followed by patients with PD without dementia and AD patients with equal severity of dementia [65]. A subsequent study revealed that the degree of cortical cholinergic deficits correlated particularly well with typical cognitive deficits found in PD-D, e.g., impaired performance on tests of attention and executive functions [66].

Some cognitive deficits, in particular in early stages, may be due to dopaminergic dysfunction, whereas dopaminergic stimulation may be detrimental in later stages [67]. In one study, reduced 18F-fluorodopa uptake in the caudate nucleus and frontal cortex correlated with impairment in tests of verbal fluency, working memory, and attention, indicating that ascending dopaminergic projections may be involved in mediating some of the cognitive deficits in PD [68]. In fluorodopa PET, bilateral impairment in the anterior cingulate area, ventral striatum, and right caudate nucleus was shown in PD patients with dementia, as compared to those without [69]. In another study, dopamine levels in neocortical areas were found to be decreased to a greater level in demented than in non-demented PD patients [70], suggesting some role for the degeneration of the mesocortical dopaminergic system. Neuronal loss was observed in ventral tegmental area as well, which provides dopaminergic input to the mesolimbic and prefrontal cortex and medial substantia nigra [71]. However, clinical experience shows that dementia does not improve with dopaminergic treatment; it may even worsen behavioral and cognitive functions, especially in demented patients. In addition, in a multi-tracer PET study, dopaminergic deficits were comparable between demented and non-demented PD patients, whereas cholinergic deficits were significantly more in demented patients [72]. These observations suggest that dopaminergic deficit is unlikely to play a major role in PD-D.

Deficits in other ascending monoaminergic systems were also suggested to be associated with cognitive impairment. Locus coeruleus, main source of noradrenergic input to the forebrain and cortex, shows neuronal loss especially in demented and depressed PD patients [73]. Degeneration in serotoninergic dorsal raphe nucleus was also suggested to be associated with dementia [74]. The association between dementia and noradrenergic or serotoninergic deficits, however, has not been consistently shown.

Neuroimaging in PD-D

For routine diagnostic structural imaging purposes, magnetic resonance imaging (MRI) is superior to computerized tomography to assess both cortical atrophy and white matter changes. Frontal, occipital, and parietal atrophy as well as an increased amount of whole brain atrophy have been described in PD-D patients compared with controls, whereas no significant gray matter loss was found in patients with PD-MCI compared to PD patients without any cognitive impairment [21]. Medial temporal lobe atrophy may be seen in PD-D patients, but it is less common and less prominent as compared to AD. Supratentorial white matter hyperintensities were suggested to be independently associated with cognitive impairment in PD-D patients [22], and an association between the volume of caudate nucleus and cognitive decline was shown in one study [75].

Novel imaging techniques have also been used in PD-D patients. In a diffusion tensor imaging study, PD-D patients showed significant reduction in fractional anisotropy (FA) in the bilateral posterior cingulate bundles compared with non-demented PD patients [76]; both FA and mean diffusivity (MD) values in the cingulate and corpus callosum showed significant correlations with cognitive parameters [76, 77]. Default mode (DM) is a resting state network detected by functional MRI; it is altered in patients with AD. DM network has been found to be preserved, whereas corticostriatal functional correlations were decreased in bilateral prefrontal regions in PD-D patients compared to control subjects [78]. In another study, however, significant decrease of DM connectivity in the right inferior frontal gyrus has been reported [79].

In functional imaging studies using radiotracers, hypometabolism in the parietal and temporal cortex can be seen in metabolic PET, similar to the pattern seen in AD; hypometabolism in the visual association areas and frontal lobe were also described. A review of rCBF SPECT studies in PD-D revealed frontal hypoperfusion or bilateral temporoparietal deficits [80]. Perfusion deficits in the precuneus and inferior lateral parietal regions have also been described in PD-D patients.

PET using N-[11C]-methyl-4-piperidyl acetate (MP4A) is a method to evaluate cholinergic innervation. PD-D patients showed a severe cholinergic deficit in various cortical regions including frontal and temporoparietal cortices [81]. Iodine-123 metaiodobenzylguanidine (^{123}I-MIBG) is a marker of postganglionic sympathetic cardiac innervation and SPECT studies with this compound demonstrate innervation deficits both in PD-D and DLB, but not in AD. The integrity of nigrostriatal dopaminergic terminals can be visualized using SPECT and markers of dopamine transporter, such as (123)I-FP-CIT. Significant reductions were found in (123)I-FP-CIT binding in the caudate and anterior and posterior putamens in subjects with DLB and PD-D compared to those with AD and controls. Both ^{123}I-MIBG and (123) I-FP-CIT SPECT methods can be used to differentiate patients with DLB or PD-D from those with AD and motor symptoms.

In PET studies with the Pittsburgh compound B (PiB), which shows amyloid burden, mean cortical amyloid load in PD-D patients was comparable to controls and non-demented PD patients [82]. In another study 83 % (10/12) of PD-D patients had "normal" PiB uptake, whereas 85 % (11/13) of DLB patients had significantly increased amyloid load in one or more cortical regions [83]. In a further PiB study, an increased cortical amyloid burden was found in DLB, but not in PD-D patients; interestingly striatal PiB retention in the DLB and PD-D groups was associated with less impaired motor function [84]. In line with these findings, only 15 % of MCI patients with PD showed increased cortical PiB binding at levels seen in patients with AD; however, cerebral amyloid load was associated with cognitive scores [85]. These findings suggest that global cortical amyloid burden is low and infrequent in PD-D compared to DLB and AD.

Diagnosis of PD-D

The clinical diagnostic criteria for PD-D have been published by the Movement Disorder Society Task Force [86], along with practical recommendations for diagnostic procedures [87]. Clinical features of PD-D are shown in Table 3.2, and diagnostic criteria for probable and possible PD-D, representing two levels of diagnostic certainty, are given in Table 3.3. Recently diagnostic criteria for mild cognitive impairment in PD (PD-MCI) have been published, also by the Task Force of Movement Disorder Society [26]. These are developed using the same structure as the PD-D criteria, and applying both sets of criteria together helps to differentiate PD patients with cognitive impairment, but no dementia from those with dementia.

The diagnosis of PD-D can be complicated by various factors, such as severe motor symptoms and dysarthria. These symptoms may make it difficult to assess if cognitive deficits are present and to what extent they contribute to impairment in daily function, a prerequisite for the diagnosis of dementia. Comorbid conditions such as depression, acute confusion (delirium) due to systemic abnormalities, or adverse effects of drugs may also mimic symptoms of dementia.

The diagnosis of dementia in PD can be subsumed into two main steps: first, ascertaining the presence of dementia, i.e., differentiating it from conditions mimicking dementia, and second, the differential diagnosis as to the etiology of dementia, i.e., if the dementia is due to the neurodegenerative process associated with PD or if it involves other etiologies such as vascular disease. Along with a detailed history elucidating the onset, course, and pattern of cognitive and behavioral symptoms, the clinical context within which these symptoms occurred and the findings from laboratory and imaging studies can be helpful in differential diagnosis.

Once other factors mimicking dementia are excluded and presence of dementia is ascertained, the second step involves differential diagnosis. In patients with established PD, this is a rather straightforward process and simply requires excluding alternative causes of dementia. If history is unclear, other conditions which can present with dementia and parkinsonism should be considered. These include cerebrovascular (in particular small vessel) disease, normal-pressure hydrocephalus, AD with drug-induced parkinsonism, DLB, and other neurodegenerative diseases such

Table 3.3 Diagnostic criteria for PD-D

Probable PD-D
A. Core features: both must be present
B. Associated clinical features:
Typical profile of cognitive deficits including impairment in at least two of the four core cognitive domains (impaired attention which may fluctuate, impaired executive functions, impairment in visuospatial functions, and impaired free recall memory which usually improves with cueing)
The presence of at least one behavioral symptom (apathy, depressed or anxious mood, hallucinations, delusions, excessive daytime sleepiness) supports the diagnosis of probable PD-D; lack of behavioral symptoms, however, does not exclude the diagnosis
C. None of the group III features present
D. None of the group IV features present
Possible PD-D
A. Core features: both must be present
B. Associated clinical features:
Atypical profile of cognitive impairment in one or more domains, such as prominent or receptive-type (fluent) aphasia or pure storage-failure-type amnesia (memory does not improve with cueing or in recognition tasks) with preserved attention
Behavioral symptoms may or may not be present
Or
C. One or more of the group III features present
D. None of the group IV features present

Reprinted with permission from Wiley, Emre et al. [86])

as corticobasal degeneration, progressive supranuclear palsy, and frontotemporal dementia with parkinsonism. A detailed history including a search for features known to be associated with PD-D, use of appropriate neuropsychological tests with assessment of all cognitive domains affected in PD-D, and review of current medication and auxiliary examinations are helpful to make the correct diagnosis.

Assessment of cognitive functions can be achieved either using structured scales or an appropriately constituted neuropsychological test battery. Several structured scales, some specifically developed for PD, can be used for screening purposes. Montreal Cognitive Assessment (MoCA) can be used as a screening instrument, and a cutoff score of 21/30 yielded a sensitivity of 90 % in PD-D patients [88]. Both MoCA and cognitive screening instruments specifically developed for PD including Mini-Mental Parkinson [89] and the Parkinson Neuropsychometric Dementia Assessment (PANDA) [90] have been shown to be more sensitive than the Mini-Mental State Examination (MMSE) to detect cognitive impairment in PD. More elaborate cognitive scales include the general purpose scales such as Mattis Dementia Rating Scale and the CAMCOG-R, as well as PD-specific scales such as SCales for Outcomes of PArkinson's disease-cognition (SCOPA-Cog) [91] and PD-Cognitive Rating Scale (PD-CRS) [92]. The presence, frequency, severity, and caregiver burden of behavioral symptoms can be assessed using a semi-structured interview or scales such as Neuropsychiatric Inventory (NPI) [93].

Management of Patients with PD-D

The first step in management is to exclude that cognitive impairment and behavioral symptoms are not due to other factors such as adverse effects of drugs, concomitant depression, systemic diseases, or metabolic abnormalities. All medication should be reviewed; drugs which can cause mental dysfunction (such as anticholinergics, tricyclic antidepressants, benzodiazepines, dopamine agonists) should be discontinued. Once other causes are excluded, the next step is to take all non-pharmacological measures and then decide if pharmacological treatment is necessary based on symptom frequency, severity, and burden. PD-D patients receive a number of medications to treat motor impairment, cognitive deficits, psychiatric symptoms, and autonomic dysfunction. Before initiating any new drug, the risk/benefit ratio should be carefully considered. In principle, one drug should be introduced at a time with low doses and titrated up as needed. Drugs to treat behavioral symptoms should be tapered and discontinued, once sufficient symptom control is obtained.

Non-pharmacological Management

Non-pharmacological measures may contribute to preserving and improving cognitive abilities. Adequate information should be provided to the patient and the family about the disease; for example, they may be less concerned when they understand that hallucinations can be part of the disease. Sufficient mental and physical activation, avoidance of aggravating factors such as too much sensory stimuli, and inappropriate environmental factors should be recommended. Physiotherapy and exercise programs should be a part of daily activities to decrease risk of falls since they are frequently associated with cognitive deficits in PD [94, 95] and common in PD-D patients.

A recent systematic review of non-pharmacological and noninvasive therapies in PD revealed no studies specifically in PD-D patients [96]. In non-demented patients although five trials showed positive results, only one study of cognitive training achieved sufficient evidence grading. The result of a small randomized controlled study demonstrated a significant benefit for cognitive training in the domains of attention, executive functions, memory, and visuospatial functions [97]. Positive effect of sudoku puzzle and computerized cognitive training was also observed in executive functions [98, 99]. Likewise, passive cycling and physical exercise were associated with improvement in executive functions [100, 101].

Pharmacological Treatment

Pharmacological treatment of patients with PD-D includes "specific" substitution treatment strategies based on neurotransmitter deficits and nonspecific treatment aimed at amelioration of behavioral symptoms.

Cholinesterase Inhibitors

Cholinergic deficits are the most consistent biochemical correlates of cognitive dysfunction in PD-D. All available ChE-Is including donepezil, rivastigmine, and galantamine have been tested in PD-D. Except for two, most of these studies have been open label with small sample sizes. One of the two large, randomized controlled trials is the EXPRESS study in which 541 patients with mild to moderate PD-D either received rivastigmine (up to 12 mg/day) or placebo over 24 weeks [102]. Both primary end points (ADAS-cog and Clinical Global Impression of Change scale) and secondary end points (MMSE, Neuropsychiatric Inventory, the clock drawing test, verbal fluency, and computer-based attention tests) showed statistically significant improvements on rivastigmine. Activities of daily living scores showed a minimal worsening from baseline in rivastigmine group, whereas those on placebo worsened statistically significantly more. Adverse events, mainly nausea and vomiting, were significantly more frequent with rivastigmine. Worsening of tremor was reported in 10 % of the patients on rivastigmine, and UPDRS motor score did not reveal any significant differences between the groups. Based on this study rivastigmine became the first specific treatment approved for the treatment of patients with mild to moderate PD-D. A patch form of rivastigmine also became available and has been approved for PD-D in several countries. Its long-term efficacy and safety as compared to capsules has been described in a large open-label prospective study, revealing no long-term safety concerns, in particular with regard to worsening of motor symptoms [103].

A post hoc analysis of computerized tests from the EXPRESS study revealed that rivastigmine improved all aspects of attention [104], and a subgroup analysis suggested that patients who had visual hallucinations at baseline may draw more benefits from cholinergic treatment, i.e., less worsening in cognitive functions as compared to placebo [105]. The EXPRESS study had a 6-month extension period during which all patients received active treatment [106]. The beneficial effects seen during the first 6 months were largely maintained, although there was some decline. Importantly, there was no evidence of worsening motor function over the course of 1-year treatment [107].

The second large randomized, controlled trial was conducted with donepezil [108], in which 550 patients with mild to moderate PD-D received either placebo, donepezil 5 mg, or donepezil 10 mg/day for 24 weeks. In the primary analysis there were no significant differences between placebo and active groups. When the country interaction was controlled for in a secondary analysis, both primary end points ADAS-cog and CIBIC-plus scores showed statistically significant superiority for 10 mg, but not for 5 mg. Statistically significant differences in favor of donepezil were also found in some secondary measures including MMSE, Brief Test of Attention, and Verbal Fluency Test, whereas there were no significant differences from placebo on the ADL scale and the behavioral scale NPI. UPDRS motor scores did not reveal any significant worsening of motor functions on donepezil. In another open-label study, the effects of donepezil on central processing speed and other attentional measures were tested over 20 weeks. Power of attention, continuity of attention, and reaction time variability were found to be improved as compared to baseline [109].

Open-label studies have suggested that galantamine may have beneficial effects in patients with PD-D [110], and there are however no randomized controlled trials in this population.

In summary, ChE-Is have been found to be efficacious in PD-D, and the strongest evidence from randomized controlled trials exists for rivastigmine. The effect size is modest: in a Cochrane meta-analysis evaluating the efficacy of ChE-Is in PD-D, 5.3 % of patients were concluded to have benefits on outcome scales, whereas 10.1 % patients on placebo demonstrated worsening, suggesting that the effect size is close to 15 % [111]. In a more recent Cochrane meta-analysis, the authors suggested that the use of ChE-Is in PD-D is associated with a positive impact on global assessment, cognitive function, behavioral disturbance, and activities of daily living scales [112]. Taking together all the evidence, patients with PD-D should be considered for treatment with a ChE-I taking in account expected benefits and risks. The doses should be slowly titrated up to therapeutic dose levels and then maintained; adverse effects such as nausea, vomiting, loss of appetite, diarrhea, and worsening of tremor should be monitored. At the usual dose range, dropout rates are in 10–31 % of patients. In addition to the relatively more common gastrointestinal adverse effects, muscle cramps, hypersalivation, rhinorrhea, lacrimation, postural hypotension, falls, bradycardia, and syncope can occur in a small proportion of patients [113]. There is no evidence-based guidance on if and when to discontinue treatment, and if such a decision is made because there is no more expectations for clinical benefits, patients should be closely monitored after discontinuation. Abrupt withdrawal of ChE-I can be associated with rapid emergence of neuropsychiatric symptoms and cognitive decline in DLB and PD-D [114]. Although reinstatement of treatment may reverse this deterioration, it is recommended that patients who are assessed as responding to ChE-I are maintained on treatment long term.

NMDA Antagonists

Memantine is an N-methyl-D-aspartate (NMDA) receptor antagonist approved for treatment of moderate to severe Alzheimer's disease. There is circumstantial evidence for glutamatergic dysfunction in PD-D. In a randomized controlled trial which included both patients with DLB and PD-D, there was a significant difference in favor of memantine in the global outcome scale, whereas MMSE and NPI did not show any differences. Patients with PD-D seem to have more benefits as compared to those with DLB [115]. An opposite finding was obtained in a larger randomized placebo-controlled trial which included 199 patients either with DLB or PD-D. In the total population, there were no statistically significant differences between memantine and placebo groups. The global outcome scale and NPI scores were significantly better under memantine in the DLB subgroup; there were no significant differences between memantine and placebo in the PD-D population, although trends were favoring memantine. The ADCS-ADL scale, Zarit caregiver burden scale, and a number of cognitive tests did not show any consistent or significant differences between active and placebo in the overall or in the either population [116].

Based on these studies it can be concluded that memantine may have mild beneficial effects in patients with Lewy body-related dementias, possibly more so in the DLB population, predominantly on the global status and behavioral symptoms.

Dopaminergic Drugs

The effects of dopaminergic medication on mental dysfunction have been scarcely studied in patients with PD-D; most formal studies have been conducted in non-demented patients. The results have been mixed describing either no effects or improvement in some and worsening in other functions [117]. In one of the few studies which specifically included demented patients, patients with PD, PD-D, or DLB were tested for cognitive functions and behavioral symptoms after acute l-dopa challenge and following 3 months of treatment. After acute challenge patients reported improvement in subjective alertness, but fluctuations increased; reaction time and accuracy remained unchanged in those with PD-D. After 3 months of treatment, neuropsychiatric scores improved both in PD and PD-D, and mean global cognitive score was better, but attention and memory scores were worse in PD patients without dementia. Reaction time became slower in those with PD-D, there were however no patients with marked deterioration, and the authors concluded that levodopa treatment is not detrimental in PD-D patients [118]. The common clinical practice suggests that dopaminergic drugs do not exert any significant benefits on cognitive and behavioral functions in PD-D patients; in particular dopamine agonists can induce or worsen psychosis or confusion.

Pharmacological Treatment of Behavioral Symptoms

Behavioral symptoms may be a source of greater distress to patients and carers than motor dysfunction [119]. Treatment with ChE-Is may exert mild benefits on some neuropsychiatric symptoms, particularly on apathy, anxiety, sleep disturbance, and delusions [110], and these benefits may be at least partly mediated through improvements in attention and cognitive processing. Since cognitive and behavioral symptoms usually coexist, the choice of a ChE-I as first-line treatment is a rationale choice, targeting both symptoms.

Aggression, agitation, and other psychotic behaviors are less likely to improve with ChE-Is. Traditional neuroleptics such as haloperidol can provoke severe neuroleptic sensitivity reactions due to their D2 receptor antagonism and are therefore contraindicated in this patient population. Such reactions are usually acute or subacute, emerging after the first few doses or following a dose increase from a previously tolerated one. These reactions or worsening of parkinsonism can be seen with second-generation ("atypical") antipsychotics such as risperidone, olanzapine, and aripiprazole. In addition, all neuroleptics can increase the risk of cerebrovascular accidents and death. Hence risk/benefit ratio should be carefully evaluated before initiating neuroleptic treatment. Although evidence base is weak, quetiapine [120, 121] can be tried as first-line treatment because of its lower risk for worsening motor symptoms. Robust evidence from randomized controlled trials to treat psychosis in PD patients, however, exists only for clozapine [122, 123]. It requires weekly blood monitoring for the first 3 months and monthly thereafter, and in addition antimuscarinic properties [124] may increase confusion in patients with dementia.

Although depression or depressive features are frequent in PD and PD-D, there have been few randomized, controlled trials of antidepressants in PD and none in PD-D. A meta-analysis of all studies in PD patients with depression showed large effect sizes, both under active and placebo, without statistically significant differences between them; increasing age and major depression predicted better response [125]. In a systematic review amitriptyline was found to be the only drug with evidence of efficacy in PD depression [126]. Albeit not large several placebo-controlled randomized trials have been conducted in PD patients with depression without dementia, desipramine and citalopram were both significantly better than placebo [127], and nortriptyline was found to be significantly better than placebo, whereas paroxetine was not [128], whereas both paroxetine and venlafaxine were significantly better than placebo in a larger randomized trial [129]. Dopamine agonist pramipexole was shown to be significantly better than placebo in a large randomized placebo-controlled trial on non-demented patients with depressive symptoms; [130] agonists, however, can worsen psychosis and cognition in PD-D patients. It should be kept in mind that all randomized controlled trials were performed in non-demented patients. There is a hint that tricyclics such as amitriptyline and nortriptyline may have larger effect sizes, and they should be, however, avoided in PD-D patients because of their anticholinergic effects and hence their potential to worsen cognition; SSRIs or SNRIs should be preferred in PD-D patients.

Excessive daytime sleepiness (EDS) and REM sleep behavior disorder (RBD) are frequent in PD-D patients [131]. In small studies clonazepam has been reported to be efficacious and well tolerated [132] in suppressing the motor features, but does not restore REM sleep atonia [133]. In a small study melatonin was beneficial, with improvement noted in 10 of 14 patients who had failed to respond to clonazepam or were unable to tolerate it [134]. Possible benefits of ChE-Is as a treatment for RBD need further study [135]. Although not specifically tested in demented PD patients, modafinil, an agent which promotes wakefulness, can be considered to treat EDS. In non-demented PD patients, modafinil was significantly better than placebo in two small randomized, placebo-controlled and one open-label study [136, 137], whereas no difference was found in another small, placebo-controlled trial [138].

Although apathy is very common and seen in the majority of PD-D patients [139], its treatment has not been well studied. In a small study, methylphenidate was reported to be beneficial [140]. In a small randomized, placebo-controlled trial in non-demented, nondepressed patients with apathy, rivastigmine given as patch significantly improved apathy score as compared to placebo [141].

References

1. Muslimovic D, Post B, Speelman JD, Schmand B. Cognitive profile of patients with newly diagnosed Parkinson disease. Neurology. 2005;65:1239–45. doi:10.1212/01.wnl.0000180516.69442.95.
2. Aarsland D, Bronnick K, Williams-Gray C, et al. Mild cognitive impairment in Parkinson disease: a multicenter pooled analysis. Neurology. 2010;75:1062–9. doi:10.1212/WNL.0b013e3181f39d0e.
3. Williams-Gray CH, Evans JR, Goris A, et al. The distinct cognitive syndromes of Parkinson's disease: 5 year follow-up of the CamPaIGN cohort. Brain. 2009;132:2958–69. doi:10.1093/brain/awp245.
4. Williams-Gray CH, Mason SL, Evans JR, et al. The CamPaIGN study of Parkinson's disease: 10-year outlook in an incident population-based cohort. J Neurol Neurosurg Psychiatr. 2013;84:1258–64. doi:10.1136/jnnp-2013-305277.
5. Aarsland D, Zaccai J, Brayne C. A systematic review of prevalence studies of dementia in Parkinson's disease. Mov Disord. 2005;20:1255–63. doi:10.1002/mds.20527.
6. Marder K, Tang MX, Cote L, et al. The frequency and associated risk factors for dementia in patients with Parkinson's disease. Arch Neurol. 1995;52:695–701.
7. De Lau LML, Schipper CMA, Hofman A, et al. Prognosis of Parkinson disease: risk of dementia and mortality: the Rotterdam study. Arch Neurol. 2005;62:1265–9. doi:10.1001/archneur.62.8.1265.
8. Hely MA, Morris JGL, Reid WGJ, Trafficante R. Sydney multicenter study of Parkinson's disease: non-L-dopa-responsive problems dominate at 15 years. Mov Disord. 2005;20:190–9. doi:10.1002/mds.20324.
9. Hely MA, Reid WGJ, Adena MA, et al. The Sydney multicenter study of Parkinson's disease: the inevitability of dementia at 20 years. Mov Disord. 2008;23:837–44. doi:10.1002/mds.21956.
10. Aarsland D, Andersen K, Larsen JP, et al. Prevalence and characteristics of dementia in Parkinson disease: an 8-year prospective study. Arch Neurol. 2003;60:387–92.
11. Buter TC, van den Hout A, Matthews FE, et al. Dementia and survival in Parkinson disease: a 12-year population study. Neurology. 2008;70:1017–22. doi:10.1212/01.wnl.0000306632.43729.24.
12. Savica R, Grossardt BR, Bower JH, et al. Incidence of dementia with Lewy bodies and Parkinson disease dementia. JAMA Neurol. 2013;70:1396–402. doi:10.1001/jamaneurol.2013.3579.
13. Levy G, Schupf N, Tang M-X, et al. Combined effect of age and severity on the risk of dementia in Parkinson's disease. Ann Neurol. 2002;51:722–9. doi:10.1002/ana.10219.
14. Pedersen KF, Larsen JP, Tysnes O-B, Alves G. Prognosis of mild cognitive impairment in early Parkinson disease: the Norwegian ParkWest study. JAMA Neurol. 2013;70:580–6. doi:10.1001/jamaneurol.2013.2110.
15. Woods SP, Tröster AI. Prodromal frontal/executive dysfunction predicts incident dementia in Parkinson's disease. J Int Neuropsychol Soc. 2003;9:17–24.
16. Alves G, Larsen JP, Emre M, et al. Changes in motor subtype and risk for incident dementia in Parkinson's disease. Mov Disord. 2006;21:1123–30. doi:10.1002/mds.20897.
17. Sollinger AB, Goldstein FC, Lah JJ, et al. Mild cognitive impairment in Parkinson's disease: subtypes and motor characteristics. Parkinsonism Relat Disord. 2010;16:177–80. doi:10.1016/j.parkreldis.2009.11.002.
18. Marion M-H, Qurashi M, Marshall G, Foster O. Is REM sleep behaviour disorder (RBD) a risk factor of dementia in idiopathic Parkinson's disease? J Neurol. 2008;255:192–6. doi:10.1007/s00415-008-0629-9.
19. Boot BP, Boeve BF, Roberts RO, et al. Probable rapid eye movement sleep behavior disorder increases risk for mild cognitive impairment and Parkinson disease: a population-based study. Ann Neurol. 2012;71:49–56. doi:10.1002/ana.22655.

20. Siderowf A, Xie SX, Hurtig H, et al. CSF amyloid {beta} 1-42 predicts cognitive decline in Parkinson disease. Neurology. 2010;75:1055–61. doi:10.1212/WNL.0b013e3181f39a78.
21. Yarnall AJ, Breen DP, Duncan GW, et al. Characterizing mild cognitive impairment in incident Parkinson disease: The ICICLE-PD study. Neurology. 2014;82:308–16. doi:10.1212/WNL.0000000000000066.
22. Lee S-J, Kim J-S, Yoo J-Y, et al. Influence of white matter hyperintensities on the cognition of patients with Parkinson disease. Alzheimer Dis Assoc Disord. 2010;24:227–33. doi:10.1097/WAD.0b013e3181d71a13.
23. Kandiah N, Mak E, Ng A, et al. Cerebral white matter hyperintensity in Parkinson's disease: a major risk factor for mild cognitive impairment. Parkinsonism Relat Disord. 2013;19:680–3. doi:10.1016/j.parkreldis.2013.03.008.
24. Ebmeier KP, Calder SA, Crawford JR, et al. Mortality and causes of death in idiopathic Parkinson's disease: results from the Aberdeen whole population study. Scott Med J. 1990;35:173–5.
25. Levy G, Tang M-X, Cote LJ, et al. Do risk factors for Alzheimer's disease predict dementia in Parkinson's disease? An exploratory study. Mov Disord. 2002;17:250–7.
26. Litvan I, Goldman JG, Tröster AI, et al. Diagnostic criteria for mild cognitive impairment in Parkinson's disease: movement disorder Society Task Force guidelines. Mov Disord. 2012;27:349–56. doi:10.1002/mds.24893.
27. Bronnick K, Ehrt U, Emre M, et al. Attentional deficits affect activities of daily living in dementia-associated with Parkinson's disease. J Neurol Neurosurg Psychiatr. 2006;77:1136–42. doi:10.1136/jnnp.2006.093146.
28. Aarsland D, Litvan I, Salmon D, et al. Performance on the dementia rating scale in Parkinson's disease with dementia and dementia with Lewy bodies: comparison with progressive supranuclear palsy and Alzheimer's disease. J Neurol Neurosurg Psychiatr. 2003;74:1215–20.
29. Costa A, Monaco M, Zabberoni S, et al. Free and cued recall memory in Parkinson's disease associated with amnestic mild cognitive impairment. PLoS One. 2014;9:e86233. doi:10.1371/journal.pone.0086233.
30. Brønnick K, Alves G, Aarsland D, et al. Verbal memory in drug-naive, newly diagnosed Parkinson's disease. The retrieval deficit hypothesis revisited. Neuropsychology. 2011;25:114–24. doi:10.1037/a0020857.
31. Weintraub D, Moberg PJ, Culbertson WC, et al. Evidence for impaired encoding and retrieval memory profiles in Parkinson disease. Cogn Behav Neurol. 2004;17:195–200.
32. Aarsland D, Brønnick K, Ehrt U, et al. Neuropsychiatric symptoms in patients with Parkinson's disease and dementia: frequency, profile and associated care giver stress. J Neurol Neurosurg Psychiatr. 2007;78:36–42. doi:10.1136/jnnp.2005.083113.
33. Fénelon G, Mahieux F, Huon R, Ziégler M. Hallucinations in Parkinson's disease: prevalence, phenomenology and risk factors. Brain. 2000;123(Pt 4):733–45.
34. Pagonabarraga J, Llebaria G, García-Sánchez C, et al. A prospective study of delusional misidentification syndromes in Parkinson's disease with dementia. Mov Disord. 2008;23:443–8. doi:10.1002/mds.21864.
35. Galvin JE, Pollack J, Morris JC. Clinical phenotype of Parkinson disease dementia. Neurology. 2006;67:1605–11. doi:10.1212/01.wnl.0000242630.52203.8f.
36. Burn DJ, Rowan EN, Minett T, et al. Extrapyramidal features in Parkinson's disease with and without dementia and dementia with Lewy bodies: a cross-sectional comparative study. Mov Disord. 2003;18:884–9. doi:10.1002/mds.10455.
37. Williams-Gray CH, Foltynie T, Brayne CEG, et al. Evolution of cognitive dysfunction in an incident Parkinson's disease cohort. Brain. 2007;130:1787–98. doi:10.1093/brain/awm111.
38. Allan LM, Ballard CG, Allen J, et al. Autonomic dysfunction in dementia. J Neurol Neurosurg Psychiatr. 2007;78:671–7. doi:10.1136/jnnp.2006.102343.
39. Boddy F, Rowan EN, Lett D, et al. Subjectively reported sleep quality and excessive daytime somnolence in Parkinson's disease with and without dementia, dementia with Lewy bodies and Alzheimer's disease. Int J Geriatr Psychiatry. 2007;22:529–35. doi:10.1002/gps.1709.

40. Huang X, Chen PC, Poole C. APOE-[epsilon]2 allele associated with higher prevalence of sporadic Parkinson disease. Neurology. 2004;62:2198–202.
41. Williams-Gray CH, Goris A, Saiki M, et al. Apolipoprotein E genotype as a risk factor for susceptibility to and dementia in Parkinson's disease. J Neurol. 2009;256:493–8. doi:10.1007/s00415-009-0119-8.
42. Tsuang D, Leverenz JB, Lopez OL, et al. APOE ε4 increases risk for dementia in pure synucleinopathies. JAMA Neurol. 2013;70:223–8. doi:10.1001/jamaneurol.2013.600.
43. Goris A, Williams-Gray CH, Clark GR, et al. Tau and alpha-synuclein in susceptibility to, and dementia in, Parkinson's disease. Ann Neurol. 2007;62:145–53. doi:10.1002/ana.21192.
44. Healy DG, Abou-Sleiman PM, Lees AJ, et al. Tau gene and Parkinson's disease: a case-control study and meta-analysis. J Neurol Neurosurg Psychiatr. 2004;75:962–5.
45. Setó-Salvia N, Clarimón J, Pagonabarraga J, et al. Dementia risk in Parkinson disease: disentangling the role of MAPT haplotypes. Arch Neurol. 2011;68:359–64. doi:10.1001/archneurol.2011.17.
46. Mata IF, Samii A, Schneer SH, et al. Glucocerebrosidase gene mutations: a risk factor for Lewy body disorders. Arch Neurol. 2008;65:379–82. doi:10.1001/archneurol.2007.68.
47. Goker-Alpan O, Lopez G, Vithayathil J, et al. The spectrum of parkinsonian manifestations associated with glucocerebrosidase mutations. Arch Neurol. 2008;65:1353–7. doi:10.1001/archneur.65.10.1353.
48. Chahine LM, Qiang J, Ashbridge E, et al. Clinical and biochemical differences in patients having Parkinson disease with vs without GBA mutations. JAMA Neurol. 2013;70:852–8. doi:10.1001/jamaneurol.2013.1274.
49. Winder-Rhodes SE, Evans JR, Ban M, et al. Glucocerebrosidase mutations influence the natural history of Parkinson's disease in a community-based incident cohort. Brain. 2013;136:392–9. doi:10.1093/brain/aws318.
50. Sironi F, Trotta L, Antonini A, et al. Alpha-Synuclein multiplication analysis in Italian familial Parkinson disease. Parkinsonism Relat Disord. 2010;16:228–31. doi:10.1016/j.parkreldis.2009.09.008.
51. Farrer M, Kachergus J, Forno L, et al. Comparison of kindreds with parkinsonism and alpha-synuclein genomic multiplications. Ann Neurol. 2004;55:174–9. doi:10.1002/ana.10846.
52. Kasten M, Kertelge L, Brüggemann N, et al. Nonmotor symptoms in genetic Parkinson disease. Arch Neurol. 2010;67:670–6. doi:10.1001/archneurol.67.6.670.
53. Emre M. What causes mental dysfunction in Parkinson's disease? Mov Disord. 2003;18 Suppl 6:S63–71. doi:10.1002/mds.10565.
54. Pletnikova O, West N, Lee MK, et al. A beta deposition is associated with enhanced cortical alpha-synuclein lesions in Lewy body diseases. Neurobiol Aging. 2005;26:1183–92. doi:10.1016/j.neurobiolaging.2004.10.006.
55. Parkkinen L, Pirttilä T, Alafuzoff I. Applicability of current staging/categorization of alpha-synuclein pathology and their clinical relevance. Acta Neuropathol. 2008;115:399–407. doi:10.1007/s00401-008-0346-6.
56. Irwin DJ, White MT, Toledo JB, et al. Neuropathologic substrates of Parkinson disease dementia. Ann Neurol. 2012;72:587–98. doi:10.1002/ana.23659.
57. Compta Y, Parkkinen L, O'Sullivan SS, et al. Lewy- and Alzheimer-type pathologies in Parkinson's disease dementia: which is more important? Brain. 2011;134:1493–505. doi:10.1093/brain/awr031.
58. Braak H, Del Tredici K, Rüb U, et al. Staging of brain pathology related to sporadic Parkinson's disease. Neurobiol Aging. 2003;24:197–211.
59. Ballard C, Ziabreva I, Perry R, et al. Differences in neuropathologic characteristics across the Lewy body dementia spectrum. Neurology. 2006;67:1931–4. doi:10.1212/01.wnl.0000249130.63615.cc.
60. Halliday G, Hely M, Reid W, Morris J. The progression of pathology in longitudinally followed patients with Parkinson's disease. Acta Neuropathol. 2008;115:409–15. doi:10.1007/s00401-008-0344-8.

61. Mattila PM, Röyttä M, Lönnberg P, et al. Choline acetyltransferase activity and striatal dopamine receptors in Parkinson's disease in relation to cognitive impairment. Acta Neuropathol. 2001;102:160–6.
62. Tiraboschi P, Hansen LA, Alford M, et al. Cholinergic dysfunction in diseases with Lewy bodies. Neurology. 2000;54:407–11.
63. Hirsch EC, Graybiel AM, Duyckaerts C, Javoy-Agid F. Neuronal loss in the pedunculopontine tegmental nucleus in Parkinson disease and in progressive supranuclear palsy. Proc Natl Acad Sci U S A. 1987;84:5976–80.
64. Kuhl DE, Minoshima S, Fessler JA, et al. In vivo mapping of cholinergic terminals in normal aging, Alzheimer's disease, and Parkinson's disease. Ann Neurol. 1996;40:399–410. doi:10.1002/ana.410400309.
65. Bohnen NI, Kaufer DI, Ivanco LS, et al. Cortical cholinergic function is more severely affected in parkinsonian dementia than in Alzheimer disease: an in vivo positron emission tomographic study. Arch Neurol. 2003;60:1745–8. doi:10.1001/archneur.60.12.1745.
66. Bohnen NI, Kaufer DI, Hendrickson R, et al. Cognitive correlates of cortical cholinergic denervation in Parkinson's disease and parkinsonian dementia. J Neurol. 2006;253:242–7. doi:10.1007/s00415-005-0971-0.
67. Kulisevsky J. Role of dopamine in learning and memory: implications for the treatment of cognitive dysfunction in patients with Parkinson's disease. Drugs Aging. 2000;16:365–79.
68. Rinne JO, Portin R, Ruottinen H, et al. Cognitive impairment and the brain dopaminergic system in Parkinson disease: [18F]fluorodopa positron emission tomographic study. Arch Neurol. 2000;57:470–5.
69. Ito K, Nagano-Saito A, Kato T, et al. Striatal and extrastriatal dysfunction in Parkinson's disease with dementia: a 6-[18F]fluoro-L-dopa PET study. Brain. 2002;125:1358–65.
70. Scatton B, Javoy-Agid F, Rouquier L, et al. Reduction of cortical dopamine, noradrenaline, serotonin and their metabolites in Parkinson's disease. Brain Res. 1983;275:321–8.
71. Rinne JO, Rummukainen J, Paljärvi L, Rinne UK. Dementia in Parkinson's disease is related to neuronal loss in the medial substantia nigra. Ann Neurol. 1989;26:47–50. doi:10.1002/ana.410260107.
72. Klein JC, Eggers C, Kalbe E, et al. Neurotransmitter changes in dementia with Lewy bodies and Parkinson disease dementia in vivo. Neurology. 2010;74:885–92. doi:10.1212/WNL.0b013e3181d55f61.
73. Jellinger KA. Morphological substrates of mental dysfunction in Lewy body disease: an update. J Neural Transm Suppl. 2000;59:185–212.
74. Jellinger KA. Pathology of Parkinson's disease. Changes other than the nigrostriatal pathway. Mol Chem Neuropathol. 1991;14:153–97.
75. Apostolova LG, Beyer M, Green AE, et al. Hippocampal, caudate, and ventricular changes in Parkinson's disease with and without dementia. Mov Disord. 2010;25:687–8. doi:10.1002/mds.22799.
76. Matsui H, Nishinaka K, Oda M, et al. Dementia in Parkinson's disease: diffusion tensor imaging. Acta Neurol Scand. 2007;116:177–81. doi:10.1111/j.1600-0404.2007.00838.x.
77. Wiltshire K, Concha L, Gee M, et al. Corpus callosum and cingulum tractography in Parkinson's disease. Can J Neurol Sci. 2010;37:595–600.
78. Seibert TM, Murphy EA, Kaestner EJ, Brewer JB. Interregional correlations in Parkinson disease and Parkinson-related dementia with resting functional MR imaging. Radiology. 2012;263:226–34. doi:10.1148/radiol.12111280.
79. Rektorova I, Krajcovicova L, Marecek R, Mikl M. Default mode network and extrastriate visual resting state network in patients with Parkinson's disease dementia. Neurodegener Dis. 2012;10:232–7. doi:10.1159/000334765.
80. Bissessur S, Tissingh G, Wolters EC, Scheltens P. rCBF SPECT in Parkinson's disease patients with mental dysfunction. J Neural Transm Suppl. 1997;50:25–30.
81. Hilker R, Thomas AV, Klein JC, et al. Dementia in Parkinson disease: functional imaging of cholinergic and dopaminergic pathways. Neurology. 2005;65:1716–22. doi:10.1212/01.wnl.0000191154.78131.f6.

82. Maetzler W, Reimold M, Liepelt I, et al. [11C]PIB binding in Parkinson's disease dementia. Neuroimage. 2008;39:1027–33. doi:10.1016/j.neuroimage.2007.09.072.
83. Edison P, Rowe CC, Rinne JO, et al. Amyloid load in Parkinson's disease dementia and Lewy body dementia measured with [11C]PIB positron emission tomography. J Neurol Neurosurg Psychiatr. 2008;79:1331–8. doi:10.1136/jnnp.2007.127878.
84. Gomperts SN, Rentz DM, Moran E, et al. Imaging amyloid deposition in Lewy body diseases. Neurology. 2008;71:903–10. doi:10.1212/01.wnl.0000326146.60732.d6.
85. Petrou M, Bohnen NI, Müller MLTM, et al. Aβ-amyloid deposition in patients with Parkinson disease at risk for development of dementia. Neurology. 2012;79:1161–7. doi:10.1212/WNL.0b013e3182698d4a.
86. Emre M, Aarsland D, Brown R, et al. Clinical diagnostic criteria for dementia associated with Parkinson's disease. Mov Disord. 2007;22:1689–707. doi:10.1002/mds.21507; quiz 1837.
87. Dubois B, Burn D, Goetz C, et al. Diagnostic procedures for Parkinson's disease dementia: recommendations from the movement disorder society task force. Mov Disord. 2007;22:2314–24. doi:10.1002/mds.21844.
88. Dalrymple-Alford JC, MacAskill MR, Nakas CT, et al. The MoCA: well-suited screen for cognitive impairment in Parkinson disease. Neurology. 2010;75:1717–25. doi:10.1212/WNL.0b013e3181fc29c9.
89. Mahieux F, Boller F, Fermanian J, Guiallard D. Mini-Mental Parkinson: first validation study of a new bedside test constructed for Parkinson's disease. Behav Neurology. 1995;8:15–22.
90. Kalbe E, Calabrese P, Kohn N, et al. Screening for cognitive deficits in Parkinson's disease with the Parkinson neuropsychometric dementia assessment (PANDA) instrument. Parkinsonism Relat Disord. 2008;14:93–101. doi:10.1016/j.parkreldis.2007.06.008.
91. Marinus J, Visser M, Verwey NA, et al. Assessment of cognition in Parkinson's disease. Neurology. 2003;61:1222–8.
92. Pagonabarraga J, Kulisevsky J, Llebaria G, et al. Parkinson's disease-cognitive rating scale: a new cognitive scale specific for Parkinson's disease. Mov Disord. 2008;23:998–1005. doi:10.1002/mds.22007.
93. Cummings JL, Mega M, Gray K, et al. The Neuropsychiatric Inventory: comprehensive assessment of psychopathology in dementia. Neurology. 1994;44:2308–14.
94. Nocera JR, Price C, Fernandez HH, et al. Tests of dorsolateral frontal function correlate with objective tests of postural stability in early to moderate stage Parkinson's disease. Parkinsonism Relat Disord. 2010;16:590–4. doi:10.1016/j.parkreldis.2010.08.008.
95. Yarnall A, Rochester L, Burn DJ. The interplay of cholinergic function, attention, and falls in Parkinson's disease. Mov Disord. 2011;26:2496–503. doi:10.1002/mds.23932.
96. Hindle JV, Petrelli A, Clare L, Kalbe E. Nonpharmacological enhancement of cognitive function in Parkinson's disease: a systematic review. Mov Disord. 2013;28:1034–49. doi:10.1002/mds.25377.
97. París AP, Saleta HG, de la Cruz Crespo Maraver M, et al. Blind randomized controlled study of the efficacy of cognitive training in Parkinson's disease. Mov Disord. 2011;26:1251–8. doi:10.1002/mds.23688.
98. Nombela C, Bustillo PJ, Castell PF, et al. Cognitive rehabilitation in Parkinson's disease: evidence from neuroimaging. Front Neurol. 2011;2:82. doi:10.3389/fneur.2011.00082.
99. Sammer G, Reuter I, Hullmann K, et al. Training of executive functions in Parkinson's disease. J Neurol Sci. 2006;248:115–9. doi:10.1016/j.jns.2006.05.028.
100. Ridgel AL, Kim C-H, Fickes EJ, et al. Changes in executive function after acute bouts of passive cycling in Parkinson's disease. J Aging Phys Act. 2011;19:87–98.
101. Cruise KE, Bucks RS, Loftus AM, et al. Exercise and Parkinson's: benefits for cognition and quality of life. Acta Neurol Scand. 2011;123:13–9. doi:10.1111/j.1600-0404.2010.01338.x.
102. Emre M, Aarsland D, Albanese A, et al. Rivastigmine for dementia associated with Parkinson's disease. N Engl J Med. 2004;351:2509–18. doi:10.1056/NEJMoa041470.
103. Emre M, Poewe W, De Deyn PP, et al. Long-term safety of rivastigmine in Parkinson disease dementia: an open-label, randomized study. Clin Neuropharmacol. 2014;37:9–16. doi:10.1097/WNF.0000000000000010.

104. Wesnes KA, McKeith I, Edgar C, et al. Benefits of rivastigmine on attention in dementia associated with Parkinson disease. Neurology. 2005;65:1654–6. doi:10.1212/01.wnl.0000184517.69816.e9.
105. Burn D, Emre M, McKeith I, et al. Effects of rivastigmine in patients with and without visual hallucinations in dementia associated with Parkinson's disease. Mov Disord. 2006;21:1899–907. doi:10.1002/mds.21077.
106. Poewe W, Wolters E, Emre M, et al. Long-term benefits of rivastigmine in dementia associated with Parkinson's disease: an active treatment extension study. Mov Disord. 2006;21:456–61. doi:10.1002/mds.20700.
107. Oertel W, Poewe W, Wolters E, et al. Effects of rivastigmine on tremor and other motor symptoms in patients with Parkinson's disease dementia: a retrospective analysis of a double-blind trial and an open-label extension. Drug Saf. 2008;31:79–94.
108. Dubois B, Tolosa E, Katzenschlager R, et al. Donepezil in Parkinson's disease dementia: a randomized, double-blind efficacy and safety study. Mov Disord. 2012;27:1230–8. doi:10.1002/mds.25098.
109. Rowan E, McKeith IG, Saxby BK, et al. Effects of donepezil on central processing speed and attentional measures in Parkinson's disease with dementia and dementia with Lewy bodies. Dement Geriatr Cogn Disord. 2007;23:161–7. doi:10.1159/000098335.
110. Aarsland D, Mosimann UP, McKeith IG. Role of cholinesterase inhibitors in Parkinson's disease and dementia with Lewy bodies. J Geriatr Psychiatry Neurol. 2004;17:164–71. doi:10.1177/0891988704267463.
111. Maidment I, Fox C, Boustani M. Cholinesterase inhibitors for Parkinson's disease dementia. Cochrane Database Syst Rev. 2006;(1):CD004747. doi:10.1002/14651858.CD004747.pub2.
112. Rolinski M, Fox C, Maidment I, McShane R. Cholinesterase inhibitors for dementia with Lewy bodies, Parkinson's disease dementia and cognitive impairment in Parkinson's disease. Cochrane Database Syst Rev. 2012;(3):CD006504. doi:10.1002/14651858.CD006504.pub2. CD006504.
113. Thomas AJ, Burn DJ, Rowan EN, et al. A comparison of the efficacy of donepezil in Parkinson's disease with dementia and dementia with Lewy bodies. Int J Geriatr Psychiatry. 2005;20:938–44. doi:10.1002/gps.1381.
114. Minett TSC, Thomas A, Wilkinson LM, et al. What happens when donepezil is suddenly withdrawn? An open label trial in dementia with Lewy bodies and Parkinson's disease with dementia. Int J Geriatr Psychiatry. 2003;18:988–93. doi:10.1002/gps.995.
115. Aarsland D, Ballard C, Walker Z, et al. Memantine in patients with Parkinson's disease dementia or dementia with Lewy bodies: a double-blind, placebo-controlled, multicentre trial. Lancet Neurol. 2009;8:613–8. doi:10.1016/S1474-4422(09)70146-2.
116. Emre M, Tsolaki M, Bonuccelli U, et al. Memantine for patients with Parkinson's disease dementia or dementia with Lewy bodies: a randomised, double-blind, placebo-controlled trial. Lancet Neurol. 2010;9:969–77. doi:10.1016/S1474-4422(10)70194-0.
117. Barker RA, Barrett J, Mason SL, Björklund A. Fetal dopaminergic transplantation trials and the future of neural grafting in Parkinson's disease. Lancet Neurol. 2013;12:84–91. doi:10.1016/S1474-4422(12)70295-8.
118. Molloy SA, Rowan EN, O'Brien JT, et al. Effect of levodopa on cognitive function in Parkinson's disease with and without dementia and dementia with Lewy bodies. J Neurol Neurosurg Psychiatr. 2006;77:1323–8. doi:10.1136/jnnp.2006.098079.
119. Aarsland D, Larsen JP, Karlsen K, et al. Mental symptoms in Parkinson's disease are important contributors to caregiver distress. Int J Geriatr Psychiatry. 1999;14:866–74.
120. Fernandez HH, Okun MS, Rodriguez RL, et al. Quetiapine improves visual hallucinations in Parkinson disease but not through normalization of sleep architecture: results from a double-blind clinical-polysomnography study. Int J Neurosci. 2009;119:2196–205. doi:10.3109/00207450903222758.
121. Morgante L, Epifanio A, Spina E, et al. Quetiapine and clozapine in parkinsonian patients with dopaminergic psychosis. Clin Neuropharmacol. 2004;27:153–6.

122. Low-dose clozapine for the treatment of drug-induced psychosis in Parkinson's disease. The Parkinson Study Group. N Engl J Med.1999;340:757–63. doi:10.1056/NEJM199903113401003.
123. Clozapine in drug-induced psychosis in Parkinson's disease. The French Clozapine Parkinson Study Group. Lancet. 1999;353:2041–2.
124. Coward DM, Imperato A, Urwyler S, White TG. Biochemical and behavioural properties of clozapine. Psychopharmacology (Berl). 1989;99(Suppl):S6–12.
125. Weintraub D, Morales KH, Moberg PJ, et al. Antidepressant studies in Parkinson's disease: a review and meta-analysis. Mov Disord. 2005;20:1161–9. doi:10.1002/mds.20555.
126. Miyasaki JM, Shannon K, Voon V, et al. Practice Parameter: evaluation and treatment of depression, psychosis, and dementia in Parkinson disease (an evidence-based review): report of the Quality Standards Subcommittee of the American Academy of Neurology. Neurology. 2006;66:996–1002. doi:10.1212/01.wnl.0000215428.46057.3d.
127. Devos D, Dujardin K, Poirot I, et al. Comparison of desipramine and citalopram treatments for depression in Parkinson's disease: a double-blind, randomized, placebo-controlled study. Mov Disord. 2008;23:850–7. doi:10.1002/mds.21966.
128. Menza M, Dobkin RD, Marin H, et al. A controlled trial of antidepressants in patients with Parkinson disease and depression. Neurology. 2009;72:886–92. doi:10.1212/01.wnl.0000336340.89821.b3.
129. Richard IH, McDermott MP, Kurlan R, et al. A randomized, double-blind, placebo-controlled trial of antidepressants in Parkinson disease. Neurology. 2012;78:1229–36. doi:10.1212/WNL.0b013e3182516244.
130. Barone P, Poewe W, Albrecht S, et al. Pramipexole for the treatment of depressive symptoms in patients with Parkinson's disease: a randomised, double-blind, placebo-controlled trial. Lancet Neurol. 2010;9:573–80. doi:10.1016/S1474-4422(10)70106-X.
131. Boeve BF, Silber MH, Ferman TJ, et al. Association of REM sleep behavior disorder and neurodegenerative disease may reflect an underlying synucleinopathy. Mov Disord. 2001;16:622–30.
132. Olson EJ, Boeve BF, Silber MH. Rapid eye movement sleep behaviour disorder: demographic, clinical and laboratory findings in 93 cases. Brain. 2000;123(Pt 2):331–9.
133. Lapierre O, Montplaisir J. Polysomnographic features of REM sleep behavior disorder: development of a scoring method. Neurology. 1992;42:1371–4.
134. Boeve BF, Silber MH, Ferman TJ. Melatonin for treatment of REM sleep behavior disorder in neurologic disorders: results in 14 patients. Sleep Med. 2003;4:281–4.
135. Di Giacopo R, Fasano A, Quaranta D, et al. Rivastigmine as alternative treatment for refractory REM behavior disorder in Parkinson's disease. Mov Disord. 2012;27:559–61. doi:10.1002/mds.24909.
136. Adler CH, Caviness JN, Hentz JG, et al. Randomized trial of modafinil for treating subjective daytime sleepiness in patients with Parkinson's disease. Mov Disord. 2003;18:287–93. doi:10.1002/mds.10390.
137. Nieves AV, Lang AE. Treatment of excessive daytime sleepiness in patients with Parkinson's disease with modafinil. Clin Neuropharmacol. 2002;25:111–4.
138. Ondo WG, Fayle R, Atassi F, Jankovic J. Modafinil for daytime somnolence in Parkinson's disease: double blind, placebo controlled parallel trial. J Neurol Neurosurg Psychiatr. 2005;76:1636–9. doi:10.1136/jnnp.2005.065870.
139. Leroi I, Pantula H, McDonald K, Harbishettar V. Neuropsychiatric symptoms in Parkinson's disease with mild cognitive impairment and dementia. Parkinsons Dis. 2012;2012:308097. doi:10.1155/2012/308097.
140. Chatterjee A, Fahn S. Methylphenidate treats apathy in Parkinson's disease. J Neuropsychiatry Clin Neurosci. 2002;14:461–2.
141. Devos D, Moreau C, Maltête D, et al. Rivastigmine in apathetic but dementia and depression-free patients with Parkinson's disease: a double-blind, placebo-controlled, randomised clinical trial. J Neurol Neurosurg Psychiatr. 2013. doi:10.1136/jnnp-2013-306439.

Chapter 4
Impulse Control Disorders

Valerie Voon

Introduction

Impulse control disorders (ICDs) or behavioral addictions in Parkinson's disease (PD) are commonly associated with dopaminergic medications occurring in 14 % of patients and can potentially have marked consequences. These behaviors include pathological gambling (PG), hypersexuality, binge eating, compulsive shopping, punding, and excessive dopaminergic medication use. Diagnostic criteria for these behaviors have been previously described [1] and broadly are defined as repeated urges and compulsive actions with associated negative consequences. The disorder of PG has now been classified in the newly published DSM-5 into the category of "Substance-Related and Addictive Disorders" and will be renamed as "gambling disorder." The reclassification is based on epidemiological, clinical, and neurobiological factors suggesting overlapping similarities with substance use disorders [2]. This chapter focuses on the epidemiology and associated factors and mechanisms including cognitive and imaging studies and treatment studies in ICDs in PD.

Epidemiology

The largest epidemiological study is the multicenter, cross-sectional North American, DOMINION study ($N=3{,}090$ patients) reporting an ICD prevalence of 13.6 % [3] (PG 5.0 %, compulsive sexual behavior 3.5 %, compulsive buying 5.7 %, and binge eating disorder 4.3 %). ICDs were more common with dopamine

V. Voon, MD, PhD
Department of Psychiatry, University of Cambridge, Addenbrookes Hospital,
Hills Road, Level E4, Box 189, Cambridge CB2 0QQ, UK
e-mail: vv247@cam.ac.uk

H. Reichmann (ed.), *Neuropsychiatric Symptoms of Movement Disorders*,
Neuropsychiatric Symptoms of Neurological Disease,
DOI 10.1007/978-3-319-09537-0_4

agonists (17.1 % vs. 6.9 %) with an odds ratio of developing an ICD on dopamine agonists at 2.72 (95 % CI 2.08–3.54). There were no differences in the frequencies of ICDs on pramipexole and ropinirole (17.7 % vs. 15.5 %, odds ratio 1.22; 95 % CI 0.94–1.57).

Although the behaviors are more common on dopamine agonists and levodopa, whether ICDs in PD and/or restless legs syndrome (RLS) subjects on dopaminergic medications occur more frequently than in the general population is less clear. In a study assessing "new-onset heightened interest or drive" of 203 PD patients compared with 190 healthy controls, 14 % of PD patients had a "heightened interest" in ICD behaviors with 3 % in gambling, whereas 0 % was reported in healthy volunteers [4]. In another Italian sample of 98 PD patients and 392 general hospital control patients, 6.1 % vs. 0.25 %, respectively, were identified with PG [5]. However, in a comparison of 115 PD patients with 115 matched healthy controls, there were no differences in the frequencies of PG (0.85 % vs. 0.85 %) [6]. Larger sample sizes and appropriate screening tools are likely required to adequately compare groups. The frequencies of these disorders are also sensitive to the setting screened. For instance, the populations of PD screened for ICDs are commonly assessed in tertiary subspecialized movement disorder centers in which more complex cases and younger populations may be referred. Along this line, the frequency of PG in PD (PG 2.9 % and problem gambling 2.1 % in North America) identified in the DOMINION study [3] may not be fully comparable to population-based frequencies of PG (PG 1.14 % and problem gambling 2.8 % based on a meta-analysis of North American reports published in 1999) [7]. The prevalence rates of ICDs in community studies in the PD population may possibly be lower and more comparable to the prevalence rates of population-based community surveys of PG in the general population. Another important issue may be that the comparison of incidence rates as new-onset ICDs without any previous history of the same age group in the general population may indeed be lower.

ICDs also occur in a diverse range of non-PD patients treated with dopaminergic medication, such as restless legs syndrome [8], progressive supranuclear palsy [9], and multiple sclerosis [10]. Furthermore, the fact that PD patients display a greater frequency of pathological gambling than patients with amyotrophic lateral sclerosis suggests that ICDs are unlikely to be caused by a chronic neurological condition [11].

Pathophysiology

That observation that ICDs only occur in a subset of PD patients argues for a role for an interaction between other factors and dopaminergic medication [3], suggesting that dopamine agonists play only a partial or interactive role and are not sufficient by themselves to result in the onset of ICDs [1, 12, 13]. Thus, other factors are likely to play a role in mediating and influencing the association between dopamine agonists and ICDs. Factors that might interact with dopamine agonists can be subdivided into

(i) the agonist preparation, the dose, and/or coadministered medications; (ii) a possible role for PD itself; and (iii) individual susceptibility [1, 12] as discussed below. This issue of interacting factors addresses the question of why one person with PD given the same medication type or dose might develop an ICD but others with PD exposed to the same drug and dose might not develop an ICD.

Medication Effects

Multiple but not all studies suggest an association between higher dopamine agonist dose and an increased risk of ICD in both subjects with PD and restless legs syndrome (RLS) [14–16]. The multicenter DOMINION study shows that "on univariate analysis the median dopamine agonist LEDD (levodopa-dose equivalent daily dose) in ICD and non-ICD patients was numerically the same (300 mg) but the interquartile range was higher for ICD patients (200–450 mg vs. 150–400 mg, overall $P=0.002$)" [3]. That a decrease in dopamine agonist dose appears to be effective in improving ICDs in many subjects also suggests a role for dose effects [17]. To adequately address the issue of the role of dopamine agonist dose, longitudinal studies are needed, many of which are underway.

The majority of PD patients are on co-medications including levodopa [3] or amantadine [18]. Both dopamine agonist (odds ratio 2.72 (95 % CI: 2.07–3.57), $P<0.001$) and levodopa use (odds ratio 1.51 (95 % CI: 1.09–2.09), $P=0.01$) were independently associated with ICDs with a higher odds ratio for dopamine agonists [3] in the DOMINION study. Coadministration of dopamine agonist and levodopa has also been shown to increase the risk of ICDs as compared to dopamine agonist monotherapy. A higher levodopa dose has also been shown to be associated with a greater risk of ICDs [3].

The association with amantadine, which has a weak antagonist effect on NMDA glutamate receptors and dopamine release, is less clear as an 8-week crossover randomized double-blind placebo-controlled trial of amantadine in 17 PD patients with PG demonstrated efficacy on symptom resolution [19]. However, amantadine was more likely to be associated with ICDs (17.6 % vs. 4.2 %, $p<0.001$) in the DOMINION study [18]. Similarly, another study also demonstrated a higher association of PG with amantadine users than nonusers (2.4 % vs. 0.6 %, $p=0.006$) in their assessment of PG frequency in 1,167 PD patients using the Minnesota Impulsive Disorders Interview [20]. Thus, the association with amantadine is less clear.

In recent congresses, the comparative frequencies of long-acting and continuous stimulation dopamine agonists and ICDs were presented [21]. 52/373 (13.9 %) of ICD cases were documented with a lower frequency on both rotigotine delivered as a transdermal patch (5.3 %) and long-acting pramipexole (6.3 %) compared to that of short-acting pramipexole (13.4 %) and ropinirole (14.9 %). The long-acting nature of the formulation may be less likely to act in a nonphysiological manner or result in sensitization effects and hence be associated with a lower risk of ICDs.

Rotigotine acts as an agonist at dopamine receptors with binding affinities at D3 and D2 receptors 2,600 and 53 times higher than dopamine (D3 > D2 > D1) [22] but is administered as a transdermal patch as a continuous delivery system (CDS) suggesting the predominant issue is that of the continuous delivery formulation rather than D3 receptor mechanisms. However, the results are not completely clear as long-acting ropinirole (14.7 %) had a similarly elevated risk. Whether the CDS nature of rotigotine is less likely to be associated with ICDs requires further confirmatory studies.

The Role of Parkinson's Disease

The role of PD in the onset of ICDs is not yet completely established. There are two possibly conflicting theories underlying a role PD might play as either facilitating or protective [1]. That ICDs occur in non-PD disorders treated with dopaminergic medications such as restless legs syndrome [8, 23, 24] suggests that PD is not absolutely necessary to onset of PG. One study that directly compared the frequency of ICDs in RLS and PD suggested that the frequency of reward-seeking behaviors was higher in PD, an effect that was no longer significant after controlling for dose differences [25]. This was suggested to be a function of higher dopaminergic medication dose in PD and the pattern of administration. Furthermore, two studies investigating the frequency of ICD in new-onset PD did not demonstrate any differences in frequency from the general population suggesting that PD by itself does not increase or decrease the frequency of ICDs [26, 27]. These observations however do not rule out a potential role for PD in facilitating or interacting with dopaminergic medications in the onset of ICDs. For instance, a recent rodent study demonstrated that a parkinsonian rodent model had greater sensitivity to rewarding effects but not motor effects of pramipexole [28]. Thus, although PD by itself is not associated with an increased expression of ICD, a factor related to PD might still interact with dopamine agonists to result in an enhanced expression of ICD. The following are examples of possible mechanisms in which PD may play a role in influencing the relationship between dopamine agonists and PD.

Overdose Hypothesis

In PD, neurodegeneration of the substantia nigra pars compacta dopaminergic cells projecting to dorsal striatal or motor regions can affect up to 70 % of dopaminergic cell bodies prior to onset of parkinsonian motor symptoms. The neurodegeneration of the more mesial dopaminergic cells, the ventral tegmental area (VTA), projecting to the ventral striatum or nucleus accumbens and ventromedial prefrontal cortex (regions implicated in limbic processes such as reward, motivation), is much more variable in PD. Thus, in PD subjects who may have greater preservation of dopaminergic cells projecting to limbic regions (ventral striatal and ventromedial prefrontal) or associative cognitive regions (caudate, orbitofrontal, or dorsolateral prefrontal cortex), treatment with dopaminergic medications targeting degenerated motor striatal regions may result in an “overdose” of otherwise intact limbic and associative regions. This “overdosing” may result in impairment of cognitive and behavioral functioning [1, 29]. The “overdose” hypothesis has been well described and supported by experimental evidence suggesting that functioning of cognition or behavior follows a U-shaped curve. Optimal functioning occurs at an optimal level of dopamine level with either higher or lower dopamine levels resulting in impairments in functioning.

PD-Related Neuropathology

Another possible role for the neurobiology of PD might include greater PD-related neuropathology (deposition of Lewy bodies or neurodegeneration in specific neural regions) related to ICDs. The issue of visual hallucinations in PD gives a very relevant analogy. For instance, visual hallucinations are common in PD occurring in 17–40 % of patients. Although visual hallucinations are clearly associated with the presence of dopaminergic medications, PD is now believed to play a clear role in the onset of hallucinations. For instance, hallucinations are associated with greater Lewy body deposition in limbic regions (amygdala, hippocampus, medial temporal) [30, 31]. Similarly, postmortem studies in PD patients with ICDs may similarly reveal greater deposition of Lewy bodies in limbic regions, thus predisposing the individual toward a greater risk for an interaction with dopamine agonists resulting in ICD symptoms. Specific subtypes of PD may be more likely to be at risk for the development of ICDs. That PG is associated with early-onset PD might also suggest that specific subtypes of PD may have a differential pattern of neurodegeneration or neurobiology [3].

Dyskinesia

A unifying view is that there is a common mechanism of action in the motor and non-motor domains of the corticostriatal circuitry, as evidenced by similarities between ICDs and levodopa-induced dyskinesias [32]. ICDs in PD are associated with an oscillatory theta-alpha activity in the ventral subthalamic nucleus along with electroencephalographic coherence with non-motor prefrontal regions. In contrast, in dyskinesias, theta-alpha activity is associated with a dorsal localization and a coherence with motor regions [33]. PD patients with punding [34] or multiple ICDs [35] also have more severe dyskinesias relative to PD controls. Taken together, this evidence supports potentially unifying neurophysiological mechanisms linking motor and behavioral side effects of dopaminergic treatment.

Apathy

A relationship between apathy (decreased motivation, interest, and emotional response to external and internal stimuli) secondary to PD has been observed with ICDs [36]. Apathy is commonly observed in PD occurring in 17–41 % of patients and is understood to be related to the neurobiology of PD [37]. In a prospective study of subthalamic stimulation in PD patients in which 17 had ICDs, the discontinuation of the dopamine agonist and marked lowering of dopaminergic medication dose was associated with an improvement in ICD in all subjects [36]. However, half of the subjects developed apathy symptoms. The authors suggest a possible relationship between those who develop ICDs on dopaminergic medications and those suffering apathy off dopaminergic medications, implicating abnormalities in ventral striatal dopaminergic functioning. Notably apathy in PD outside of the context of subthalamic stimulation is likely much more complex involving other neurotransmitters including acetylcholine and norepinephrine.

Cognitive Deficits

Cognitive deficits in PD may facilitate the onset of ICDs [38, 39]. PD patients without ICDs were shown to have elevated delay discounting scores (tendency to select immediate smaller rewards over delayed larger rewards) both on and off medications [39]. Elevated delay discounting is associated with ICDs in the general population [40, 41], and three studies of PD patients with ICDs, particularly PG or compulsive shopping, demonstrated elevated delay discounting compared to PD controls without ICDs [35, 42, 43]. Delay discounting is a known predictive risk factor for cocaine dependence in rodents. Rodents who have higher delay discounting at baseline are more likely to escalate into cocaine acquisition and compulsive drug-seeking behaviors than those with lower delay discounting scores at baseline [44, 45]. Thus, the facts that elevated delay discounting (i) is a known predictor for substance dependence, (ii) is increased in ICDs in the general population and in ICDs in PD, and (iii) is increased in PD patients at baseline might suggest a potential interaction between a cognitive deficit in PD and dopamine agonists in the development of ICDs [38].

Individual Susceptibility Factors

There are multiple known factors that contribute to the pathophysiology of PG in the general population that have also been demonstrated to be associated with PG in the PD population. The papers reporting associated factors with PG in the general population have been systematically assessed and ranked for level of evidence in a review by Johansson et al. in 2009 [46]. In this review, associated factors for PG in the general population are ranked by level of evidence (well established: more than two studies to support conclusions; probable: 1–2 studies). The following discusses the identified factors associated with PG in the general population as discussed in this review and compared evidence from the literature on factors associated with PG in the PD population. That the associated factors are similar between PG in the general population and in PD suggests a similar underlying individual vulnerability.

Age and Gender

PG in the general population is associated with younger age and male gender (2:1 male to female ratio) based on level 1 supportive evidence [46]. Similarly, PG in PD is associated with younger age in multiple studies and definitively demonstrated as an independent associated factor for PG in PD in the DOMINION study [3]. Although there were no gender differences in PG in PD in the DOMINION study, males were more likely to express hypersexuality and women to express binge eating and compulsive shopping [3].

Depression

Depression is identified as a probable risk factor for PG in the general population [46] with a genetic link postulated between the two disorders [47]. In a survey of 7,869 individuals from the Vietnam Era Twin Registry (middle-aged men), the odds ratio for major depression was elevated for PG (OR 4.06). Thirty-four percent of the genetic variance for each disorder contributed to that of the other with the best-fitting model estimating that 100 % of the overlap between PG and MD was genetic [47]. Furthermore, the likelihood of major depression predicting the onset of PG has been reported at 6.6 based on data from the US National Comorbidity Survey Replication study [48]. Similarly, the DOMINION study identified higher depression scores in both the cross-sectional and case-control study as an independent risk factor in the association of ICDs in PD patients [3, 35].

Substance Use Disorders

Alcohol and other substance use disorders have level 1 evidence to support an association with PG in the general population [46] with a genetic link postulated between alcohol use disorders and PG [49]. Substance use disorders such as alcohol or drug abuse, alcohol or drug dependence, or nicotine dependence have an odds ratio predicting the onset of PG of 5.4, 8.8, and 1.9, respectively, based on the US National Comorbidity Survey Replication study [48]. In a twin study of genetics, 12–20 % of the genetic variation and 3–8 % of the non-shared environmental risk for PG was accounted for by the risk for alcohol dependence [49].

Although the DOMINION cross-sectional study identified an increased association with a family history of alcohol use disorder with PG, following multivariate analysis this factor was not identified as an independent risk factor suggesting that it is closely linked to another associated factor (e.g., current smoking or family history of gambling) [3, 12]. In a smaller study of 21 PD and PG patients compared to 42 PD controls, a personal or immediate family history of alcohol use disorders (rather than current alcohol use) was assessed. This factor along with novelty seeking and younger age of PD onset predicted PG at 83.7 % and accounted for 62 % of the variance [50]. Current alcohol use as measured using the alcohol-use disorders identification test (AUDIT) was not associated with PG in either the cross-sectional or case-control arms of the DOMINION study. In contrast, current cigarette smoking was identified as an independent factor associated in PG in both arms of the DOMINION study [3, 12]. In a study of restless legs syndrome and ICDs, a premorbid history of experimental drug use was also highlighted as an independent associated factor [23].

Family History of Gambling

Twin studies suggest possible genetic factors underlying PG. In PG-affected subjects, 8 % of first-degree relatives compared to 2 % of first-degree relatives in unaffected controls had a lifetime history of PG [51]. In the Vietnam Era Twin Registry study, 23 % of monozygotic co-twins and 10 % of dizygotic male co-twins had a lifetime history of PG [52] which modeling suggested was attributed to shared genetic rather than environmental factors [49]. In the recent community-based Australian Twin Registry study, the variation in the risk for disordered gambling due to genetic influences was 49.2 %, whereas no evidence for shared environmental influences contributed to the variation in risk [53].

PG in PD patients is also associated with a greater likelihood of a family history of gambling problems as an independent factor predicting the onset of PG in the DOMINION study [3]. Similarly, in a study of RLS and ICDs, a family history of gambling problems was identified as an independent associated factor [23]. These studies highlight the role of genetic and environmental factors in mediating the relationship between dopamine agonists and PG.

Personality and Temperamental Traits

PG in the general population is associated with greater impulsivity and novelty and sensation seeking as probable risk factors [46]. PG is also associated with more personality disorders, specifically antisocial personality disorder, as a probable risk factor [46]. For instance, in a study by Slutske et al. of the Vietnam Era Twin Registry data, subjects with a history of PG had higher prevalence rates of antisocial personality disorder (odds ratio = 6.4) which precedes the onset of PG symptoms [54]. PG is also significantly associated with delinquency, criminal, and illegal activity with level 1 supportive evidence [46]. Similarly, PG and compulsive shopping subjects in the PD population have higher scores on novelty seeking and impulsivity questionnaires as demonstrated in the case-control arm of the DOMINION study [35].

Social Factors

The relationship between marital status and PG in the general population is less clear with both being married and being single identified as associated factors [46]. Proximity and availability of gambling are identified as an associated factor for PG in the general population with level 1 supportive evidence [46]. In the cross-sectional arm of the DOMINION study, ICDs were independently associated with being unmarried and living in the United States as compared to Canada [3]. The latter association may be mediated by greater availability of casinos in the United States or by differences in medication practices. Thus, these individual susceptibility factors may modify the relationship between dopamine agonists and the expression of ICDs in PD.

Neural Mechanisms

The following section discusses possible cognitive, neural, and molecular mechanisms that underlie the expression of ICDs in PD.

Reward Processing

Dopamine mediates reward-related processing playing a role in the initial acquisition and the subsequent craving and compulsive use in substance use disorders. Phasic ventral striatal dopamine is triggered by unexpected receipt of reward and shifts to the cue predicting reward after associative learning [55] and, along with glutamate, underlies formation of conditioned responses. Converging human and primate studies have demonstrated that phasic dopamine encodes discrepancies between rewards received and those predicted, thus acting as a teaching signal signifying a prediction error [55].

In rodents, pramipexole acts similarly to methamphetamine, but not saline control, to promote conditioned place preference or learning to associate a context with a reward [28]. Higher doses of pramipexole were required to achieve the same rewarding effect in sham rodents as compared to the lower doses required in parkinsonian rodents, but there were no differences in locomotor responses. The authors suggested that PD may play a role in enhancing responsiveness to the rewarding but not the motor effects of pramipexole. Dopamine replacement therapy may influence physiological function via either exogenous tonic dopaminergic stimulation or interference with the endogenous, physiological, phasic pattern of striatal dopamine release. In response to conditioned cues or to a gambling task, PD + ICD patients demonstrate increased ventral striatal dopamine release as measured using (^{11}C)raclopride. Similarly, in response to conditioned cues or to unexpected and anticipated rewards, PD + ICD patients demonstrated increased ventral striatal activity [56–58]. DAs in PD patients with either problem gambling or compulsive shopping were shown to enhance the rate of learning from gain-specific outcomes [56] although not all studies demonstrate this effect [59]. Using a reinforcement learning computational approach that models reward prediction error activity to assess fMRI blood oxygen level-dependent (BOLD) response and indirectly assess phasic dopaminergic activity, DAs were shown to increase ventral striatal activity to prediction error in ICD, signifying a "better-than-expected outcome" and enhanced reward prediction. These results are most consistent with the early acquisition stage and also are relevant to forming learned associations with cues.

Incentive Salience

The incentive motivation theory hypothesizes that dopamine alters nucleus accumbens sensitivity to incentive processing, such that motivational value is assigned to cues associated with rewards, making them desirable in their own right [60]. Using (^{11}C)raclopride PET imaging, PD patients with mixed ICDs were shown to have a heightened striatal dopamine release to heterogeneous reward-related visual cues as compared to levodopa or neutral cues [58]. Similarly, using fMRI, PD patients with hypersexuality were shown to have greater ventral striatal activity to sexual cues as compared to those without hypersexuality, an effect that correlated with an index of subjective sexual desire or wanting but not liking [61]. These findings were suggested to be in support of an incentive salience process. Similarly, activation of the ventral striatum in response to gambling-related cues was demonstrated in a small fMRI study in PD patients with ICDs [62]. These studies are consistent with studies in cocaine dependence demonstrating greater striatal dopamine release in response to cocaine cues [63].

Risk and Uncertainty

Pathological behavioral choices are associated with both positive and negative financial, social, and occupational outcomes, thus consistent with definitions of risky (with known probabilities) or uncertain (with unknown probabilities) choices. In rodent studies, pramipexole increases probabilistic discounting or the preference for the risky choice. This increase in risk taking occurs irrespective of the presence of the parkinsonian model of 6-OHDA injected in the dorsolateral striatum [64]. Similarly, d-amphetamine impaired task performance on a rodent gambling task modeled on the Iowa gambling task which measures risk taking under uncertainty [65].

Two studies focusing on risk anticipation without outcome demonstrate that DAs increase risk taking in PD patients with ICDs [59, 66]. This risk-taking bias appears to be unrelated to loss aversion and is accompanied by lower ventral striatal, orbitofrontal, and anterior cingulate activity [66]. The lower ventral striatal activity is consistent with an fMRI study of PD patients with ICDs using the balloon analogue risk task (BART) that examines uncertainty with feedback [67]. Similarly, ICD subjects tested using the BART demonstrate greater risk taking on medication as compared to off medication [68].

A recent study has proposed that the findings of greater reflection impulsivity (or decisions under uncertainty without adequate information sampling) [69], delay discounting (selection of the immediate salient lower reward over the possibly more uncertain delayed reward) [35, 43], and novelty seeking in the context of uncertainty [70] may reflect underlying uncertainty about mapping future actions into rewards [71].

Behavioral Regulation and Impulsivity

Some evidence for impaired "top-down" prefrontal regulation is beginning to emerge. Using H_2O PET, in PD patients with pathological gambling engaged in a probabilistic gambling task, apomorphine challenge was associated with decreased activity in circuits involved in behavioral regulation, including the lateral orbitofrontal cortex and rostral cingulate cortex [72]. Similarly, a resting state single-photon emission tomography (SPECT) study in PD patients with pathological gambling demonstrated decreased functional connectivity between the striatum and the anterior cingulate cortex, the latter being a region involved in negative feedback and conflict detection [73]. Impulsivity, defined as a lack of behavioral inhibition, has motor and decisional subtypes. Impulsive choice is characterized by a preference for small, immediate, rewards, instead of larger, delayed rewards. Enhanced impulsive choice has been demonstrated in PD patients with ICDs using delay discounting tasks with hypothetical long delayed monetary rewards [35, 43] and real-time short delay monetary rewards [35]. In one study, impaired delay discounting with intact reward incentive performance in PD patients with ICDs was interpreted as evidence for a potential impairment in waiting for the delayed reward, rather than an enhanced incentive toward the immediate reward [43]. Alternatively, impulsive choice normally demonstrates a magnitude effect whereby lower impulsive choices accompany increasing reward magnitude. This magnitude effect in delay discounting is less pronounced in PD patients with ICDs, suggesting that dopamine agonists may be associated with greater subjective devaluation of the delayed, higher reward magnitude [35], resulting in greater impulsivity toward the smaller, immediate choice.

With respect to other forms of impulsivity, DAs in PD patients with ICDs appear to enhance the rapidity of decision-making, also known as reflection impulsivity, suggesting that the long-term negative consequences may not be as carefully considered as they otherwise would be [42]. Impulsive PD patients do not perform differently to non-impulsive PD patients on the Stroop color word test [59] that probes inhibition of prepotent responses and response selection associated with anterior cingulate function.

Lateral Prefrontal Cortex Function

Visuospatial working memory tested "on" medication was impaired in medicated PD patients with ICD compared with those without [42]. Similarly, PD patients with ICD both when "on" and "off" medications have a significantly reduced digit span compared with PD and control groups [59]. These results suggest that dorsolateral corticostriatal circuitry in PD with ICD might be similarly affected by "overdose" from exogenous dopamine when "on" medication and possibly from endogenous dopamine when "off" medication.

Molecular Mechanisms

Dopamine Transporter Levels

Two studies have demonstrated decreased striatal dopamine transporter (DAT) levels in PD patients with ICDs compared to those without [74, 75]. Dopamine reuptake via DAT, a membrane-spanning protein located in the axon terminals, is the primary mechanism by which striatal dopamine is removed from the synaptic cleft and dopamine neurotransmission regulated and terminated. These findings may help explain the observation of enhanced ventral striatal activity and enhanced dopamine release in PD + ICD patients in response to conditioned cues or to unexpected and anticipated rewards [56–58]. Impaired clearance of dopamine may play a role in extending the physiological effect of dopamine at the synaptic terminal.

The binding levels of (^{123}I)FP-CIT may reflect either lower DAT levels or greater dopaminergic nerve terminal degeneration. However, there is no clear clinical evidence for a greater decrease in dopaminergic terminals in PD + ICD patients relative to PD controls [75] suggesting that the lower binding levels might either reflect greater sensitivity to medication-related DAT downregulation or baseline trait differences and hence higher dopaminergic activity. Lower DAT levels with similar nerve terminal density suggest that extracellular dopamine neurotransmission can be enhanced both in distance from the synaptic cleft and duration of action.

Multiple substances of abuse, such as methamphetamine, cocaine, and alcohol, can differentially affect the regulation of DAT. For instance, methamphetamine and alcohol are associated with decreased DAT density as measured using PET imaging and DAT ligands [76, 77] particularly in early abstinence (<6 months) with some degree of recovery after prolonged abstinence (12–16 months) [78, 79] In contrast to the effects of substances of abuse, DAT regulation by Levodopa or dopamine agonists, if any, appears to be modest, and its effect might be dependent on its use in early versus late PD or as monotherapy versus co-therapy. Although any regulation of DAT by antiparkinsonian medications appears to be modest [80–91], PD + ICD patients may be differentially sensitive to regulatory mechanisms of DAT expression (e.g., D2 autoreceptor, TAAR1, protein kinase A and C) [81] compared to PD controls. A mechanism implicating DAT downregulation would also suggest that symptom improvement following discontinuation of the dopamine agonist would have a delayed time course. This may also play a role in the observation of enhanced dopamine withdrawal symptoms (DAWS) observed following dopamine agonist discontinuation in PD patients with ICDs [82].

D2/D3 Autoreceptor Downregulation and Increase in Gain

Although acute dopamine agonist (pramipexole) administration in rodents has been shown to decrease the proportion of spontaneously firing dopaminergic neurons, chronic dopamine agonists normalize this proportion of firing neurons mediated via D2/D3 autoreceptor downregulation [83]. Furthermore, chronic levodopa administration in a parkinsonian rodent model has been shown to increase the proportion of spontaneously firing dopaminergic neurons, secondary to D2/D3 autoreceptor downregulation [84]. These spontaneously firing dopaminergic neurons are the neurons that are capable of phasic activity in response to a stimulus (e.g., the unconditioned rewarding stimulus, conditioned stimulus, a gambling task) [85]. Thus, increasing the proportion of spontaneously firing neurons effectively increases the gain and proportion of dopamine neurons capable of phasically responding to a stimulus. Preliminary evidence exists that PD patients with ICDs have decreased sensitivity of the D2/D3 autoreceptor in the midbrain as measured using (^{11}C)FLB-457 PET [86]. In this study, PD controls on dopamine agonists demonstrated decreased D2/D3 midbrain autoreceptor binding to a gamble task as compared to a control task, consistent with the feedback regulation of endogenous dopamine released in the gamble task. In contrast, PD patients with ICDs on dopamine agonists failed to demonstrate a difference suggesting decreased sensitivity of the D2/D3 autoreceptor. Thus, the enhanced dopamine levels observed in PD + ICD may be related to impaired regulatory feedback.

Dopamine Receptor Subtypes

Dopamine D3 receptors are predominantly expressed in the ventral striatum, and they mediate reward, emotional, and cognitive processes. Pramipexole and ropinirole, two widely used non-ergot DAs, have greater D2/D3 selectivity relative to D1. That concurrent levodopa use with a DA increases the odds of developing an ICD [3] is consistent with a primate study demonstrating that levodopa administration results in ectopic induction of dorsal striatal D3 receptors [87].

Genetic Polymorphisms

Genetic polymorphisms may also contribute to ICD susceptibility. Evaluation of dopamine and glutamate receptors and serotonin transporter gene polymorphisms identified D3 dopamine receptor p.S9G and GRIN2B c.366C > G as a risk factor for ICDs in PD [88].

Diagnosis

Patients and caregivers should be warned about the risk of development of ICDs at treatment onset and actively questioned on follow-up. Patients with a premorbid history of substance or behavioral addiction may be at a greater risk for the development of these disorders. The validated screening tool, questionnaire for impulsive-compulsive disorders in Parkinson's disease (QUIP), has >80 % sensitivity and specificity and can be completed in 5 min [89]. Given the low positive predictive value (21–59 %), clinical interview should follow a positive screening result. The QUIP is valid also when completed by the patient's informant [90].

Treatment

Pharmacotherapy

Observational follow-up studies suggest that a decrease or discontinuation of the DA, if tolerated, may be efficacious for some patients. PD patients with ICDs will be more sensitive to dopamine agonist withdrawal symptoms (DAWS) [82]. A recent crossover randomized trial demonstrated efficacy of amantadine [19]; however, a contradicting report of increased risk of ICDs associated with amantadine [3] suggests its role is not yet established. Cognitive behavioral therapy has been shown in a randomized wait list control with standard medical care to improve global symptom severity [91]. Naltrexone, an opioid antagonist, which has been shown to be effective in the management of PG in the general population, was effective in a case study involving 3 PD patients with PG [92]. Other case reports have also reported preliminary efficacy with valproate [93] and clozapine [94].

Deep Brain Stimulation

There is as yet no clear consensus regarding the role of DBS for preoperative ICD and compulsive medication use. ICD behaviors have been reported to improve, remain unchanged, or worsen after surgery [95]. De novo onset of ICDs has also been reported [96]. In two retrospective case series, mixed ICD behaviors were reported primarily to remain unchanged or worsen following bilateral STN DBS or unilateral STN or GPi DBS. For instance, in one of the retrospective bilateral STN and GPi DBS case series that included both ICDs and compulsive medication use, postoperative worsening of symptoms was associated with the lack of preoperative recognition of the disorder and high dopaminergic medication dose [95]. In another retrospective unilateral STN DBS case series, only two of seven subjects with preoperative ICD improved, with no clear relationship to medication dose [97]. That there were no significant changes in medication dosage following the unilateral DBS may be an important limiting factor. Compulsive medication use in 5 patients persisted in the postoperative stage. In this same case series, 17 of 159 patients developed new-onset ICD behaviors, although the exact nature of these behaviors was not reported. In contrast, other small retrospective studies have suggested that ICD can resolve after STN DBS and could become a new indication for surgery in this target [98, 99]. In a prospective study of 17 patients with preoperative ICDs treated with bilateral STN DBS, using systematic preoperative and postoperative evaluation of ICD and systematic discontinuation of dopamine agonists, all ICD behaviors ceased [36]. In this study, however, preoperative overall appetitive behavior changed into an overall more apathetic mode of functioning, which might mitigate the beneficial effect on ICD [36]. Thus, careful preoperative behavioral assessment and management of postoperative medications are crucial.

Overall, although ICDs can occur after surgery, the case reports suggest that their occurrence, particularly that of pathological gambling or compulsive shopping, is rare. This may differ for the behaviors of binge eating and hypersexuality. The existing data suggest that, with careful preoperative and postoperative assessment and management, there is a role for STN DBS in the management of ICD in patients in whom medication changes are ineffective or poorly tolerated. Transient postoperative worsening might occur early in the postoperative stage. STN DBS allows a greater decrease in dopaminergic medication dose relative to GPi DBS and enables a discontinuation of the dopamine agonist. However, patients may be reluctant to decrease their dopaminergic medication. Patients with ICD may also be at greater risk of DAWS, requiring careful titration of medications [100], and of postoperative suicidal behaviors [101].

References

1. Voon V, Potenza MN, Thomsen T. Medication-related impulse control and repetitive behaviors in Parkinson's disease. Curr Opin Neurol. 2007;20(4):484–92.
2. Leeman RF, Potenza MN. Similarities and differences between pathological gambling and substance use disorders: a focus on impulsivity and compulsivity. Psychopharmacology (Berl). 2012;219(2):469–90.
3. Weintraub D, Koester J, Potenza MN, Siderowf AD, Stacy M, Voon V, et al. Impulse control disorders in Parkinson disease: a cross-sectional study of 3090 patients. Arch Neurol. 2010;67(5):589–95.
4. Giladi N, Weitzman N, Schreiber S, Shabtai H, Peretz C. New onset heightened interest or drive for gambling, shopping, eating or sexual activity in patients with Parkinson's disease: the role of dopamine agonist treatment and age at motor symptoms onset. J Psychopharmacol. 2007;21(5):501–6.
5. Avanzi M, Baratti M, Cabrini S, Uber E, Brighetti G, Bonfa F. Prevalence of pathological gambling in patients with Parkinson's disease. Mov Disord. 2006;21(12):2068–72.
6. de Chazeron I, Llorca PM, Chereau-Boudet I, Blanc O, Perriot J, Ouchchane L, et al. Hypersexuality and pathological gambling in Parkinson's disease: a cross-sectional case-control study. Mov Disord. 2011;26(11):2127–30.

7. Shaffer HJ, Hall MN, Vander BJ. Estimating the prevalence of disordered gambling behavior in the United States and Canada: a research synthesis. Am J Public Health. 1999;89(9):1369–76.
8. Cornelius JR, Tippmann-Peikert M, Slocumb NL, Frerichs CF, Silber MH. Impulse control disorders with the use of dopaminergic agents in restless legs syndrome: a case-control study. Sleep. 2010;33(1):81–7.
9. O'Sullivan SS, Djamshidian A, Ahmed Z, Evans AH, Lawrence AD, Holton JL, et al. Impulsive-compulsive spectrum behaviors in pathologically confirmed progressive supranuclear palsy. Mov Disord. 2010;25(5):638–42.
10. Evans AH, Butzkueven H. Dopamine agonist-induced pathological gambling in restless legs syndrome due to multiple sclerosis. Mov Disord. 2007;22(4):590–1.
11. Wicks P, MacPhee GJ. Pathological gambling amongst Parkinson's disease and ALS patients in an online community (PatientsLikeMe.com). Mov Disord. 2009;24(7):1085–8.
12. Voon V, Mehta AR, Hallett M. Impulse control disorders in Parkinson's disease: recent advances. Curr Opin Neurol. 2011;24(4):324–30.
13. Voon V, Fox SH. Medication-related impulse control and repetitive behaviors in Parkinson disease. Arch Neurol. 2007;64(8):1089–96.
14. Dodd ML, Klos KJ, Bower JH, Geda YE, Josephs KA, Ahlskog JE. Pathological gambling caused by drugs used to treat Parkinson disease. Arch Neurol. 2005;62(9):1377–81.
15. Driver-Dunckley E, Samanta J, Stacy M. Pathological gambling associated with dopamine agonist therapy in Parkinson's disease. Neurology. 2003;61(3):422–3.
16. Weintraub D, Siderowf AD, Potenza MN, Goveas J, Morales KH, Duda JE, et al. Association of dopamine agonist use with impulse control disorders in Parkinson disease. Arch Neurol. 2006;63(7):969–73.
17. Mamikonyan E, Siderowf AD, Duda JE, Potenza MN, Horn S, Stern MB, et al. Long-term follow-up of impulse control disorders in Parkinson's disease. Mov Disord. 2008;23(1):75–80.
18. Weintraub D, Sohr M, Potenza MN, Siderowf AD, Stacy M, Voon V, et al. Amantadine use associated with impulse control disorders in Parkinson disease in cross-sectional study. Ann Neurol. 2010;68(6):963–8.
19. Thomas A, Bonanni L, Gambi F, Di Iorio A, Onofrj M. Pathological gambling in Parkinson disease is reduced by amantadine. Ann Neurol. 2010;68(3):400–4.
20. Lee JY, Kim HJ, Jeon BS. Is pathological gambling in Parkinson's disease reduced by amantadine? Ann Neurol. 2011;69(1):213–4; author reply 4-5.
21. Rizos A, Kessel B, Henriksen T, Røkenes KK, Martin A, Koch I, et al., editors. Impulse control disorder/behaviour related to prolonged release oral and transdermal dopamine agonists: a comparative European multicenter survey 16th International Congress of Parkinson's disease and Movement Disorders. Dublin; 2012.
22. Scheller D, Ullmer C, Berkels R, Gwarek M, Lubbert H. The in vitro receptor profile of rotigotine: a new agent for the treatment of Parkinson's disease. Naunyn Schmiedebergs Arch Pharmacol. 2009;379(1):73–86.
23. Voon V, Schoerling A, Wenzel S, Ekanayake V, Reiff J, Trenkwalder C, et al. Frequency of impulse control behaviours associated with dopaminergic therapy in restless legs syndrome. BMC Neurol. 2011;11:117.
24. Pourcher E, Remillard S, Cohen H. Compulsive habits in restless legs syndrome patients under dopaminergic treatment. J Neurol Sci. 2010;290(1–2):52–6.
25. Ondo WG, Lai D. Predictors of impulsivity and reward seeking behavior with dopamine agonists. Parkinsonism Relat Disord. 2008;14(1):28–32.
26. Weintraub D, Papay K, Siderowf A. Screening for impulse control symptoms in patients with de novo Parkinson disease: a case-control study. Neurology. 2013;80(2):176–80.
27. Antonini A, Siri C, Santangelo G, Cilia R, Poletti M, Canesi M, et al. Impulsivity and compulsivity in drug-naive patients with Parkinson's disease. Mov Disord. 2011;26(3):464–8.

28. Riddle JL, Rokosik SL, Napier TC. Pramipexole- and methamphetamine-induced reward-mediated behavior in a rodent model of Parkinson's disease and controls. Behav Brain Res. 2012;233(1):15–23.
29. Cools R. Dopaminergic modulation of cognitive function-implications for L-DOPA treatment in Parkinson's disease. Neurosci Biobehav Rev. 2006;30(1):1–23.
30. Harding AJ, Broe GA, Halliday GM. Visual hallucinations in Lewy body disease relate to Lewy bodies in the temporal lobe. Brain. 2002;125(Pt 2):391–403.
31. Papapetropoulos S, McCorquodale DS, Gonzalez J, Jean-Gilles L, Mash DC. Cortical and amygdalar Lewy body burden in Parkinson's disease patients with visual hallucinations. Parkinsonism Relat Disord. 2006;12(4):253–6.
32. Voon V, Fernagut PO, Wickens J, Baunez C, Rodriguez M, Pavon N, et al. Chronic dopaminergic stimulation in Parkinson's disease: from dyskinesias to impulse control disorders. Lancet Neurol. 2009;8(12):1140–9.
33. Rodriguez-Oroz MC, Lopez-Azcarate J, Garcia-Garcia D, Alegre M, Toledo J, Valencia M, et al. Involvement of the subthalamic nucleus in impulse control disorders associated with Parkinson's disease. Brain. 2011;134(Pt 1):36–49.
34. Silveira-Moriyama L, Evans AH, Katzenschlager R, Lees AJ. Punding and dyskinesias. Mov Disord. 2006;21(12):2214–7.
35. Voon V, Sohr M, Lang AE, Potenza MN, Siderowf AD, Whetteckey J, et al. Impulse control disorders in Parkinson disease: a multicenter case-control study. Ann Neurol. 2011;69(6):986–96.
36. Lhommee E, Klinger H, Thobois S, Schmitt E, Ardouin C, Bichon A, et al. Subthalamic stimulation in Parkinson's disease: restoring the balance of motivated behaviours. Brain. 2012;135(Pt 5):1463–77.
37. Dujardin K, Defebvre L. Apathy in Parkinson disease: what are the underlying mechanisms? Neurology. 2012;79(11):1082–3.
38. Voon V, Dalley JW. Parkinson disease: impulsive choice-Parkinson disease and dopaminergic therapy. Nat Rev Neurol. 2011;7(10):541–2.
39. Milenkova M, Mohammadi B, Kollewe K, Schrader C, Fellbrich A, Wittfoth M, et al. Intertemporal choice in Parkinson's disease. Mov Disord. 2011;26(11):2004–10.
40. Andrade LF, Petry NM. Delay and probability discounting in pathological gamblers with and without a history of substance use problems. Psychopharmacology (Berl). 2012;219(2):491–9.
41. Petry NM. Pathological gamblers, with and without substance use disorders, discount delayed rewards at high rates. J Abnorm Psychol. 2001;110(3):482–7.
42. Voon V, Reynolds B, Brezing C, Gallea C, Skaljic M, Ekanayake V, et al. Impulsive choice and response in dopamine agonist-related impulse control behaviors. Psychopharmacology (Berl). 2010;207(4):645–59.
43. Housden CR, O'Sullivan SS, Joyce EM, Lees AJ, Roiser JP. Intact reward learning but elevated delay discounting in Parkinson's disease patients with impulsive-compulsive spectrum behaviors. Neuropsychopharmacology. 2010;35(11):2155–64.
44. Belin D, Mar AC, Dalley JW, Robbins TW, Everitt BJ. High impulsivity predicts the switch to compulsive cocaine-taking. Science. 2008;320(5881):1352–5.
45. Anker JJ, Perry JL, Gliddon LA, Carroll ME. Impulsivity predicts the escalation of cocaine self-administration in rats. Pharmacol Biochem Behav. 2009;93(3):343–8.
46. Johansson A, Grant JE, Kim SW, Odlaug BL, Gotestam KG. Risk factors for problematic gambling: a critical literature review. J Gambl Stud. 2009;25(1):67–92.
47. Potenza MN, Xian H, Shah K, Scherrer JF, Eisen SA. Shared genetic contributions to pathological gambling and major depression in men. Arch Gen Psychiatry. 2005;62(9):1015–21.
48. Kessler RC, Hwang I, LaBrie R, Petukhova M, Sampson NA, Winters KC, et al. DSM-IV pathological gambling in the National Comorbidity Survey Replication. Psychol Med. 2008;38(9):1351–60.

49. Slutske WS, Eisen S, True WR, Lyons MJ, Goldberg J, Tsuang M. Common genetic vulnerability for pathological gambling and alcohol dependence in men. Arch Gen Psychiatry. 2000;57(7):666–73.
50. Voon V, Thomsen T, Miyasaki JM, de Souza M, Shafro A, Fox SH, et al. Factors associated with dopaminergic drug-related pathological gambling in Parkinson disease. Arch Neurol. 2007;64(2):212–6.
51. Black DW, Monahan PO, Temkit M, Shaw M. A family study of pathological gambling. Psychiatry Res. 2006;141(3):295–303.
52. Eisen SA, Lin N, Lyons MJ, Scherrer JF, Griffith K, True WR, et al. Familial influences on gambling behavior: an analysis of 3359 twin pairs. Addiction. 1998;93(9):1375–84.
53. Slutske WS, Zhu G, Meier MH, Martin NG. Genetic and environmental influences on disordered gambling in men and women. Arch Gen Psychiatry. 2010;67(6):624–30.
54. Waldman ID, Slutske WS. Antisocial behavior and alcoholism: a behavioral genetic perspective on comorbidity. Clin Psychol Rev. 2000;20(2):255–87.
55. Schultz W, Dayan P, Montague PR. A neural substrate of prediction and reward. Science. 1997;275(5306):1593–9.
56. Voon V, Pessiglione M, Brezing C, Gallea C, Fernandez HH, Dolan RJ, et al. Mechanisms underlying dopamine-mediated reward bias in compulsive behaviors. Neuron. 2010;65(1):135–42.
57. Steeves TD, Ko JH, Kideckel DM, Rusjan P, Houle S, Sandor P, et al. Extrastriatal dopaminergic dysfunction in tourette syndrome. Ann Neurol. 2010;67(2):170–81.
58. O'Sullivan SS, Wu K, Politis M, Lawrence AD, Evans AH, Bose SK, et al. Cue-induced striatal dopamine release in Parkinson's disease-associated impulsive-compulsive behaviours. Brain. 2011;134(Pt 4):969–78.
59. Djamshidian A, Jha A, O'Sullivan SS, Silveira-Moriyama L, Jacobson C, Brown P, et al. Risk and learning in impulsive and nonimpulsive patients with Parkinson's disease. Mov Disord. 2010;25(13):2203–10.
60. Robinson TE, Berridge KC. The neural basis of drug craving: an incentive-sensitization theory of addiction. Brain Res Brain Res Rev. 1993;18(3):247–91.
61. Politis M, Loane C, Wu K, O'Sullivan SS, Woodhead Z, Kiferle L, et al. Neural response to visual sexual cues in dopamine treatment-linked hypersexuality in Parkinson's disease. Brain. 2013;136(Pt 2):400–11.
62. Frosini D, Pesaresi I, Cosottini M, Belmonte G, Rossi C, Dell'Osso L, et al. Parkinson's disease and pathological gambling: results from a functional MRI study. Mov Disord. 2010;25(14):2449–53.
63. Volkow ND, Wang GJ, Telang F, Fowler JS, Logan J, Childress AR, et al. Cocaine cues and dopamine in dorsal striatum: mechanism of craving in cocaine addiction. J Neurosci. 2006;26(24):6583–8.
64. Rokosik SL, Napier TC. Pramipexole-induced increased probabilistic discounting: comparison between a rodent model of Parkinson's disease and controls. Neuropsychopharmacology. 2012;37(6):1397–408.
65. Zeeb FD, Robbins TW, Winstanley CA. Serotonergic and dopaminergic modulation of gambling behavior as assessed using a novel rat gambling task. Neuropsychopharmacology. 2009;34(10):2329–43.
66. Voon V, Gao J, Brezing C, Symmonds M, Ekanayake V, Fernandez H, et al. Dopamine agonists and risk: impulse control disorders in Parkinson's disease. Brain. 2011;134(Pt 5):1438–46.
67. Rao H, Mamikonyan E, Detre JA, Siderowf AD, Stern MB, Potenza MN, et al. Decreased ventral striatal activity with impulse control disorders in Parkinson's disease. Mov Disord. 2010;25(11):1660–9.
68. Claassen DO, van den Wildenberg WP, Ridderinkhof KR, Jessup CK, Harrison MB, Wooten GF, et al. The risky business of dopamine agonists in Parkinson disease and impulse control disorders. Behav Neurosci. 2011;125(4):492–500.

69. Djamshidian A, Sanotsky Y, Matviyenko Y, O'Sullivan SS, Sharman S, Selikhova M, et al. Increased reflection impulsivity in patients with ephedrone-induced Parkinsonism. Addiction. 2013;108(4):771–9.
70. Djamshidian A, O'Sullivan SS, Wittmann BC, Lees AJ, Averbeck BB. Novelty seeking behaviour in Parkinson's disease. Neuropsychologia. 2011;49(9):2483–8.
71. Averbeck BB, Djamshidian A, O'Sullivan SS, Housden CR, Roiser JP, Lees AJ. Uncertainty about mapping future actions into rewards may underlie performance on multiple measures of impulsivity in behavioral addiction: evidence from Parkinson's disease. Behav Neurosci. 2013;127(2):245–55.
72. van Eimeren T, Pellecchia G, Cilia R, Ballanger B, Steeves TD, Houle S, et al. Drug-induced deactivation of inhibitory networks predicts pathological gambling in PD. Neurology. 2010;75(19):1711–6.
73. Cilia R, Cho SS, van Eimeren T, Marotta G, Siri C, Ko JH, et al. Pathological gambling in patients with Parkinson's disease is associated with fronto-striatal disconnection: a path modeling analysis. Mov Disord. 2011;26(2):225–33.
74. Cilia R, Ko JH, Cho SS, van Eimeren T, Marotta G, Pellecchia G, et al. Reduced dopamine transporter density in the ventral striatum of patients with Parkinson's disease and pathological gambling. Neurobiol Dis. 2010;39(1):98–104.
75. Voon V, Rizos A, Chakravartty R, Mulholland N, Robinson S, Howell NA, Harrison N, Vivian G, Ray Chaudhuri K. Impulse control disorders In Parkinson's disease: decreased dopamine transporter levels. J Neurol Neurosurg Psychiatry. 2014;85(2):148–52.
76. Sekine Y, Iyo M, Ouchi Y, Matsunaga T, Tsukada H, Okada H, et al. Methamphetamine-related psychiatric symptoms and reduced brain dopamine transporters studied with PET. Am J Psychiatry. 2001;158(8):1206–14.
77. McCann UD, Wong DF, Yokoi F, Villemagne V, Dannals RF, Ricaurte GA. Reduced striatal dopamine transporter density in abstinent methamphetamine and methcathinone users: evidence from positron emission tomography studies with [11C]WIN-35,428. J Neurosci. 1998;18(20):8417–22.
78. Volkow ND, Chang L, Wang GJ, Fowler JS, Franceschi D, Sedler M, et al. Loss of dopamine transporters in methamphetamine abusers recovers with protracted abstinence. J Neurosci. 2001;21(23):9414–8.
79. Laine TP, Ahonen A, Torniainen P, Heikkila J, Pyhtinen J, Rasanen P, et al. Dopamine transporters increase in human brain after alcohol withdrawal. Mol Psychiatry. 1999;4(2):189–91, 04-5.
80. Guttman M, Stewart D, Hussey D, Wilson A, Houle S, Kish S. Influence of L-dopa and pramipexole on striatal dopamine transporter in early PD. Neurology. 2001;56(11):1559–64.
81. Schmitt KC, Reith ME. Regulation of the dopamine transporter: aspects relevant to psychostimulant drugs of abuse. Ann N Y Acad Sci. 2010;1187:316–40.
82. Rabinak CA, Nirenberg MJ. Dopamine agonist withdrawal syndrome in Parkinson disease. Arch Neurol. 2010;67(1):58–63.
83. Chernoloz O, El Mansari M, Blier P. Sustained administration of pramipexole modifies the spontaneous firing of dopamine, norepinephrine, and serotonin neurons in the rat brain. Neuropsychopharmacology. 2009;34(3):651–61.
84. Harden DG, Grace AA. Activation of dopamine cell firing by repeated L-DOPA administration to dopamine-depleted rats: its potential role in mediating the therapeutic response to L-DOPA treatment. J Neurosci. 1995;15(9):6157–66.
85. Grace AA. Dopamine system dysregulation by the hippocampus: implications for the pathophysiology and treatment of schizophrenia. Neuropharmacology. 2012;62(3):1342–8.
86. Ray NJ, Miyasaki JM, Zurowski M, Ko JH, Cho SS, Pellecchia G, et al. Extrastriatal dopaminergic abnormalities of DA homeostasis in Parkinson's patients with medication-induced pathological gambling: a [11C] FLB-457 and PET study. Neurobiol Dis. 2012;48(3):519–25.
87. Bordet R, Ridray S, Carboni S, Diaz J, Sokoloff P, Schwartz JC. Induction of dopamine D3 receptor expression as a mechanism of behavioral sensitization to levodopa. Proc Natl Acad Sci U S A. 1997;94(7):3363–7.

88. Lee JY, Lee EK, Park SS, Lim JY, Kim HJ, Kim JS, et al. Association of DRD3 and GRIN2B with impulse control and related behaviors in Parkinson's disease. Mov Disord. 2009;24(12):1803–10.
89. Weintraub D, Hoops S, Shea JA, Lyons KE, Pahwa R, Driver-Dunckley ED, et al. Validation of the questionnaire for impulsive-compulsive disorders in Parkinson's disease. Mov Disord. 2009;24(10):1461–7.
90. Papay K, Mamikonyan E, Siderowf AD, Duda JE, Lyons KE, Pahwa R, et al. Patient versus informant reporting of ICD symptoms in Parkinson's disease using the QUIP: validity and variability. Parkinsonism Relat Disord. 2011;17(3):153–5.
91. Okai D, Askey-Jones S, Samuel M, O'Sullivan SS, Chaudhuri KR, Martin A, et al. Trial of CBT for impulse control behaviors affecting Parkinson patients and their caregivers. Neurology. 2013;80(9):792–9.
92. Bosco D, Plastino M, Colica C, Bosco F, Arianna S, Vecchio A, et al. Opioid antagonist naltrexone for the treatment of pathological gambling in Parkinson disease. Clin Neuropharmacol. 2012;35(3):118–20.
93. Sriram A, Ward HE, Hassan A, Iyer S, Foote KD, Rodriguez RL, et al. Valproate as a treatment for dopamine dysregulation syndrome (DDS) in Parkinson's disease. J Neurol. 2013;260(2):521–7.
94. Hardwick A, Ward H, Hassan A, Romrell J, Okun MS. Clozapine as a potential treatment for refractory impulsive, compulsive, and punding behaviors in Parkinson's disease. Neurocase. 2012;19(6):587–91.
95. Lim SY, O'Sullivan SS, Kotschet K, Gallagher DA, Lacey C, Lawrence AD, et al. Dopamine dysregulation syndrome, impulse control disorders and punding after deep brain stimulation surgery for Parkinson's disease. J Clin Neurosci. 2009;16(9):1148–52.
96. Smeding HM, Goudriaan AE, Foncke EM, Schuurman PR, Speelman JD, Schmand B. Pathological gambling after bilateral subthalamic nucleus stimulation in Parkinson disease. J Neurol Neurosurg Psychiatry. 2007;78(5):517–9.
97. Moum SJ, Price CC, Limotai N, Oyama G, Ward H, Jacobson C, et al. Effects of STN and GPi deep brain stimulation on impulse control disorders and dopamine dysregulation syndrome. PLoS One. 2012;7(1):e29768.
98. Ardouin C, Voon V, Worbe Y, Abouazar N, Czernecki V, Hosseini H, et al. Pathological gambling in Parkinson's disease improves on chronic subthalamic nucleus stimulation. Mov Disord. 2006;21(11):1941–6.
99. Witjas T, Baunez C, Henry JM, Delfini M, Regis J, Cherif AA, et al. Addiction in Parkinson's disease: impact of subthalamic nucleus deep brain stimulation. Mov Disord. 2005;20(8):1052–5.
100. Nirenberg MJ. Dopamine agonist withdrawal syndrome and non-motor symptoms after Parkinson's disease surgery. Brain. 2010;133(11):e155; author reply e6.
101. Voon V, Krack P, Lang AE, Lozano AM, Dujardin K, Schupbach M, et al. A multicentre study on suicide outcomes following subthalamic stimulation for Parkinson's disease. Brain. 2008;131(Pt 10):2720–8.

Chapter 5
Influence of Dietary Constituents on Motor and Non-motor Symptoms in Parkinson's Disease

Matthias Löhle and Heinz Reichmann

Introduction

Parkinson's disease (PD) is a progressive neurodegenerative disorder, which affects about 1 % of the population over the age of 65 [1, 2] and is pathologically characterized by a progressive loss of dopaminergic cells of the nigrostriatal pathway [3, 4]. Despite considerable efforts to unravel the pathogenesis of PD, the actual trigger for the degeneration of dopaminergic and other neurotransmitter systems in PD remains unknown, which hampers the development of causative and neuroprotective treatments [5]. Numerous population-based studies have tried to identify environmental and lifestyle factors that may influence the risk for PD in order to dissect the source and potential treatments for the disease. These studies have found that smoking, coffee, and alcohol drinking lower the risk to develop PD, whereas pesticide exposure and well-water drinking are associated with a greater risk for the disease (see [6] for review). Moreover, it has been recently suggested that nicotine-containing edibles of the *Solanaceae* species, such as peppers, tomatoes, and potatoes, may reduce the risk for PD [7]. Interestingly, a potential involvement of dietary factors in the pathogenesis PD is now also supported by experimental findings from a mouse model, in which chronic, low-dose intragastric administration of the pesticide rotenone was able to reproduce the typical progression of alpha-synuclein pathology in the central nervous system seen in PD [8].

M. Löhle, MD (✉) • H. Reichmann, MD, PhD
Department of Neurology, Dresden University of Technology,
Fetscherstrasse 74, Dresden D-01307, Germany
e-mail: matthias.loehle@uniklinikum-dresden.de;
Heinz.Reichmann@uniklinikum-dresden.de

H. Reichmann (ed.), *Neuropsychiatric Symptoms of Movement Disorders*,
Neuropsychiatric Symptoms of Neurological Disease,
DOI 10.1007/978-3-319-09537-0_5

In contrast to numerous risk studies on the impact of environmental factors on the incidence of PD, little is known about the symptomatic effects of dietary factors in patients that have already been diagnosed with the disease, which makes it hard for treating physicians to recommend specific diets to PD patients. The following chapter therefore aims to investigate scientific evidence from previous studies on the effects of dietary components on motor and non-motor symptoms of the disease. Given the multitude of food constituents that have been suggested to have beneficial effects on PD based on preclinical studies, we will concentrate on those food components, which have also been examined in clinical trials.

Antioxidants

Coenzyme Q10

One very popular dietary supplement and potent antioxidant is coenzyme Q10 (CoQ10 or ubiquinone), an electron acceptor bridging mitochondrial complexes I/II and III, which has been suggested to have potential therapeutic value in PD since mitochondrial dysfunction plays an important role in the pathogenesis of the disease [9]. After an initial 3-month open-label trial with 200 mg CoQ10 per day in ten mildly affected PD patients had found no improvement of motor symptoms [10], a parallel-group, placebo-controlled, double-blind trial in 28 PD patients suggested that daily oral administration of 360 mg CoQ10 over 4 weeks provides a mild symptomatic benefit on PD symptoms and improves color vision, but not motor function [11] (Table 5.1). We performed a multicenter, randomized, double-blind, placebo-controlled, stratified, parallel-group, single-dose trial with nanoparticular CoQ10 at a dosage of 300 mg per day, but did not find any symptomatic effects in 131 patients with midstage Parkinson's disease [12]. Nonetheless, a randomized, double-blind, calibrated futility clinical trial of CoQ10 in early untreated PD suggested that further study into disease-modifying capabilities of this component may be warranted [13]. Just recently, a placebo-controlled, double-blind clinical trial, in which 600 participants with early PD were randomly assigned to placebo, 1,200 mg/day of CoQ10 or 2,400 mg/day of CoQ10, however did not find any proof that the component would slow disease progression [14]. Based on the data presented above, there is currently no scientific evidence for an effect of CoQ10 on motor or non-motor symptoms of PD and hence no reason to recommend supplementation of CoQ10 to PD patients.

Creatine

Creatine is a naturally occurring bioenergetic compound, which is mainly taken up with meat, is essential for adenosine triphosphate (ATP) homeostasis, and has been demonstrated to have neuroprotective properties in animal models of PD [25].

Table 5.1 Randomized, double-blind, clinical trials into effects of dietary constituents on motor and non-motor symptoms of Parkinson's disease [11, 12, 14–24]

Substance	Study reference	n^a	Duration	Outcome
Antioxidants				
Coenzyme Q10	Müller et al. [11]	28	4 weeks	Mild effect on the total UPDRS and improved color vision, but no effect on motor function as measured by the UPDRS part III
	Storch et al. [12]	131	3 months	No effect on UPDRS parts II/III in midstage PD
	Parkinson Study Group [14]	600	16 months	No effect on total UPDRS in early PD
Creatine	Bender et al. [15]	60	2 years	No effect on total UPDRS, but antidepressant effect on UPDRS part I and lower requirement for dopaminergic agents
	NINDS [16, 17]	1,741	Aborted	Outcomes not reported yet, but interim analysis revealed no effect
Methylxanthines				
Caffeine	Postuma et al. [18]	61	6 weeks	Improvement on UPDRS part III and total UPDRS, but no improvement of daytime somnolence, depression, or quality of life
Natural sources of biogenic amines				
Mucuna pruriens	Katzenschlager et al. [19]	8	Single dose	Faster onset of effect on the UPDRS and longer on time without dyskinesias in comparison to conventional levodopa
Chocolate	Wolz et al. [20]	26	Single dose	No effect of dark chocolate on the UPDRS part III motor score in comparison to cocoa-free white chocolate
Polyphenols				
EGCG	Chan et al. [21]	410	12 months	Improvement on the total UPDRS compared to baseline, but no proof of neuroprotective effects
Polyunsaturated fatty acids				
Fish oil (DHA)	Da Silva et al. [22]	31	3 months	Improvement of depressive symptoms on the MADRS compared to baseline and placebo

(continued)

Table 5.1 (continued)

Substance	Study reference	n^a	Duration	Outcome
Vitamins				
Vitamin D	Suzuki et al. [23]	114	12 months	Prevention of deterioration on Hoehn and Yahr stage and UPDRS part II and improvement of subscores on PDQ-39, but no effect on motor function as measured by UPDRS part III or cognition
Vitamin E	Parkinson Study Group [24]	800	14±6 months	No delaying effect on disability requiring symptomatic treatment

EGCG (-)-epigallocatechin-3-gallate, *DHA* docosahexaenoic acid, *UPDRS* Unified Parkinson's Disease Rating Scale, *MADRS* Montgomery-Asberg Depression Rating Scale, *PDQ*-39 39-item Parkinson's disease questionnaire
[a]Number of randomized patients

After a randomized, double-blind, futility clinical trial in 200 patients with early PD had suggested that creatine should be investigated as a candidate to alter the long-term course of the disease [26], the National Institute of Neurological Disorders and Stroke (NINDS) initiated a large multicenter, double-blind, parallel-group, placebo-controlled phase III long-term study (LS-1) in patients with early, treated PD, in which 1,741 participants were randomized to treatment with either 10 g of creatine per day or matching placebo [16]. Unfortunately, the LS-1 study was stopped by the NINDS recently after an interim analysis had shown that it would be futile to continue the study since longer patient follow-up was unlikely to demonstrate a statistically significant difference between creatine and placebo [17]. Similarly, an earlier placebo-controlled and randomized pilot trial in 60 patients with early PD in Germany had demonstrated that oral creatine treatment over 2 years had no effect on overall scores of the Unified Parkinson's Disease Rating Scale (UPDRS) or dopamine transporter single-photon emission computed tomography [15]. However, this trial also revealed that creatine treatment reduced the dosages required for dopamine-replacement therapy and led to a lower UPDRS part 1 subscore, which was attributed to an antidepressant effect of this substance [15]. Although a study in major depression has indicated that creatine may lead to an augmentation of the response to antidepressant treatment with selective serotonin reuptake inhibitors [27], creatine supplementation should not be advocated as adjunctive antidepressant treatment for parkinsonian patients at the present, since corresponding studies still need to reproduce similar effects in PD patients.

Methylxanthines

Caffeine

Caffeine, a methylated xanthine that, for example, is found in coffee beans, tea leaves, and kola nuts, has been repeatedly suggested to have neuroprotective effects in PD, after numerous epidemiological studies had shown that coffee drinking is associated with a lower risk for PD [28]. Animal models of PD indicate that the advantageous effects of caffeine in PD may be mediated by antagonistic effects on the A_{2A} subtypes of adenosine receptors [29], which are predominantly expressed in the striatum [30] and co-localized with dopaminergic D2 receptors, inhibiting effects of dopaminergic transmission [31, 32].

After an open-label, 6-week dose-escalation study in 25 PD patients had found potential improvements in motor symptoms and daytime sleepiness with 400 mg caffeine per day, Postuma et al. conducted a 6-week randomized, placebo-controlled trial evaluating the effects of 100–200 mg caffeine twice daily on daytime somnolence, motor severity, and other non-motor features in 61 PD patients suffering from daytime sleepiness indicated by values of more than 10 points on the Epworth Sleepiness Scale [18]. In this study, caffeine led to a nonsignificant reduction of daytime sleepiness and did not improve sleep quality, depression, or quality of life but was associated with a significant improvement of motor function documented by a 3.2-point and 4.7-point reduction on the UPDRS part III and the total UPDRS, respectively. Moreover, anticipated side effects such as anxiety, irritability, insomnia, or worsening of action tremor were not reported more in caffeine-treated patients than in controls demonstrating good tolerability of this treatment. Although the results of this trial are in contrast to negative results of two older small-scale studies [33, 34] and still must be confirmed in separate longer-term trials, these advantageous experiences with caffeine are indeed encouraging and should prompt further research with this compound.

Natural Sources of Amino Acids and Biogenic Amines

Plants of the Mucuna *Genus*

It is already known for long that L-DOPA, the most effective antiparkinsonian agent, can also be found in several plants of the *Mucuna* genus, such as the broad bean *Vicia faba* or the velvet bean *Mucuna pruriens*, which are endemic in India and Central and South America and contain considerable amounts of natural L-DOPA [35]. After Ayurvedic medicine had already described positive effects of *Mucuna* on Kampavata [35], a disease with similarities to PD, three open-label studies involving between 18 and 60 patients reported significant improvements of PD symptoms with mean dosages of 45 g/day of *Mucuna* seed powder extract

Table 5.2 Chocolate and non-chocolate sweet consumption in patients with Parkinson's disease and household controls [44]

	PD patients	Household controls	*P* values
No. of subjects	274	234	
Sweet consumption (grams/week)			
Chocolate (mean ± SD)	100.3 ± 105.3	57.3 ± 78.1	<0.0001
Non-chocolate sweets (mean ± SD)	207.1 ± 206.9	192.5 ± 184.0	0.4542

(containing about 1,500 mg L-DOPA) [36–38]. These open-label studies were followed by a double-blind, clinical, and pharmacological study in 8 PD patients, which found a more rapid onset of action and longer *on* time with 30 g of a *M. pruriens* suspension compared to a standard dose of 200/50 mg L-DOPA/carbidopa without concomitant increase in dyskinesias [19]. Although this small pilot study suggested superior bioavailability with *M. pruriens* than with standard L-DOPA formulations and hence would have merited further investigation, its results still await confirmation by larger and longer-term studies.

Cocoa and Chocolate

Another natural source of amino acids and biogenic amines are cocoa-containing foods such as dark chocolate, which contains tyrosine, phenylalanine, tryptophan, tyramine, and β-phenylethylamine (β-PEA). Especially β-PEA may be of interest for PD, since this biogenic amine can cross the blood-brain barrier and in animal studies has shown to increase dopamine release into the synaptic cleft [39, 40]. Moreover, chocolate contains methylated xanthines, such as theobromine and caffeine, as well as flavonols, which are most likely responsible for its beneficial effects on cardiovascular disease and stroke [41–43].

Potential benefits of chocolate in PD gained our interest after we observed during ward rounds that PD patients always seemed to have chocolate at their bedside. Following this observation, we initiated a questionnaire study, in which we evaluated 498 PD patients and their partners for consumption of chocolate and non-chocolate sweets, changes in chocolate consumption during the disease course, and depressive symptoms [44]. This study revealed that consumption of chocolate was significantly higher in PD patients compared to controls, whereas consumption of non-chocolate sweets was similar in both groups (Table 5.2). Our observation prompted us to wonder whether cocoa-containing chocolate would indeed have symptomatic effects in PD. In a monocenter, investigator-blinded crossover study using cacao-free white chocolate as placebo comparator, we thus examined the effects of a single dose of 200 g dark chocolate containing 80 % of cocoa on the UPDRS motor score after 1 and 3 h in 26 subjects with moderate PD without motor fluctuations [20]. In this study, dark chocolate did not show significant improvement over white cacao-free chocolate on motor function, which however needs to be interpreted with caution since we only used a single dose of chocolate, did not investigate the content of amino acids and biogenic amines in the administered chocolate, and did not assess potential effects on non-motor aspects of PD. At the present, we are therefore conducting another trial aiming to investigate potential effects of cocoa-containing chocolate on motor and non-motor symptoms of PD over a period of 1 week in order to account for a potential delay of uptake due to gastroparesis.

Polyphenols

Polyphenols can be found in various foods and food products, especially fruits and vegetables, coffee, green and black tea, olives, and olive oil [45]. Polyphenols have been shown to elicit anticarcinogenic, anti-inflammatory, antimutagenic, antithrombotic, and most importantly antioxidant effects [46]. Although other polyphenolic compounds, such as curcumins and baicalein, were also suggested to have neuroprotective properties in cell cultures and animal models of PD, we will concentrate on catechins in green tea, which also underwent clinical testing.

Catechins in Green Tea

Several epidemiological studies were able to demonstrate that tea drinking is associated with a lower risk to develop PD [47–50]. Green tea contains various polyphenolic compounds, among them catechins such as (-)-epicatechin, (-)-epicatechin-3-gallate, (-)-epigallocatechin and (-)-epigallocatechin-3-gallate (EGCG). EGCG is the most abundant catechin in green tea [51] and suggested to have neuroprotective properties in PD as pretreatment with both green tea extracts, and EGCG has been shown to prevent N-methyl-4-phenyl-1,2,3,6-tetrahydropyridine (MPTP)-induced dopaminergic neurodegeneration in mice [52]. Following numerous positive studies in cell cultures as well as toxic and inflammatory animal models of neurodegenerative diseases, EGCG and other catechins are now assumed to be multimodal-acting, brain-permeable, neuroprotective substances that do not only serve as antioxidants and iron chelators but also have beneficial effects on various signaling pathways, in particular the protein kinase C pathway (see [53] for review). Consequently, the Michael J. Fox Foundation decided to support a study led by Piu Chan to evaluate whether green tea polyphenols were also capable to slow disease progression in patients with early PD [21]. In this multicenter, double-blind, randomized, placebo-controlled, delayed-start study in China, 410 untreated patients with early PD were randomized to receive one of three doses of green tea polyphenols (0.4, 0.8 or 1.2 g daily) or matching placebo and evaluated with safety measures and the UPDRS over a period of 12 months. Placebo-treated patients were switched to the highest dose of green tea polyphenols after 6 months. Although the results of this study have unfortunately not been officially published to date, the website of the Michael J. Fox foundation reports that treatment with green tea polyphenols led to a significant improvement on the total UPDRS compared to baseline after 6 months, whereas there was no difference between the early- and delayed-start group after 12 months [21]. These results would argue for an advantageous effect of green tea polyphenols on PD symptoms but also against neuroprotective properties, which would be in keeping with a previous retrospective study that did not identify disease-modifying effects of tea consumption in PD patients [54]. Since the results of the study of Chan et al. have not been published and still need to be reproduced by others, there is to date however no sufficient clinical proof to advocate green tea consumption to PD patients.

Polyunsaturated Fatty Acids

Polyunsaturated fatty acids (PUFAs) can be divided into two distinct groups according to the position of the first double bond in relation to the terminal methyl group. n-3 PUFAs and n-6 PUFAs are derived from the precursors alpha-linoleic (ALA) and linoleic acid, respectively, which both are essential to humans and cannot be synthesized de novo. One of the most important n-3 PUFAs is docosahexaenoic acid (DHA), which in the blood is mainly bound to albumin and after crossing the blood-brain barrier can be integrated into phospholipid bilayers of brain cells, where it increases membrane fluidity and contributes to optimal function of receptors and channels (see [55] for review). Although the liver has the potential to convert ALA into DHA, in vivo studies have shown that this endogenous source for the supply of DHA to the brain is rather limited compared to dietary intake of preformed DHA [56], thereby emphasizing the importance of sufficient uptake of DHA from food sources, for example, oily fish.

Various epidemiological studies have suggested that n-3 PUFAs may lower the risk for PD. In the Rotterdam Study, which investigated the interplay between the intake of unsaturated fatty acids and incident PD in a cohort of 5,289 subjects free of dementia and parkinsonism, higher PUFA intake was associated with a significantly lower risk for PD [57]. Despite not directly addressing PUFAs, another study has similarly shown that adherence to a diet with high intakes of fruit, vegetables, and fish can also significantly lower the risk to develop PD [58]. Moreover, it has been demonstrated that higher adherence to Mediterranean diet, which is known to be rich in n-3 PUFAs, is associated with reduced odds for PD, whereas lower adherence to Mediterranean diet was associated with an earlier PD age at onset [59].

Although n-3 PUFA supplementation has been shown to have symptomatic and potentially neuroprotective effects in rodent models of PD [60, 61] and to significantly reduce dyskinesias in MPTP-treated monkeys without altering the antiparkinsonian effect of levodopa [62], no clinical study has been investigating whether PUFAs would be effective to ameliorate motor symptoms of PD. Nevertheless, one clinical study has examined whether n-3 PUFA supplementation could have advantageous effects on depression in PD. In this double-blind, placebo-controlled trial, 31 patients with PD and major depression were assigned to two groups that either received fish oil (containing n-3 fatty acids) or mineral oil capsules [22]. After 3 months of treatment, patients that had been treated with fish oil showed a significant reduction of depressive symptoms on the Montgomery-Asberg Depression Rating Scale in comparison to baseline as well as in comparison to PD patients that had been treated with mineral oil capsules. High-performance liquid chromatography analysis of fatty acid profile moreover revealed an increase of DHA in the erythrocyte membrane of patients taking fish oil, but not in patients that had been treated with mineral oil capsules. Although the results of this pilot study are encouraging, they need to be interpreted with caution since there was no difference between groups on the Beck Depression Inventory, which may be attributed to a significant placebo response on this scale. Despite effects of PUFAs on motor symptoms are unknown and the scientific rationale for supplementation of PUFAs in PD is still insufficient, we would argue that adherence to a healthy, Mediterranean-type diet may still be suggested to PD patients given the beneficial effects of this diet on cerebrovascular disease [63].

Vitamins

Vitamins C and E

One of the earliest attempts to investigate potential effects of vitamins in PD was performed by Fahn with an open-label pilot study in 15 patients suffering from early PD, who were recommended to take 3,000 mg ascorbate (vitamin C) and 3,200 IU alpha-tocopherol (vitamin E) per day [64]. The outcome of the trial was the time until patients needed symptomatic treatment with levodopa. This small study found that the combination of vitamins C and E extended the time until levodopa was needed by 2.5 years, which suggested a disease-modifying effect of both vitamins on the disease. However, the small size of the study, the lack of a control group, and its open-label design hamper the interpretation of this study. A much larger, placebo-controlled, and double-blind clinical trial was the Deprenyl and Tocopherol Antioxidative Therapy of Parkinson (DATATOP) trial, which evaluated disease-modifying capabilities of selegiline (deprenyl), a monoamine oxidase type B inhibitor, and tocopherol (vitamin E) in 800 patients with early PD [24]. In this study, treatment with 2,000 IU tocopherol per day did not lead to a delay in the need for additional symptomatic treatment. The lack of therapeutic effect of vitamin E in the DATATOP study is in agreement with epidemiological studies that did not find a significant influence of antioxidative vitamins on the incidence of PD [65, 66], whereas other studies have found that the risk for PD was reduced with higher vitamin C [67] and vitamin E intake [68–71]. Taken together, scientific evidence on the effects of vitamins C and E in PD is however not sufficient to generally recommend supplementation to patients. Given that both vitamins seem to have positive effects on cognitive function in elderly people (see [72] for review), substitution of vitamins C and E should however be considered in those patients, in whom dietary uptake with vegetables and fruits is insufficient.

Vitamin D

Several studies have demonstrated that serum concentrations of 25-hydroxy vitamin D, the primary circulating form of vitamin D, are lower in PD patients than in age-matched healthy controls [73, 74]. Recently, a cross-sectional and longitudinal case-control study has revealed that unrecognized vitamin D deficiency is common in PD patients and that low 25-hydroxy-vitamin D3 as well as total 25-hydroxy-vitamin D levels are correlated with higher total UPDRS scores [75]. Conversely, higher plasma vitamin D levels have shown to be associated with better cognition and better mood in PD patients without dementia [76].

Surprisingly, only one intervention study with vitamin D supplementation in PD has been published until today. In this double-blind, randomized, placebo-controlled study, 114 PD patients were randomly assigned to receive vitamin D3 supplements (1,200 IU/day) or placebo for 12 months. All participants were evaluated with Hoehn and Yahr (HY) staging, UPDRS, and mini-mental state examination and asked to complete the EQ-5D and the 39-item Parkinson's disease questionnaire (PDQ-39) to assess quality of life [23]. Compared to placebo, daily supplementation with vitamin D3 for 12 months significantly prevented the deterioration of PD as measured with the HY stage, UPDRS part II (activities of daily living), and the total UPDRS and led to an improvement on some parts of the PDQ-39, whereas motor function measured by the UPDRS part III as well as cognitive function measured with the MMSE remained unchanged. Although the positive effects of vitamin D supplementation in this study may have been due to unspecific effects of vitamin D on muscle strength and balance [77] and still need to be reproduced by larger studies, it is advisable to examine the vitamin D status in PD patients and to start substitution whenever necessary, especially since PD patients have a lower bone mineral density [78] and are more prone to falls than age-matched controls [79]. Aside from motor function, future studies should also evaluate whether vitamin D supplementation is indeed accompanied by beneficial effects on cognition and mood as has been suggested by a recent study, in which higher vitamin D concentrations were associated with better verbal memory and verbal fluency and lower depression scores in non-demented PD patients [76].

Conclusion

Taken together, clinical studies on the influence of food components on motor and non-motor symptoms in PD have so far yielded largely inconclusive or negative results, which on the first look may argue against further pursuit of alimentary approaches for symptomatic treatment of the disease. In our opinion, there is however still enough rationale for future research into this matter. At first, it needs to be acknowledged that some substances, such as caffeine and DHA, have indeed shown to have advantageous effects on motor function and non-motor symptoms of PD. Secondly, some of the negative results of previous studies must be interpreted in the light of their limited sample size and short study length, which may have prevented them from detecting potential effects on disease outcomes. Thirdly, almost all studies have concentrated on investigating single dietary components and consequently have been dependent on a single mechanism of action, e.g., antioxidative properties. In a disease with relatively slow progression and assumedly multiple underlying pathomechanisms such as PD, it may be more promising for future studies to choose a multifaceted approach and to combine multiple substances with different modes of action in order to achieve symptomatic efficacy or even disease modification. Due to their low cost, wide availability, and good tolerability, dietary components therefore remain an interesting and attractive subject for future research in PD.

Conflicts of Interest Matthias Löhle was supported by a seed grant of the Center for Regenerative Therapies Dresden (CRTD) and received honoraria for presentations from Boehringer Ingelheim, GlaxoSmithKline, MEDA Pharma, and UCB Pharma. Heinz Reichmann was acting on advisory boards and gave lectures and received research grants from Abbott, AbbVie, Bayer Health Care, Boehringer Ingelheim, Britannia, Cephalon, Desitin, GSK, Lundbeck, Medtronic, Merck Serono, Novartis, Orion, Pfizer, TEVA, UCB Pharma, and Valeant. No funding was provided for the preparation of this manuscript.

References

1. de Lau LM, Giesbergen PC, de Rijk MC, et al. Incidence of parkinsonism and Parkinson disease in a general population: the Rotterdam Study. Neurology. 2004;63(7):1240–4.
2. Driver JA, Logroscino G, Gaziano JM, et al. Incidence and remaining lifetime risk of Parkinson disease in advanced age. Neurology. 2009;72(5):432–8.
3. Lang AE, Lozano AM. Parkinson's disease. First of two parts. N Engl J Med. 1998;339(15):1044–53.
4. Olanow CW, Tatton WG. Etiology and pathogenesis of Parkinson's disease. Annu Rev Neurosci. 1999;22:123–44.
5. Löhle M, Reichmann H. Clinical neuroprotection in Parkinson's disease – still waiting for the breakthrough. J Neurol Sci. 2010;289(1–2):104–14.
6. Noyce AJ, Bestwick JP, Silveira-Moriyama L, et al. Meta-analysis of early nonmotor features and risk factors for Parkinson disease. Ann Neurol. 2012;72(6):893–901.
7. Nielsen SS, Franklin GM, Longstreth WT, et al. Nicotine from edible Solanaceae and risk of Parkinson disease. Ann Neurol. 2013;74(3):472–7.
8. Pan-Montojo F, Anichtchik O, Dening Y, et al. Progression of Parkinson's disease pathology is reproduced by intragastric administration of rotenone in mice. PLoS One. 2010;5(1):e8762.
9. Shults CW. Therapeutic role of coenzyme Q(10) in Parkinson's disease. Pharmacol Ther. 2005;107(1):120–30.
10. Strijks E, Kremer HP, Horstink MW. Q10 therapy in patients with idiopathic Parkinson's disease. Mol Asp Med. 1997;18(Suppl):S237–40.

11. Muller T, Buttner T, Gholipour AF, et al. Coenzyme Q10 supplementation provides mild symptomatic benefit in patients with Parkinson's disease. Neurosci Lett. 2003;341(3):201–4.
12. Storch A, Jost WH, Vieregge P, et al. Randomized, double-blind, placebo-controlled trial on symptomatic effects of coenzyme Q(10) in Parkinson disease. Arch Neurol. 2007;64(7):938–44.
13. NINDS NET-PD Investigators. A randomized clinical trial of coenzyme Q10 and GPI-1485 in early Parkinson disease. Neurology. 2007;68(1):20–8.
14. The Parkinson Study Group Q. E. Investigators, Beal MF, Oakes D, et al. A randomized clinical trial of high-dosage coenzyme Q10 in early Parkinson disease: no evidence of benefit. JAMA Neurol. 2014;71(5):543–52.
15. Bender A, Koch W, Elstner M, et al. Creatine supplementation in Parkinson disease: a placebo-controlled randomized pilot trial. Neurology. 2006;67(7):1262–4.
16. Elm JJ, NINDS NET-PD Investigators. Design innovations and baseline findings in a long-term Parkinson's trial: the National Institute of Neurological Disorders and Stroke Exploratory Trials in Parkinson's Disease Long-Term Study-1. Mov Disord. 2012;27(12):1513–21.
17. National Institute of Neurological Disorders and Stroke. Statement on the Termination of NET-PD LS-1 Study. 2013 [11 Sept 2013]. Available from: http://www.ninds.nih.gov/news_and_events/news_articles/pressrelease_NET-PD_LS-1_study_termination_09112013.htm.
18. Postuma RB, Lang AE, Munhoz RP, et al. Caffeine for treatment of Parkinson disease: a randomized controlled trial. Neurology. 2012;79(7):651–8.
19. Katzenschlager R, Evans A, Manson A, et al. Mucuna pruriens in Parkinson's disease: a double blind clinical and pharmacological study. J Neurol Neurosurg Psychiatry. 2004;75(12):1672–7.
20. Wolz M, Schleiffer C, Klingelhofer L, et al. Comparison of chocolate to cacao-free white chocolate in Parkinson's disease: a single-dose, investigator-blinded, placebo-controlled, crossover trial. J Neurol. 2012;259(11):2447–51.
21. The Michael J. Fox Foundation. Parkinson's funded grant: ability to slow disease progression and safety and tolerability of green tea polyphenols in early Parkinson's disease. Available from: http://www.michaeljfox.org/foundation/grant-detail.php?grant_id=187.
22. da Silva TM, Munhoz RP, Alvarez C, et al. Depression in Parkinson's disease: a double-blind, randomized, placebo-controlled pilot study of omega-3 fatty-acid supplementation. J Affect Disord. 2008;111(2–3):351–9.
23. Suzuki M, Yoshioka M, Hashimoto M, et al. Randomized, double-blind, placebo-controlled trial of vitamin D supplementation in Parkinson disease. Am J Clin Nutr. 2013;97(5):1004–13.
24. Parkinson Study Group. Effects of tocopherol and deprenyl on the progression of disability in early Parkinson's disease. N Engl J Med. 1993;328(3):176–83.
25. Matthews RT, Ferrante RJ, Klivenyi P, et al. Creatine and cyclocreatine attenuate MPTP neurotoxicity. Exp Neurol. 1999;157(1):142–9.
26. NINDS NET-PD Investigators. A randomized, double-blind, futility clinical trial of creatine and minocycline in early Parkinson disease. Neurology. 2006;66(5):664–71.
27. Lyoo IK, Yoon S, Kim TS, et al. A randomized, double-blind placebo-controlled trial of oral creatine monohydrate augmentation for enhanced response to a selective serotonin reuptake inhibitor in women with major depressive disorder. Am J Psychiatry. 2012;169(9):937–45.
28. Hernan MA, Takkouche B, Caamano-Isorna F, et al. A meta-analysis of coffee drinking, cigarette smoking, and the risk of Parkinson's disease. Ann Neurol. 2002;52(3):276–84.
29. Chen JF, Xu K, Petzer JP, et al. Neuroprotection by caffeine and A(2A) adenosine receptor inactivation in a model of Parkinson's disease. J Neurosci. 2001;21(10):RC143.
30. Svenningsson P, Le Moine C, Fisone G, et al. Distribution, biochemistry and function of striatal adenosine A2A receptors. Prog Neurobiol. 1999;59(4):355–96.
31. Benarroch EE. Adenosine and its receptors: multiple modulatory functions and potential therapeutic targets for neurologic disease. Neurology. 2008;70(3):231–6.
32. Fredholm BB, Svenningsson P. Adenosine-dopamine interactions: development of a concept and some comments on therapeutic possibilities. Neurology. 2003;61(11 Suppl 6):S5–9.
33. Kartzinel R, Shoulson I, Calne DB. Studies with bromocriptine: III. Concomitant administration of caffeine to patients with idiopathic parkinsonism. Neurology. 1976;26(8):741–3.

34. Shoulson I, Chase T. Caffeine and the antiparkinsonian response to levodopa or piribedil. Neurology. 1975;25(8):722–4.
35. Manyam BV. Paralysis agitans and levodopa in "Ayurveda": ancient Indian medical treatise. Mov Disord. 1990;5(1):47–8.
36. Vaidya AB, Rajagopalan TG, Mankodi NA, et al. Treatment of Parkinson's disease with the cowhage plant-Mucuna pruriens Bak. Neurol India. 1978;26(4):171–6.
37. HP-200 in Parkinson's Disease Study Group. An alternative medicine treatment for Parkinson's disease: results of a multicenter clinical trial. J Altern Complement Med. 1995;1(3):249–55.
38. Nagashayana N, Sankarankutty P, Nampoothiri MR, et al. Association of L-DOPA with recovery following Ayurveda medication in Parkinson's disease. J Neurol Sci. 2000;176(2):124–7.
39. Dyck LE. Release of monoamines from striatal slices by phenelzine and beta-phenylethylamine. Prog Neuropsychopharmacol Biol Psychiatry. 1983;7(4–6):797–800.
40. McQuade PS, Wood PL. The effects of beta-phenylethylamine on tyramine and dopamine metabolism. Prog Neuropsychopharmacol Biol Psychiatry. 1983;7(4–6):755–9.
41. Buijsse B, Feskens EJ, Kok FJ, et al. Cocoa intake, blood pressure, and cardiovascular mortality: the Zutphen elderly study. Arch Intern Med. 2006;166(4):411–7.
42. Buijsse B, Weikert C, Drogan D, et al. Chocolate consumption in relation to blood pressure and risk of cardiovascular disease in German adults. Eur Heart J. 2010;31(13):1616–23.
43. Larsson SC, Virtamo J, Wolk A. Chocolate consumption and risk of stroke: a prospective cohort of men and meta-analysis. Neurology. 2012;79(12):1223–9.
44. Wolz M, Kaminsky A, Lohle M, et al. Chocolate consumption is increased in Parkinson's disease. Results from a self-questionnaire study. J Neurol. 2009;256(3):488–92.
45. D'Archivio M, Filesi C, Vari R, et al. Bioavailability of the polyphenols: status and controversies. Int J Mol Sci. 2010;11(4):1321–42.
46. Urquiaga I, Leighton F. Plant polyphenol antioxidants and oxidative stress. Biol Res. 2000;33(2):55–64.
47. Hu G, Bidel S, Jousilahti P, et al. Coffee and tea consumption and the risk of Parkinson's disease. Mov Disord. 2007;22(15):2242–8.
48. Tanaka K, Miyake Y, Fukushima W, et al. Intake of Japanese and Chinese teas reduces risk of Parkinson's disease. Parkinsonism Relat Disord. 2011;17(6):446–50.
49. Checkoway H, Powers K, Smith-Weller T, et al. Parkinson's disease risks associated with cigarette smoking, alcohol consumption, and caffeine intake. Am J Epidemiol. 2002;155(8):732–8.
50. Tan EK, Tan C, Fook-Chong SM, et al. Dose-dependent protective effect of coffee, tea, and smoking in Parkinson's disease: a study in ethnic Chinese. J Neurol Sci. 2003;216(1):163–7.
51. Weinreb O, Mandel S, Amit T, et al. Neurological mechanisms of green tea polyphenols in Alzheimer's and Parkinson's diseases. J Nutr Biochem. 2004;15(9):506–16.
52. Levites Y, Weinreb O, Maor G, et al. Green tea polyphenol (-)-epigallocatechin-3-gallate prevents N-methyl-4-phenyl-1,2,3,6-tetrahydropyridine-induced dopaminergic neurodegeneration. J Neurochem. 2001;78(5):1073–82.
53. Mandel SA, Amit T, Kalfon L, et al. Targeting multiple neurodegenerative diseases etiologies with multimodal-acting green tea catechins. J Nutr. 2008;138(8):1578S–83.
54. Kandinov B, Giladi N, Korczyn AD. The effect of cigarette smoking, tea, and coffee consumption on the progression of Parkinson's disease. Parkinsonism Relat Disord. 2007;13(4):243–5.
55. Bousquet M, Calon F, Cicchetti F. Impact of omega-3 fatty acids in Parkinson's disease. Ageing Res Rev. 2011;10(4):453–63.
56. Brenna JT, Salem Jr N, Sinclair AJ, et al. alpha-Linolenic acid supplementation and conversion to n-3 long-chain polyunsaturated fatty acids in humans. Prostaglandins Leukot Essent Fatty Acids. 2009;80(2-3):85–91.
57. de Lau LM, Bornebroek M, Witteman JC, et al. Dietary fatty acids and the risk of Parkinson disease: the Rotterdam study. Neurology. 2005;64(12):2040–5.
58. Gao X, Chen H, Fung TT, et al. Prospective study of dietary pattern and risk of Parkinson disease. Am J Clin Nutr. 2007;86(5):1486–94.

59. Alcalay RN, Gu Y, Mejia-Santana H, et al. The association between Mediterranean diet adherence and Parkinson's disease. Mov Disord. 2012;27(6):771–4.
60. Bousquet M, Saint-Pierre M, Julien C, et al. Beneficial effects of dietary omega-3 polyunsaturated fatty acid on toxin-induced neuronal degeneration in an animal model of Parkinson's disease. FASEB J: Off Pub Fed Am Soc Exp Biol. 2008;22(4):1213–25.
61. Cansev M, Ulus IH, Wang L, et al. Restorative effects of uridine plus docosahexaenoic acid in a rat model of Parkinson's disease. Neurosci Res. 2008;62(3):206–9.
62. Samadi P, Gregoire L, Rouillard C, et al. Docosahexaenoic acid reduces levodopa-induced dyskinesias in 1-methyl-4-phenyl-1,2,3,6-tetrahydropyridine monkeys. Ann Neurol. 2006;59(2):282–8.
63. Chowdhury R, Stevens S, Gorman D, et al. Association between fish consumption, long chain omega 3 fatty acids, and risk of cerebrovascular disease: systematic review and meta-analysis. BMJ. 2012;345:e6698.
64. Fahn S. A pilot trial of high-dose alpha-tocopherol and ascorbate in early Parkinson's disease. Ann Neurol. 1992;32(Suppl):S128–32.
65. Logroscino G, Marder K, Cote L, et al. Dietary lipids and antioxidants in Parkinson's disease: a population-based, case-control study. Ann Neurol. 1996;39(1):89–94.
66. Scheider WL, Hershey LA, Vena JE, et al. Dietary antioxidants and other dietary factors in the etiology of Parkinson's disease. Mov Disord. 1997;12(2):190–6.
67. Hellenbrand W, Boeing H, Robra BP, et al. Diet and Parkinson's disease. II: a possible role for the past intake of specific nutrients. Results from a self-administered food-frequency questionnaire in a case-control study. Neurology. 1996;47(3):644–50.
68. Zhang SM, Hernan MA, Chen H, et al. Intakes of vitamins E and C, carotenoids, vitamin supplements, and PD risk. Neurology. 2002;59(8):1161–9.
69. de Rijk MC, Breteler MM, den Breeijen JH, et al. Dietary antioxidants and Parkinson disease. The Rotterdam study. Arch Neurol. 1997;54(6):762–5.
70. Golbe LI, Farrell TM, Davis PH. Case-control study of early life dietary factors in Parkinson's disease. Arch Neurol. 1988;45(12):1350–3.
71. Golbe LI, Farrell TM, Davis PH. Follow-up study of early-life protective and risk factors in Parkinson's disease. Mov Disord. 1990;5(1):66–70.
72. Martin A, Youdim K, Szprengiel A, et al. Roles of vitamins E and C on neurodegenerative diseases and cognitive performance. Nutr Rev. 2002;60(10 Pt 1):308–26.
73. Evatt ML, Delong MR, Khazai N, et al. Prevalence of vitamin d insufficiency in patients with Parkinson disease and Alzheimer disease. Arch Neurol. 2008;65(10):1348–52.
74. Evatt ML, DeLong MR, Kumari M, et al. High prevalence of hypovitaminosis D status in patients with early Parkinson disease. Arch Neurol. 2011;68(3):314–9.
75. Ding H, Dhima K, Lockhart KC, et al. Unrecognized vitamin D3 deficiency is common in Parkinson disease: Harvard biomarker study. Neurology. 2013;81(17):1531–7.
76. Peterson AL, Murchison C, Zabetian C, et al. Memory, mood, and vitamin d in persons with Parkinson's disease. J Park Dis. 2013;3(4):547–55.
77. Muir SW, Montero-Odasso M. Effect of vitamin D supplementation on muscle strength, gait and balance in older adults: a systematic review and meta-analysis. J Am Geriatr Soc. 2011;59(12):2291–300.
78. van den Bos F, Speelman AD, Samson M, et al. Parkinson's disease and osteoporosis. Age Ageing. 2013;42(2):156–62.
79. Cole MH, Silburn PA, Wood JM, et al. Falls in Parkinson's disease: kinematic evidence for impaired head and trunk control. Mov Disord. 2010;25(14):2369–78.

Chapter 6
Psychosis in Parkinson's Disease

Ilia Bountouni, Panagiotis Zis, K. Ray Chaudhuri, and Anette Schrag

Introduction

Psychosis is one of the most disabling non-motor symptoms of Parkinson's disease (PD). Non-motor symptoms are common, occur at higher prevalence than in age-matched controls, and have significant impact on quality of life [1]. In the present chapter, we will consider the psychopathology, the epidemiology, the pathophysiology, the risk factors, the prognosis, and the management of psychotic features in PD. Before doing so, we provide the historical background of psychosis in PD (PDPsy).

I. Bountouni, MRCPsych, MD
Department of Psychiatry, South London and Maudsley NHS Trust, Lewisham University Hospital, Lewisham High Street, Lewisham, London SE13 6LH, England, UK
e-mail: ilia.bountouni@slam.nhs.uk

P. Zis, MRCPsych, MSc, PhD
Department of Neurology, National Parkinson Foundation International Centre of Excellence, King's College Hospital, Denmark Hill, London SE5 9RS, UK
e-mail: takiszis@gmail.com

K.R. Chaudhuri, DSc MD FRCP (Edin) FRCP (Lond)
National Parkinson Foundation International Centre of Excellence, Kings College Hospital and Kings College, Kings Neuroscience Research and Development, DeNDroN, London South, UK

Movement Disorders Society Non Motor Study Group, Denmark Hill, London SE5 9RS, UK
e-mail: chaudhuriray@hotmail.com

A. Schrag, FRCP, PhD (✉)
Department of Clinical Neurosciences, Institute of Neurology, Royal Free Campus, University College London, Rowland Hill Street, London NW3 2PF, UK
e-mail: a.schrag@ucl.ac.uk

H. Reichmann (ed.), *Neuropsychiatric Symptoms of Movement Disorders*, Neuropsychiatric Symptoms of Neurological Disease,
DOI 10.1007/978-3-319-09537-0_6

Historical Background

In James Parkinson's original description of the disease he concluded, "...by the absence of any injury to the senses and to the intellect, we are taught that the morbid state does not extend to the encephalon" [2]. This view of PD as a process that spares the intellectual and psychological functioning was held for many decades.

Especially in the era before the discovery of levodopa treatment, reports regarding psychotic symptoms in PD were limited. Initial reports were regarding patients suffering from parkinsonism who developed psychotic symptoms. In 1882, Ball probably referred to the signs of rapid eye movement (REM) sleep behavior disorder in postencephalitic parkinsonism when describing a man with visual and auditory hallucinations occurring only at nighttime [3]. In 1906, Regis categorized the mental disorders associated with parkinsonism and specifically mentioned hallucinations as a symptom associated with advanced disease [4].

One of the first reports of psychotic symptoms in "paralysis agitans" was in 1923, when Jackson presented a case series of patients with prominent symptoms of psychosis [5]. Early features, such as sleep disturbance, withdrawal from social situations, and suspiciousness, were also mentioned. In this report, more dramatic symptoms such as paranoid delusions and hallucinations that were "generally limited to the organic sensations and tactile sense" were also discussed [5]. In 1949, Mjönes described two patients with tactile hallucinations, one of which also had visual and auditory hallucinations [6]. In 1950, Schwab described a number of psychiatric symptoms including "paranoia" and "schizoid reactions" [7].

Thus, it appears that psychotic features may be an inherent though rare part of the disease itself [8]. However, a number of these cases reported might have had secondary forms of parkinsonism, especially postencephalitic [9].

In the levodopa treatment era, it became apparent that various psychiatric syndromes were occurring with a much higher frequency in treated patients than in untreated patients [9]. Even in the first reports, it was highlighted that apart from higher levodopa dose, psychotic symptoms were much more likely to occur in patients with certain predisposing characteristics, including older age, cognitive impairment, and premorbid psychiatric pathology [10–12]. Newer reports added in these other predisposing factors such as depression, sleep disorders, and visual impairment [13–16]. However, risk factors are discussed in more detail in a separate section.

Signs and Symptoms

The basic psychopathological terms and their correspondent definitions that will be used in this chapter are summarized in Table 6.1

Psychotic symptoms have long been recognized as a feature of PD as well as a complication of PD therapies. PDPsy can occur in non-demented subjects but is also a common feature in patients with PD dementia (PDD) and in patients with

Table 6.1 Summary of the basic psychopathological terms and their correspondent definitions [17, 18]

Term	Definition
Illusions	Misinterpretations of real perception stimuli
Hallucinations	Spontaneous aberrant perceptions without a physical stimulus
Elementary auditory hallucinations	Unstructured sounds, for example, rattles or whistling
Elementary visual hallucinations	Crudely formed flashes of light or color
Complex visual hallucinations	Range from more organized patterns and shapes to full visual perceptions of people and scenes
Passage hallucination	The sensation of a person or animal passing in the periphery of someone's visual field
Sense of presence	The vivid feeling that somebody is present nearby when nobody is actually there

Table 6.2 Characteristics of psychosis in Parkinson's disease [24, 25, 28]

Psychotic feature in PD	Clinical profile in PD	Prevalence
Psychosis	Encompasses hallucinations, delusions, and the "minor" phenomena of illusions, "passage hallucinations," and "sense of presence"	26–60 % [24, 25]
Visual hallucinations	Abnormal visual perceptions without a physical stimulus. Typically stereotyped, and colorful images of familiar people or animals. Associated with older age, duration of PD, cognitive impairment, depression, and sleep disturbances [25, 26]. May be more likely to occur during times of low ambient stimulation and share some characteristics of hallucinations in the visually impaired [27]	13–50 % [24, 28]
Delusions	False, fixed, idiosyncratic beliefs that are maintained despite evidence to the contrary. Often paranoid delusions pertaining to spousal infidelity or fear of abandonment. Distinct from clinical profile of schizophrenia as delusions of thought insertion or broadcasting and delusions of grandeur or of external control and religiosity, which are hallmarks of schizophrenia, are rarely seen in PD psychosis [29]	3–7 % [24, 25]

dementia with Lewy bodies (DLB). PDPsy is known to reduce quality of life and increases caregiver distress [19]. It is an independent risk factor for poor prognosis, nursing home placement, and development of dementia [20, 21], and it is also associated with increased risk of mortality [20, 22, 23]. The characteristics of PDPsy are summarized in Table 6.2.

The prevalence and severity of hallucinations, the commonest manifestation of PDPsy, increase over time [30]. Higher levels of thought disorder and hallucinations are positively associated with disease severity and impairment. Features of PDPsy are more common in late-stage disease but can occur throughout the disease course [31, 32]. Early hallucinations occurring before or shortly after starting a dopaminergic treatment in a patient with a recent diagnosis of PD may be part of the DLB syndrome [33]. However, the cutoff between both conditions, although theoretically well defined, may be more difficult to establish in clinical practice, and the phenomenology of visual hallucinations linked to PD and DLB is similar [34].

Mental disturbances in PD range from comparatively subtle symptoms such as non-disturbing visual hallucinations, vivid dreams, and mild illusions to a psychotic state with disturbing hallucinations and paranoid frightening psychotic delusions [35]. The classic hallucinations in long-term treated PD are usually chronic and repetitive in their content.

Diagnostic Criteria

Diagnostic criteria for psychosis in PD have been proposed by a NINDS/NIMH working group [36]. These require the presence of at least one of illusions, false sense of presence, hallucinations, or delusions, a primary diagnosis based on UK brain bank criteria for PD; symptoms occurring after the onset of PD, symptoms that are recurrent or continuous for at least 1 month, and the psychotic symptoms are not better accounted for by another cause of parkinsonism such as DLB. Furthermore, Duvoisin's classical description perfectly illustrates the panoply of psychotic phenomena in PD patients [37]: "…Visual illusions are especially frequent. Familiar objects may be mistaking for something else. The patient may mention seeing worms on the floor, whereas actually there is a design in the flooring, which is misinterpreted because the pattern seems to move. Spectral illusions generally of a benign if not pleasant character are experienced. There may be hallucinations of people or animals roaming around the house … Complex scenes with a group of people wandering around, having a party … seem to go about their business without disturbing the patient. Patients may experience these visions for long periods of time but are afraid to mention them to anyone for fear of being thought 'crazy'. Finally, however the patient reacts, angrily ordering the strangers out of the house, accusing them of stealing…" [37].

Visual Illusions and Hallucinations

Establishing the time of the first true visual hallucinations may be difficult as they may begin insidiously, out of seemingly normal heightened perceptions, misperceptions (illusions), and very fleeting impressions with preserved insight that cause no concern to the patients. Even after patients recognize the hallucinations as a false perception, many remain hesitant to admit them to family members [38]. The awareness of the presence of another person ("sensation de presence" or "Anwesenheit") and the sensation of movement in the peripheral visual field ("sensation de passage") were first described in PD in 1982 [39]. Fénelon et al. systematically investigated them as presumably prehallucinatory symptoms [18]. Isolated occurrence was noted in 14 % and combined occurrence with formed hallucinations in another 9 % of the patients. PD patients also frequently misinterpret nonliving objects, especially moving ones as living beings.

These illusions may be facilitated by dim light and/or reduced vigilance and attentiveness during drowsiness. Their frequency has been rarely investigated separately, because in systematic interviews it is often difficult for the PD patient to differentiate illusions from visual hallucinations [40, 41]. Most studies therefore combine illusions with visual hallucinations as a single phenomenon.

The content and contextual framework of the prototypic or core hallucinatory syndrome has been investigated by different research groups, and similar descriptive core features have been reported [29, 41, 42]. Patients with hallucinations typically report visual hallucinations that represent human beings, animals, or both, often mobile, appearing in scenes of short duration, lasting often only seconds. They are usually moving, doing otherwise appropriate activities without disturbing the patient. By their repetitive and stereotyped character, the visual hallucination figures become familiar to the patient, who, as a bystander, observes them with amused interest (the "marketplace effect") [43]. The patients never involve themselves in the activities of the hallucinations. Favored by dim light or reduced vigilance, visual hallucinations appear suddenly, without any known trigger or voluntary effort. They also vanish suddenly, sometimes when the patient tries to check their reality by approaching or touching them. It is notable that simple visual hallucinations, consisting in elementary geometrical patterns, are uncommon in PD [34]. Visual hallucinations are not regularly bound to the same motoric state ("on" or "off") and have no direct temporal relation to antiparkinsonian medication ingestion. Often a given visual hallucination occurs when the PD patient is in a specific environmental setting. Real objects may contribute to the scene by being mistaken in an illusionary way. Visual hallucinations often have blurred borders but have neither color predominance nor a specific localization to a field of vision (lateral vs. central) [43].

Affectively, patients usually express little concern about the visual hallucinations, although in two studies some patients found themselves anxious or depressed when a few felt terrified [18, 44]. Full-blown psychotic decompensation with secondary frightening paranoid delusion, without any insight, was a rare phenomenon in these studies [43]. Comparative prevalence and phenomenology at day- or nighttime have not been extensively studied, although one report found that diurnal visual hallucinations were more common than nocturnal visual hallucinations, with 46 % of patients indicating only diurnal visual hallucinations, 13 % only nocturnal visual hallucinations, and 41 % both types [41]. Another study with continuous polysomnographic recording found that in 20 hallucinating patients, 14 patients experienced visual hallucinations during daytime, 8 during a "wakeful state," 5 during a twilight state, and 1 on awaking from napping in the afternoon. In contrast, four patients developed visual hallucinations upon awakening at night [45].

Hallucinations in Other Sensory Modalities

Auditory hallucinations may be elementary (ringing, knocks, etc.) or, more often, complex. The voice content is neutral or incomprehensible, but it can also be threatening [46, 47] and nonetheless differs from the pejorative or threatening auditory hallucinations of schizophrenia [18, 46]. Auditory hallucinations may constitute the "soundtrack" of visual hallucinations, with the patient hearing the conversation of unreal persons. Auditory hallucinations variably occur together with visual hallucinations and are less likely to be seen in isolation [46, 48]. Tactile hallucinations [49] involve contact with small animals, although they do not usually generate the belief of infestation. They may also manifest as the feeling of being touched by someone. Olfactory and gustatory hallucinations have only been reported in series and case reports [42]. Both olfactory and tactile hallucinations can be experienced as very unpleasant and long-lasting [49–51].

Multimodal Hallucinations

Patients experiencing visual hallucinations may also experience nonvisual hallucinations, although they often do not report them. When focusing on new-onset hallucinations, it has been shown that elderly patients were more likely to have multimodal hallucinations than pure visual hallucinations, suggesting that age and ageing processes may influence the phenomenology of hallucinations [52]. Nonvisual hallucinations are mostly accompanied by visual hallucinations [53]. Most patients have retained insight of their hallucinations although when severe and in the context of cognitive impairment insight may fluctuate or be lost [18, 42].

Delusions

Delusions are false beliefs that are maintained despite evidence of the contrary. Delusions affect about 8 % of treated patients with PD [54, 55]. They are usually paranoid in nature and commonly involve suspicions of spousal infidelity. Other paranoid themes include people stealing money, intruders living in the house, or nurses planning harmful plots. In contrast to this, thought broadcasting, ideas of reference, loosened associations, and "negative symptoms," which are all commonly found in schizophrenics, are not a feature of PD-associated psychosis [55].

Paranoid thoughts such as spousal infidelity are a common theme, although grandiose, somatic, persecutory, and religious delusions have also been documented [56]. Recent research suggests that the occurrence of delusions, as opposed to hallucinations, may be related to younger age at onset of PD and psychotic symptoms [57].

Delirium

Delirium with concomitant hallucinations can be found in PD patients, especially with advanced age [55]. When being part of a toxic delirium, hallucinations occur in the context of a clouded sensorium. Sometimes it starts as nocturnal confusion or "sundowning," which when left untreated can also affect the patient's behavior during the day. An associated problem is that the sleep cycle is often inverted [55].

In this syndrome, patients usually show signs of distractibility, agitation, myoclonus, paratonia. It may occur with systemic disease, in the context of fever, infection, or renal failure, and with medications including anticholinergic treatment or amantadine [58]. In the perioperative state, especially when PD patients receive pain medications, there is also a significantly increased risk of a confusional state with hallucinations [59]. In cases of anticholinergic toxic effects, visual hallucinations are accompanied by dry skin, urinary retention, and mydriasis [60]. In general, the hallucinations clear when the underlying medical condition is treated.

Epidemiology

Establishing the prevalence of neuropsychiatric disorders in PD is complicated by the symptomatic overlap between the somatic features of the neuropsychiatric and underlying movement disorder, differences in the phenomenology of these disorders in PD and the general population, frequently coexisting cognitive problems, psychiatric side effects of dopaminergic medication, the presence of motor and non-motor fluctuations, and the different diagnostic frameworks available. Thus, estimates of prevalence of neuropsychiatric disorders in PD vary considerably in published studies [61].

With regard to reports about hallucinations and psychosis in PD, one of the limitations of the published studies is their difference in study design, data collection, and study population. In addition, most studies utilized non-validated scales or arbitrary definitions of symptoms [35, 62, 63]. Furthermore, PD patients may not report visual hallucinations when completing self-report screening questionnaires.

For example, in a community-based sample, there was a 25 % lifetime prevalence [64] of psychotic phenomena compared with nearly 50 % in some clinic-based samples [18, 65]. Some studies have focused only on hallucinations and did not assess illusions or delusions [46, 66]. In spite of the limitations presented, several studies have reported a cross-sectional prevalence of psychosis in the range of 25–30 % [68, 69, 71–75]. The estimated prevalence of formed visual hallucinations has been recorded as 22–38 %, of minor psychotic symptoms (illusions of presence, passage, and visual illusions) as 17–72 %, of auditory hallucinations as 0–22 %, and of delusions as 1–7 %. Tactile, somatic, and olfactory hallucinations are relatively rare and usually not systematically sought. Lifetime prevalence of reported visual hallucinations was 50 % in a large retrospective autopsy study in pathologically proven PD (445 patients) [61]. Longitudinal studies have reported that the proportion of hallucinating PD patients increases with disease duration. In a 4-year prospective longitudinal study, 33 % of the patients had visual hallucinations at baseline, 44 % at 18 months, and 63 % at 48 months [66]. Having hallucinations at baseline or at any given assessment was a strong predictor of continued hallucinations at all follow-up evaluations, demonstrating the chronicity of the hallucinatory syndrome. The evolution of the so-called "benign" hallucinations, defined as hallucinations with retained insight, has also been investigated. Unlike the name suggested, after 3 years, 81 % of the patients had hallucinations with loss of insight, if no specific treatment was initiated [65].

Pathophysiology

There has been considerable interest in identifying risk factors for developing psychotic symptoms in Parkinson's disease. Not all patients will develop them, and it appears that a variety of factors, both intrinsic and extrinsic, contribute to their occurrence [56]. In this section, we are reviewing the role of neurotransmitters that research has identified as facilitating the emergence of psychotic symptoms in PD.

Role of Dopamine

As early as in 1978, Moskowitz postulated a pharmacological kindling model to suggest enhanced sensitivity of dopaminergic receptors after chronic treatment with levodopa. Thus, excess dopamine from medications could overflow onto supersensitive receptors, inducing psychotic signs [77]. Since then extensive research has taken place in order to examine the relationship between dopamine and altered perceptions [78].

It is well recognized that dopaminergic agonists (such as amphetamines) can induce psychotic states [79] and that dopamine D2 receptor antagonists (such as haloperidol) are effective antipsychotics [78]. All PD medications (not just levodopa) have been implicated in the appearance of psychotic features, and these features often remit after drug therapy has been reduced or eliminated [80].

Excessive dopaminergic activity, probably in mesocortical and mesolimbic systems, appears to play a role in the generation of hallucinations. This action may be mediated by dopamine's influence on glutamatergic systems [81]. There are experimental suggestions that chronic stimulation may cause persistent sensitization of dopamine receptors, leading to dysfunction of limbic structures responsible for assigning emotional and hedonic significance to sensory input. This dysfunction may result in misattributions of internal stimuli having originated from the external sensory world [82] causing thus psychotic phenomena [83, 84].

However, several observations have challenged the hypothesis that psychotic symptoms represent a medication-induced toxic syndrome [43]. Not only there are reports of hallucinations in PD patients before dopaminergic drugs became available [85], but also studies of hallucinating PD patients have demonstrated that psychosis severity and medication doses are poorly correlated [42]. Moreover, Goetz showed that in predisposed patients, high-dose intravenous levodopa does not provoke visual hallucinations in a predefined clinical setting [86].

Role of Serotonin

Serotonin (5-HT) is another monoamine neurotransmitter, and it is also thought to play a role in producing psychotic symptoms. The body of evidence for serotonin's involvement parallels that for dopamine. Therefore, agonists at the 5-HT2 receptor can induce hallucinations, and 5-HT receptors antagonists (like novel antipsychotics) can ameliorate psychosis [87]. The efficacy of atypical antipsychotic, such as clozapine and quetiapine, without worsening motor function, has been partly attributed to their affinity to 5-HT receptors. However, the exact relationship between serotonergic systems and PD-related psychosis remains unclear [78].

Role of Acetylcholine

Although the role of acetylcholine is still under investigation, neuropathological studies of patients with DLB indicate that levels of choline acetyltransferase were lower and the ratio of 5-hydroxyindoleacetic acid to choline acetyltransferase was higher in hallucinating patients than in patients without hallucinations [88]. Moreover, marked degeneration of cholinergic neurons is evident in the brains of PD patients which is possibly even greater compared to what is seen in patients with Alzheimer's dementia [89, 90].

The possible role of acetylcholine in psychotic features is also supported by research that showed that after effectively treating hallucinations by reducing anticholinergic and/or dopaminergic agents, acetylcholine blockade may induce PD-related hallucinations. It was hypothesized that the responsible mechanism involves acetylcholine's reciprocal relationship with dopamine in limbic cortex [80]. Finally, another hypothesis is that as PD causes degeneration of cholinergic pedunculopontine neurons, which control rapid eye movement (REM) sleep, hallucinations may be fragments of dreams that are released from the usual cholinergic inhibition [88]. However, sleep dysregulation is discussed separately below.

Risk Factors

Apart from the role of dopaminergic treatment as a risk factor for developing psychotic features in PD, which has been reviewed above, other risk factors may contribute to the development of psychotic features in PD as discussed in this section.

Age and Disease Duration

Older age has been shown to be a risk factor of developing psychosis in PD [67], and psychotic symptoms in PD typically occur later in the course of the disease. On average, symptoms are reported 10 or more years after the initial diagnosis [91]. Moreover, psychotic symptoms tend to recur and worsen over time [92] as disease progresses and have been correlated to PD severity [61].

Cognitive Impairment

Dementia is an important risk factor for psychosis in PD, and severity of dementia and severity of psychosis are correlated [76, 93]. Psychosis may be an early indicator of beginning cognitive decline. Recently, it was suggested that the hippocampus is a neural substrate underlying the occurrence of psychosis, sleep disturbance, and cognitive impairment in PD patients [93]. However, if psychosis occurs in the early stages of PD, it is particularly important to consider other diagnoses, specifically dementia with Lewy bodies (DLB). In one study, all patients identified as having early-onset (within 3 months of initiating levodopa therapy) hallucinations were later found to carry a diagnosis other than or in addition to Parkinson's disease that could account for their psychotic symptoms [31].

Lewy Body Distribution

Lewy body deposition has long been known to be associated with dementia in Parkinson's disease, which has been identified as risk factor for PD psychosis. One study found a strong correlation between the distribution of Lewy bodies in the temporal lobe, specifically in the amygdale and parahippocampus, and well-formed visual hallucinations in Lewy body diseases such as DLB and Parkinson's disease dementia [94]. These temporal lobe Lewy bodies were also associated with an earlier onset of hallucinations. A large-scale autopsy study of 788 cases of parkinsonism showed a high specificity of visual hallucinations for Lewy body diseases (92.9 %) [95]. A recent clinicopathological comparison of 10 PD patients with a history of visual hallucinations and 10 PD controls revealed a significantly greater Lewy body burden in the amygdala and cortical areas in the hallucinating patients [96].

Sleep Disorders

Psychosis in PD has also been linked to sleep disturbances such as insomnia [97] and daytime sleepiness [98], which are common in PD. The "continuum hypothesis" of psychosis in PD asserts that sleep disturbances in PD lead to altered dream phenomena, which later lead to frank daytime hallucinations and delusions. Indeed, these early phenomena occur frequently in PD. A study found that 48 % of PD patients experienced some sort of altered dream phenomena such as vivid dreams, nightmares, and reports suggestive of REM disorder or night terrors [99]. 30.7 % of patients in an early retrospective study were reported to experience vivid dreams [77]. One study designed to test the continuum hypothesis found that sleep fragmentation, altered dream phenomena, and hallucinations/illusions were not independent; however, no interaction was found between sleep fragmentation and hallucinations/illusions, which the authors explained by suggesting that the three phenomena are distinct but often overlapping [99].

A prominent view of the relationship between sleep disturbances and PD psychosis involves a disruption in rapid eye movement (REM) sleep. Polysomnographic studies of Parkinson's patients have found a relationship between visual hallucinations and short, fragmented REM sleep. Specifically, patients experiencing hallucinations evidenced lower sleep efficiency and reduced total REM sleep time and percentage, as compared to patients not experiencing hallucinations [100]. Visual hallucinations in PD have been purported by some to represent narcolepsy-like phenomena involving the intrusion of REM dream imagery into the waking state [101]. This intrusion may be related to a reduction in acetylcholine, which leads to the disinhibition of the dream images and their release into the waking state [88].

Visual Processing Deficits

Research has suggested that PD patients who experience visual hallucinations may also suffer from deficits in visual processing. These patients have been found to have lower visual acuity [42], deficits in color and contrast recognition [102], and greater ocular pathology [18], including cataracts, retinal disease, and glaucoma, as compared to non-hallucinating PD patients. Dopamine deficiency at the level of the retina is also found in PD [103] and has been linked to the occurrence of visual hallucinations in both dementia with DLB [104] and PD [105]. These deficits may serve to facilitate the onset of visual hallucinations in PD.

While structural MRI studies of hallucinating PD patients have yielded little insight into specific occipital lobe or deep white matter lesions [106], more recent studies have used fMRI to identify functional abnormalities in the processing of visual stimuli among hallucinating patients. Specifically, Stebbins et al. found that hallucinating PD patients indexed more frontal (Brodmann areas 44, 6) and subcortical (caudate nucleus) activation and less visual cortical activation than non-hallucinating PD patients [107]. The authors postulated that PD patients with hallucinations suffer from a weakening of retinal–striatal–cortical signals, which may lead to the disinhibition of "top-down" processing and the subsequent release of internally generated images into areas that normally represent externally generated percepts. Another fMRI study documented a similar pattern of increased activation of visual association cortex (Brodmann area 19) coupled with decreased activation of primary visual cortex (Brodmann area 17) in PD patients experiencing visual hallucinations [108]. Barnes et al. report deficient reality monitoring in PD patients with hallucinations in that these patients were more likely than non-hallucinating PD patients and elderly controls to believe that mental images were real external stimuli [109]. Currently, studies are underway to determine the effects of pharmacological treatments for hallucinations on functional visual networks. Gallagher et al. report that higher overall cortical Lewy body counts, particularly in areas implicated in visual perception and executive function, such as the middle frontal and middle temporal gyri, transentorhinal, and anterior cingulate cortices, were associated with visual hallucinations [110]. These data were in support of a unifying hypothesis proposed by Goetz that included impaired visual input and central visual processing, impaired brain stem regulation of sleep–wake cycle with fluctuating vigilance, intrusion of rapid eye movement dream imagery into wakefulness and emergence of internally generated imagery, cognitive dysfunction, and influence of pharmacological treatments [43].

Genetics

Recent research has increasingly attended to genetic contributions to Parkinson's disease and its associated neuropsychiatric symptoms. Family history of dementia appears to be a significant risk factor for the development of hallucinations in patients with PD [70]. Furthermore, preliminary evidence suggests that certain genetic profiles may be associated with the development of psychosis in PD. For example, studies have identified the APOE epsilon4 allele as a significant risk factor for drug-induced visual hallucinations in PD [111] and an earlier appearance of psychosis in PD [112]. However, other studies have failed to document an association between APOE4 and PD psychosis [113, 114]. More recently, a postmortem analysis reported an association between PD-related hallucinations and the tau H1H1 genotype [115]. Further research is necessary to elucidate the role of genetics in the expression of psychotic symptoms in PD.

Deep Brain Stimulation (DBS) Surgery

Many researchers have noted that DBS surgery may improve psychotic symptoms in Parkinson's disease, which is presumed to be due to the resultant reduction in dopaminergic medications [116]. However, there have also been reports of stimulation-induced psychotic symptoms as well as transient manic psychosis following DBS surgery, which may be more common in older patients [117–119].

Others

Other risk factors reported for Parkinson's disease psychosis include family history of depression, severe olfactory impairment [120], and autonomic dysfunction [121]. A recent study suggested that PD patients who show a blunted circadian blood pressure rhythm are more likely to develop psychosis than those whose BP decreases normally at night [23]. A recent case crossover study reported that elevation of plasma CRP is also another independent risk factor for psychosis in PD [122]. Finally, it is always important to consider that hallucinations can occur in the context of other conditions, e.g., confusion due to systemic infection or mood congruent hallucinations in the context of severe depression.

Prognosis

Course

Psychotic symptoms in PD typically occur later in the disease. On average, symptoms are reported 10 or more years after the initial diagnosis [91, 92]. In its early stages, psychosis in PD occurs within a context of a clear sensorium and retained insight [123]. Psychotic symptoms tend to recur and worsen over time, and insight may be lost [92]. Psychosis in PD has often been conceptualized as occurring along a continuum in that experiences such as vivid dreaming and illusions herald more frank hallucinations and delusions, which ultimately lead to florid psychosis and dementia [77]. However, recent evidence suggests that this conceptualization may not be accurate [99]. While the specific course of PD psychosis remains to be adequately described, it seems clear that psychotic symptoms, once present, are persistent and distressing.

Thus, the existence of hallucinations at baseline is also a strong predictor of their presence at follow-up evaluations [64]. Some studies documented no differences in hallucinations between patients who received treatment compared to those who did not, and many treated patients were still experiencing hallucinations at long-term follow-up [21, 64]. Other reports suggest that many patients receiving antipsychotic treatment experience continued efficacy, especially those who responded to their medication early on [124]. However, there is little data to suggest that antipsychotic treatment improves long-term functional outcome.

Once patients initiate antipsychotic therapy, continued treatment may be necessary to maintain symptom control and avoid exacerbation of psychosis. One study that attempted to wean psychosis-free PD patients off of their antipsychotic medications was aborted after enrolling only six patients (with an average antipsychotic exposure of 20 months) because five out of the six subjects experienced "rebound psychosis" [125]. Furthermore, three out of these five patients experienced a worsening of psychotic episodes (compared to their original psychotic episode that prompted antipsychotic use) in the form of paranoid delusions or threatening auditory hallucinations. This experience, which is also congruent with anecdotal evidence and the authors' experiences, also provides support for the efficacy of antipsychotic medications at least in some patients. Additional research is needed to confirm the efficacy and necessary treatment duration with antipsychotic treatment.

Prognostic Indicators

The prognostic value of psychosis and hallucinations in PD varies depending upon when symptoms are seen during the disease course. If symptoms are evident at time of diagnosis or very early on in the disease, then a preexisting psychiatric disorder or another parkinsonian syndrome such as DLB is likely to be present, and additional symptoms of such disorders may manifest [31].

When psychotic features arise later in the disease course, they may suggest additional complications such as cognitive impairment [126] and weight loss [127] or may be a manifestation of concomitant depression with mood congruent hallucinations. They are also associated with negative outcome variables such as caregiver distress [19], nursing home placement [20], and mortality [128]. Kempster and colleagues surveyed 129 case records from donors with pathologically proven PD. These cases were separated into five groups according to age at death, thus comparing patients who reached the advanced stage of the disease at different ages. Four milestones of advanced disease (frequent falls, visual hallucinations, dementia, and need for residential care) occurred at a similar time, approximately 5 years from death in each group. There were no significant differences in disease duration across these age groupings, nor were there differences in the severity and distribution of Lewy body and other pathologies. Once this advanced disease stage was reached, survival was similar in all groups [129].

Psychotic symptomatology has been considered by some to represent a "harbinger to cognitive decline" [13] as PD patients who present with visual hallucinations are more likely to develop cognitive impairments later on [21, 56, 126]. Psychosis and cognitive decline often co-occur, and both have been related to the development of the other.

A case control study identified hallucinations as the primary factor differentiating PD patients who were placed in a nursing home from those who were not, whereas motor and cognitive impairment did not differ between the groups [128]. In a 2-year follow-up study, the authors found that 100 % of nursing home PD patients had died [130]. Recent reports have documented more conservative nursing home mortality rates, which have been attributed in part to the increasingly common use of atypical antipsychotic agents for the treatment of psychosis [21, 124]. However, the finding that hallucinations and other psychotic phenomena are predictive of negative outcome has been well replicated and underscores the importance of both treating PD psychosis as well as its utility as a prognostic indicator. When psychosis and dementia coexist in PD, it is perhaps the greatest limiting factor for the optimal treatment of motor symptoms.

Management

The management of psychosis is dependent upon an understanding of the pathophysiology, which is due to a complex mixture of intrinsic and extrinsic factors. Intrinsic factors (such as the neurochemical changes in dopaminergic, serotonergic, and cholinergic systems) increase the likelihood of misinterpretation of visual images and the development of delusions [131]. In the presence of extrinsic factors (such as PD medications), the development of psychosis also becomes more likely [131].

1st Step: Identify and Treat Other Potential Conditions

Before treating psychosis in PD, it is important to rule out underlying medical illnesses as the cause of the symptoms in the context of delirium. For example, urinary and pulmonary infections, metabolic and endocrine imbalances, cerebral hypoperfusion states, and psychosocial stressors can lead to delirium and psychotic symptoms, especially in geriatric patients [78]. In addition, severe depression may lead to mood-congruent, distressing hallucinations, which can improve with antidepressant treatment alone.

2nd Step: Optimize the Environment

Similarly to the management of delirium, a team of healthcare professionals who are familiar to the patient suffering from PD psychosis should be involved. It is important to avoid moving people within and between wards or rooms unless absolutely necessary [132]. Optimizing the environment will reduce the likelihood of visual misinterpretations. Environmental interventions are designed to reduce or eliminate factors that exacerbate delirium. They include providing an optimal level of environmental stimulation (such as optimal lighting), reducing sensory impairments (such as loud noises), and providing environmental cues that facilitate orientation (such as a clock on the wall).

Contrary to schizophrenic patients, PD patients frequently use self-driven coping strategies for dealing with their psychotic symptoms such as visual techniques (including better focusing on the hallucinatory object, focusing at another object, or looking away from the hallucination), cognitive techniques (related to the patient's self-initiated reactions that do not involve other people, consciously noting that the hallucinations are not real or purposefully reassuring oneself that they will resolve shortly), and interactive techniques, relying on discussions with family and other caregivers to gain comfort and reassurance as well as verification of the non-reality of the hallucinations [44]. Therefore, cognitive training in such techniques may improve the psychotic symptoms.

3rd Step: Changing PD Treatment

PD medications contribute to psychosis through effects on both the dopaminergic and cholinergic systems with the latter exacerbating an existing cholinergic dysfunction. Stopping all potentially offending antiparkinsonian drugs is usually not an option for most patients, although dose reduction can frequently be accomplished with amelioration of hallucinations and little loss of drug-related benefit. Antiparkinsonian drugs can be reduced or stopped in reverse order starting from the last medication introduced before occurrence of hallucinations and continuing based on the potential of the drug to cause hallucinations. A stepwise approach to the consideration of withdrawal of medication is recommended [131]. Anticholinergics and tricyclics (which have anticholinergic properties) should be withdrawn first [133], followed by careful reduction or gradual withdrawal of other monoamine oxidase-B inhibitors, amantadine, and dopamine agonists. In severe cases, the basis of management is maintaining the patient on the minimum amount of antiparkinsonian medication focusing on levodopa as the main treatment [131]. Figure 6.1 summarizes the suggested order for withdrawal of medications in psychosis in PD.

4th Step: Specific Management

Clozapine is a dibenzodiazepine that binds to D1 mesolimbic receptors with relative sparing of striatal dopamine receptors. It has prominent activity at D4 dopamine receptors and is an antagonist at adrenergic, cholinergic, histaminergic, and serotonergic receptors. Clozapine has been shown to be effective for psychosis in PD [134]. However, it can cause granulocytopenia in 1–2 % of patients, and weekly to biweekly blood counts are required on treatment. The risk of clozapine-induced leukopenia or agranulocytosis decreases exponentially over time, and the likelihood of developing fatal granulocytopenia beyond 6 months of clozapine treatment is low [135]. It is important to start at a low dose, either 6.25 or 12.5 mg once a day. Most patients will only require 25 mg and do not require doses beyond 50 mg. There are concerns about possible anticholinergic side effects in larger doses,

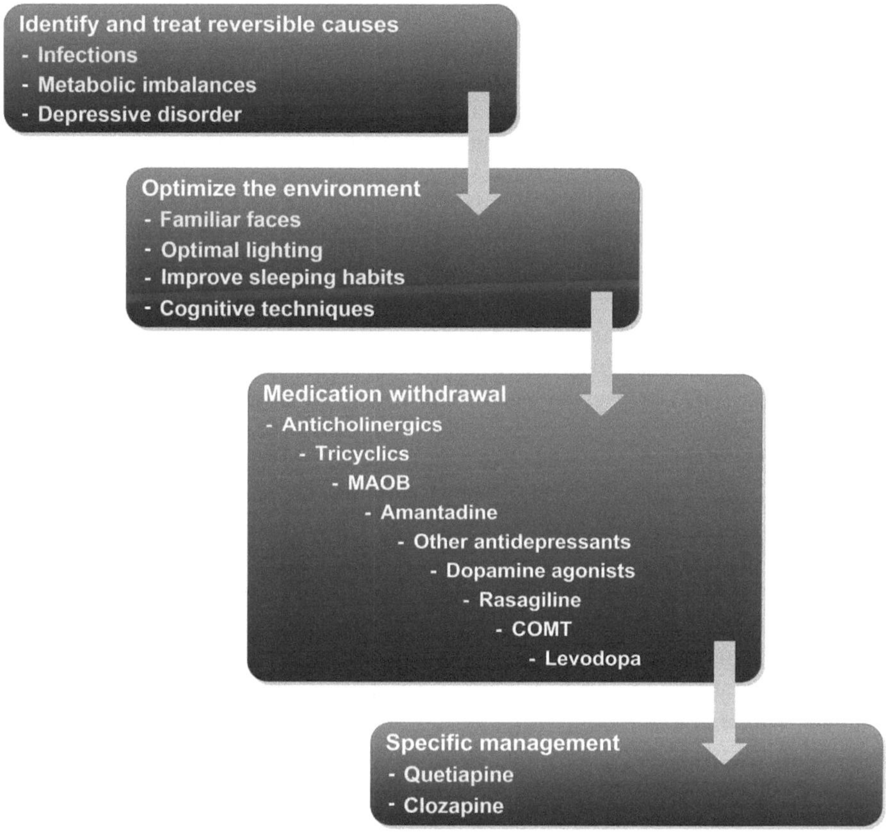

Fig. 6.1 Suggested management of psychosis in PD, including the order of withdrawal of medication

but in practice, these are avoided in the smaller doses in PD [136]. Clozapine is metabolized through the cytochrome system with inhibitors of metabolism clozapine levels [137, 138].

Quetiapine is an atypical dibenzothiazepine structurally similar to clozapine. As clozapine, quetiapine also does not appear to worsen parkinsonism to the same degree as other atypical neuroleptics such as risperidone and olanzapine or the typical neuroleptics such as haloperidol. The use of quetiapine in clinical practice is well established, and it is by far the most widely used antipsychotic for dopaminergic-induced psychosis. However, there are inconsistent study data regarding the effectiveness of quetiapine. Although several open label studies reported that quetiapine is effective for treatment of psychosis in patients with PD and two single-blind randomized trials [137] comparing quetiapine and clozapine reported they were equally effective, only one of five small randomized controlled trials found benefit for quetiapine compared with placebo [139]. In community studies, quetiapine was reported to have a lower risk of cardiovascular death compared to other atypical agents, with an absence of a dose–response effect in relation to the risk of death [140]. Moreover, studies in nursing homes have shown a lower risk of cerebrovascular incidents or infections compared to other antipsychotics [141]. Small doses of quetiapine should be used in older people starting at 25 mg just once a day. It is important to remember that quetiapine is metabolized through the cytochrome system [142] with inhibitors of this system (such as diltiazem and clarithromycin) increasing quetiapine levels and inducers of metabolism (such as carbamazepine), reducing levels [138].

Other drugs that have been studied regarding their efficacy in managing psychotic features in PD include antipsychotics and cholinesterase inhibitors. Olanzapine was rated in the MDS 2011 report as not efficacious, with an unacceptable risk of exacerbating parkinsonism, and clinically not useful [143]. The efficacy of other antipsychotics (including risperidone, aripiprazole, ziprasidone, and melperone) and cholinesterase inhibitors (including rivastigmine, donepezil, and galantamine) has only been reported based in open label studies, case series, or single case reports [56, 144]. Subanalyses of a double-blind, placebo-controlled study in PD dementia [145] suggested that rivastigmine was more effective in some cognitive and behavioral measures in patients experiencing hallucinations compared to patients not experiencing hallucinations [146]. Thus, there is some support for the use of cholinesterase inhibitors for the treatment of psychosis in cognitively impaired PD patients, which are commonly used in this setting, but evidence for their use in treating psychosis in non-demented PD is lacking [144].

Recently, the experimental antipsychotic agent pimavanserin was found to be significantly better than placebo at reducing PD-related psychosis in a 6-week double-blind randomized placebo-controlled trial of 199 patients with Parkinson's disease psychosis. Antipsychotic treatments were not permitted during the study, but controlled antiparkinsonian medication or deep brain stimulation was allowed. Eligible participants entered a 2-week non-pharmacological lead-in phase to limit the placebo response, after which they were randomly allocated (1:1) to receive pimavanserin 40 mg per day or matched placebo. The primary outcome was antipsychotic benefit as assessed by central, independent raters with the Parkinson's disease-adapted scale for assessment of positive symptoms (SAPS-PD). Pimavanserin was associated with a −5.79 decrease in SAPS-PD scores. Pimavanserin was well tolerated and was not associated with worsening of motor symptoms or other adverse effects. The investigators concluded that pimavanserin, though not clinically available yet, may benefit patients with Parkinson's disease psychosis for whom few other treatment options exist. Further studies are needed to confirm the long-term safety and efficacy of pimavanserin [147].

Finally, it is important to consider that psychotic symptoms may be attributable to a preexisting psychiatric disorder such as major depression or another parkinsonian syndrome such as DLB.

Case Scenarios

Case Report 1 This report describes presence hallucinations in a patient with PD [39].

A 71-year-old woman had had tremor-predominant Parkinson's disease diagnosed 2 years previously, with no cognitive impairment. She received levodopa, mianserin, and lorazepam for an anxiety disorder. She had daily presence hallucinations for approximately 6 months before inclusion. The patient lived alone and had a sister living somewhere else. During the night or when awakening in the morning, she repeatedly had the vivid sensation that her sister was lying beside her in the bed. She knew that this was not possible and she did not see her, but she used to lift the top sheet to check that her sister was not there. Later in the morning, when passing near her bed, she often again had the feeling that her sister was there and she had to check again. Each episode lasted only a few seconds.

Case Report 2 This report describes passage hallucinations [39].

A 59-year-old man had received levodopa and bromocriptine for Parkinson's disease diagnosed 3 years previously. In the evening, while clearing away the tables and chairs, he often had the brief impression of a mouse passing on the right. He turned his head to the right but could not see anything.

Case Report 3 This report describes formed visual hallucinations in the context of cognitive impairment in PD [39].

A 71-year-old man had had Parkinson's disease for 8 years and was taking levodopa. His motor symptoms and signs were mild to moderate, and he was independent in all daily activities. However, the patient also had developed cognitive impairment about 4 years after the onset of motor symptoms. Hallucinations had started during a therapeutic trial of a dopaminergic agonist but had not subsided after the agonist was withdrawn. They consisted of characters that commonly took the form of small ill-formed devils with a blurred face and a changing size. They moved rapidly in "a sort of haze." During an episode of lumbar pain, the patient described these characters as armed with blades and was "butchering" his back. However, in most instances, the hallucinations of devils were not frightening and were well tolerated. The patient said that he had become familiar with them, that their lives were now intermingled with his own, and that it was like "living in a fantasy novel" or a "parallel world." The patient repeatedly stated that he was aware of the unreality of the visions but admitted that he would occasionally speak to them because they "looked so real." Visual hallucinations occurred daily, predominantly at night, and the characters seemed to be "scared" and "scattered" by light, a noise, or a sudden wave of the hand. The patient also experienced presence hallucinations: "it's a presence behind me; I try to catch it by turning round but I never see its face."

Case Report 4 This report describes rare auditory hallucinations in PD psychosis [39].

A 68-year-old-woman had received a diagnosis of Parkinson's disease 18 years previously. She was taking levodopa, bromocriptine, piribedil, and amantadine. She had subtle cognitive impairment and has also felt depressed. She had experienced presence hallucinations (of an unidentified person) for the last 6 months. In one instance, she saw her deceased son with another person. Her son distinctly said to her: "take care of yourself."

Case Report 5 This report highlights the importance of monitoring and screening the psychotic symptoms in patients treated with oral dopamine agonists, especially in elderly patients [148].

The patient was an 89-year-old man with a 6-year history of PD. Two years previously, he had been started on amantadine and selegiline. Three months later, pramipexole (0.25 mg/day) had been added to his treatment regimen to combat his persistent tremor and bradykinesia, and the dosage was increased to 0.5 mg/day in 2 weeks. One month after the dosage was titrated to 0.5 mg/day, visual hallucinations (VH) developed. He could see faces of people and ghosts in different sizes and colors. The occurrence of VH was mostly limited to nighttime, when he was fully conscious and aware, but he did not inform the others about these symptoms. In terms of his prominent motor symptoms, pramipexole was titrated up to 2.25 mg/day 5 months before this admission. After 2 months on this regimen, he experienced an increased frequency of complex VH and also had olfactory hallucinations, delusions of being poisoned, delusions of persecution, and destructive behaviors. All these psychotic symptoms persisted under normal consciousness. Amantadine and selegiline were discontinued. Pramipexole was decreased to 1.5 mg/day, and quetiapine 25 mg/day was prescribed. However, all the psychotic symptoms remained the same for 1 week under the regimen. He was then admitted, and pramipexole was discontinued. Due to his vivid psychotic symptoms and agitation, quetiapine was increased gradually to 300 mg/day in 10 days. Three weeks after admission, his psychotic symptoms gradually resolved. After discharge, quetiapine dosage was reduced gradually without psychotic exacerbation. In addition, no antiparkinsonian drug was used for his tremor and bradykinesia, which were reported as tolerable.

Case Report 6 The following case illustrates the challenge of advanced Parkinson's disease in schizophrenic patient on neuroleptic treatment. Differentiating between drug-induced parkinsonism and idiopathic Parkinson's disease is recommended by presynaptic nuclear imaging (e.g. FP-CIT SPECT) [149].

A 74-year-old man with no dementia was previously diagnosed with paranoid schizophrenia and repeatedly treated with first- and second-generation antipsychotics. Ten years ago, parkinsonism was first noticed, and antipsychotic treatment was switched to clozapine (62.5 mg/day). As the patient refused to take clozapine in the course of the disease, it was replaced by olanzapine (5 mg/day). Additionally, he received L-DOPA (400 mg/day) and pramipexole (4 mg/day) to treat parkinsonism. He responded well to treatment but later developed on/off fluctuations and peak-dose dyskinesias, wherefore a treatment with amantadine (200 mg/day) was initiated.

He then rapidly developed severe delusions. On admission, he was floridly psychotic but also disabled by severe on/off fluctuation and peak-dose dyskinesias. As there was some doubt concerning the diagnosis of idiopathic Parkinson's disease, FP-CIT SPECT was performed, and it showed bilaterally marked reduction of striatal dopamine transporter binding in the putamen. Pramipexole and amantadine were stopped, and quetiapine (125 mg/day) was added to the drug regimen, which led to marked improvement of the mental state. However, motor symptoms became worse. The total dose of L-DOPA was increased to 500 mg in combination with entacapone, and the intervals between the doses were shortened (five times 100 mg, every 3–4 h) whereby good motor control was achieved.

References

1. Chaudhuri KR, Martinez-Martin P, Schapira AH, Stocchi F, Sethi K, Odin P, Brown RG, Koller W, Barone P, MacPhee G, Kelly L, Rabey M, MacMahon D, Thomas S, Ondo W, Rye D, Forbes A, Tluk S, Dhawan V, Bowron A, Williams AJ, Olanow CW. International multicenter pilot study of the first comprehensive self-completed nonmotor symptoms questionnaire for Parkinson's disease: the NMSQuest study. Mov Disord. 2006;21(7):916–23.
2. Parkinson J. An essay on the shaking palsy. London: Neely and Jones; 1817.
3. Ball B. De l'insanité dans la paralysie agitante. Encéphale. 1882;2:22–32.
4. Regis E. Precis de Psychiatrie. Paris: Gaston Doiz; 1906.
5. Jackson JA, Free GBM, Pike HV. The psychic manifestations in paralysis agitans. Arch Neurol Psychiatry. 1923;10:680–4.
6. Mjönes H. Paralysis agitans, A clinical and genetic study. Copenhagen: Ejnar Munksgaard; 1949.
7. Schwab RS, Fabing HD, Prichard JS. Psychiatric symptoms and syndromes in Parkinson's disease. Am J Psychiatry. 1950;107:901–7.
8. Fenelon G, Goetz CG, Karenberg A. Hallucinations in Parkinson disease in the prelevodopa era. Neurology. 2006;66:93–8.
9. Molho ES. Drug-induced psychosis: terminology, history, and frequency. In: Factor SA, Weiner WJ, editors. Parkinson's disease: diagnosis and clinical management. New York: Demos Medical Publishing; 2002.
10. Jenkins RB, Groh RH. Mental symptoms in Parkinsonian patients with L-dopa. Lancet. 1970;2:177–80.
11. Damasio AR, Lobo-Antunes J, Macedo C. Psychiatric aspects in Parkinsonism treated with L-dopa. J Neurol Neurosurg Psychiatry. 1971;34:502–7.
12. Goodwin FK. Psychiatric side effects of levodopa in man. JAMA. 1971;218:1915–20.
13. Sanchez-Ramos JR, Ortoll R, Paulson GW. Visual hallucinations associated with Parkinson's disease. Arch Neurol. 1996;53:1265–8.
14. Aarsland D, Larsen JP, Cummings JL, Laake K. Prevalence and clinical correlates of psychotic symptoms in Parkinson's disease. Arch Neurol. 1999;56:595–601.
15. Quelhas R. Psychiatric care in Parkinson's disease. J Psychiatr Pract. 2013;19(2):118–41.
16. Lepore FE. Visual loss as a causative factor in visual hallucinations associated with Parkinson's disease. Arch Neurol. 1997;54:799.
17. Oyebode F. Sims symptoms in the mind: an introduction to descriptive psychopathology. 4th ed. Edinburgh: Saunders Elsevier; 2008.
18. Fénelon G, Mahieux F, Huon R, Ziegler M. Hallucinations in Parkinson's disease. Prevalence, phenomenology and risk factors. Brain. 2000;123:733–45.

19. Aarsland D, Larsen JP, Karlsen K, Lim NG, Tandberg E. Mental symptoms in Parkinson's disease are important contributors to caregiver distress. Int J Geriatr Psychiatry. 1999;14:866–74.
20. Aarsland D, Larsen JP, Tandberg E, Laake K. Predictors of nursing home placement in Parkinson's disease: a population-based, prospective study. J Am Geriatr Soc. 2000;48:938–42.
21. Factor SA, Feustel PJ, Friedman JH, Comella CL, Goetz CG, Kurlan R, Parsa M, Pfeiffer R, Parkinson Study Group. Longitudinal outcome of Parkinson's disease patients with psychosis. Neurology. 2003;60:1756–61.
22. Aarsland D, Brønnick K, Ehrt U, De Deyn PP, Tekin S, Emre M, Cummings JL. Neuropsychiatric symptoms in patients with Parkinson's disease and dementia: frequency, profile and associated care giver stress. J Neurol Neurosurg Psychiatry. 2007;78:36–42.
23. Stuebner E, Vichayanrat E, Low DA, Mathias CJ, Isenmann S, Haensch C-A. Nocturnal blood pressure, non-dipping and psychosis in Parkinson's disease. J Neurol Sci, 2013;333(e75–e76):0022–510X.
24. Chaudhuri KR, Martinez-Martin P. Quantitation of non-motor symptoms in Parkinson's disease. Eur J Neurol. 2008;15 Suppl 2:2–7.
25. Berardelli A, Wenning GK, Antonini A, Berg D, Bloem BR, Bonifati V, Brooks D, Burn DJ, Colosimo C, Fanciulli A, Ferreira J, Gasser T, Grandas F, Kanovsky P, Kostic V, Kulisevsky J, Oertel W, Poewe W, Reese JP, Relja M, Ruzicka E, Schrag A, Seppi K, Taba P, Vidailhet M. EFNS/MDS-ES recommendations for the diagnosis of Parkinson's disease. Eur J Neurol. 2013;20:16–34.
26. Mack J, Rabins P, Anderson K, Goldstein S, Grill S, Hirsch ES, Lehmann S, Little JT, Margolis RL, Palanci J, Pontone G, Weiss H, Williams JR, Marsh L. Prevalence of psychotic symptoms in a community-based Parkinson disease sample. Am J Geriatr Psychiatry. 2012;20:123–32.
27. Fénelon G, Alves G. Epidemiology of psychosis in Parkinson's disease. J Neurol Sci. 2010;289:12–7.
28. Barnes J, Connelly V, Wiggs L, Boubert L, Maravic K. Sleep patterns in Parkinson's disease patients with visual hallucinations. Int J Neurosci. 2010;120:564–9.
29. Barnes J, David AS. Visual hallucinations in Parkinson's disease: a review and phenomenological survey. J Neurol Neurosurg Psychiatry. 2001;70:727–33.
30. Goetz CG, Ouyang B, Negron A, Stebbins GT. Hallucinations and sleep disorders in PD Ten-year prospective longitudinal study. Neurology. 2010;75:1773–9.
31. Goetz CG, Vogel C, Tanner CM, Stebbins GT. Early dopaminergic drug-induced hallucinations in parkinsonian patients. Neurology. 1998;51:811–4.
32. Khoo TK, Yarnall AJ, Duncan GW, Coleman S, O'Brien JT, Brooks DJ, Barker RA, Burn DJ. The spectrum of nonmotor symptoms in early Parkinson disease. Neurology. 2013;80:276–81.
33. McKeith IG, Dickson DW, Lowe J, Emre M, O'Brien JT, Feldman H, Cummings J, Duda JE, Lippa C, Perry EK, Aarsland D, Arai H, Ballard CG, Boeve B, Burn DJ, Costa D, Del Ser T, Dubois B, Galasko D, Gauthier S, Goetz CG, Gomez-Tortosa E, Halliday G, Hansen LA, Hardy J, Iwatsubo T, Kalaria RN, Kaufer D, Kenny RA, Korczyn A, Kosaka K, Lee VM, Lees A, Litvan I, Londos E, Lopez OL, Minoshima S, Mizuno Y, Molina JA, Mukaetova-Ladinska EB, Pasquier F, Perry RH, Schulz JB, Trojanowski JQ, Yamada M, Consortium on DLB. Diagnosis and management of dementia with Lewy bodies: third report of the DLB Consortium. Neurology. 2005;65:1863–72.
34. Mosimann UP, Rowan EN, Partington CE, Collerton D, Littlewood E, O'Brien JT, Burn DJ, McKeith IG. Characteristics of visual hallucinations in Parkinson disease dementia and dementia with Lewy bodies. Am J Geriatr Psychiatry. 2006;14:153–60.
35. Thanvi BR, Lo TC, Harsh DP. Psychosis in Parkinson's disease. Postgrad Med J. 2005;81:644–6.

36. Ravina B, Marder K, Fernandez HH, Friedman JH, McDonald W, Murphy D, Aarsland D, Babcock D, Cummings J, Endicott J, Factor S, Galpern W, Lees A, Marsh L, Stacy M, Gwinn-Hardy K, Voon V, Goetz C. Diagnostic criteria for psychosis in Parkinson's disease: report of an NINDS, NIMH work group. Mov Disord. 2007;22:1061–8.
37. Duvoisin RC. Parkinson's disease. A guide for patient and family. Raven: New York; 1991.
38. Haeske-Dewick HC. Hallucinations in Parkinson's disease: characteristics and associated features. Int J Geriatr Psych. 1995;10:487–95.
39. Thompson C. Anwesenheit: psychopathology and clinical associations. Br J Psychiatry. 1982;141:628–30.
40. Graham JM, Gruenewald RA, Sagar HJ. Hallucinosis in idiopathic Parkinson's disease. J Neurol Neurosurg Psychiatry. 1997;63:434–40.
41. Diederich NJ, Pieri V, Goetz CG. Die visuellen Halluzinationen des Parkinson-Patienten und das Charles Bonnet Syndrom. Eine phänomenologische und pathogenetische Gegenüberstellung. Fortschr Neurol Psychiat. 2000;68:129–36.
42. Holroyd S, Currie L, Wooten GF. Prospective study of hallucinations and delusions in Parkinson's disease. J Neurol Neurosurg Psychiatry. 2001;70:734–8.
43. Goetz CG, Diederich NJ, Fenelon G. Psychosis in Parkinson's disease. In: Chaudhuri KR, editor. Non-motor symptoms of Parkinson's disease. New York: Oxford University Press; 2009.
44. Diederich NH, Pieri V, Goetz CG. Coping strategies for visual hallucinations in Parkinson's disease. Mov Disord. 2003;18:831–8.
45. Manni R, Pacchetti C, Terzaghi M, Sartori I, Mancini F, Nappi G. Hallucinations and sleep-wake cycle in PD: a 24-h continuous polysomnographic study. Neurology. 2002;59:1979–81.
46. Inzelberg R, Kipervasser S, Korczyn AD. Auditory hallucinations in Parkinson's disease. J Neurol Neurosurg Psychiatry. 1998;64:533–5.
47. Factor SA, Molho ES. Threatening auditory hallucinations and Cotard syndrome in Parkinson disease. Clin Neuropharmacol. 2004;27:205–7.
48. Marsh L, Williams JR, Rocco M, Grill S, Munro C, Dawson TM. Psychiatric comorbidities in patients with Parkinson disease and psychosis. Neurology. 2004;63:293–300.
49. Fénelon G, Thobois S, Bonnet AM, Broussolle E, Tison F. Tactile hallucinations in Parkinson's disease. J Neurol. 2002;12:1699–703.
50. Jiménez-Jiménez FJ, Ortí-Pareja M, Gasalla T, Tallón-Barranco A, Cabrera-Valdivia F, Fernández-Lliria A. Cenesthetic hallucinations in a patient with Parkinson's disease. J Neurol Neurosurg Psychiatry. 1997;63:120.
51. Sandyk R. Olfactory hallucinations in Parkinson's disease. S Afr Med J. 1981;60:950.
52. Goetz CG, Wuu J, Curgian LM, Leurgans S. Hallucinations and sleep disorders in PD: six-year prospective longitudinal study. Neurology. 2005;64:81–6.
53. Chou KL, Messing S, Oakes D, Feldman PD, Breier A, Friedman JH. Drug induced psychosis in Parkinson disease: phenomenology and correlations among psychosis rating instruments. Clin Neuropharmacol. 2005;28:215–9.
54. Klawans H. Levodopa-induced psychosis. Psychiatr Ann. 1978;8:447–71.
55. Rabey JM. Hallucinations and psychosis in Parkinson's disease. Parkinsonism Relat Disord. 2009;15 Suppl 4:S105–10.
56. Zahodne LB, Fernandez HH. A review of the pathophysiology and treatment of psychosis in Parkinson's disease. Drugs Aging. 2008;25(8):665–82.
57. Kiziltan G, Ozekmekci S, Ertan S, Ertan T, Erginoz E. Relationship between age and subtypes of psychotic symptoms in Parkinson's disease. J Neurol. 2007;254(4):448–52.
58. De Smet Y, Ruberg M, Serdaru M, Dubois B, Lhermitte F, Agid Y. Confusion, dementia and anticholinergics in Parkinson's disease. J Neurol Neurosurg Psychiatry. 1982;45:1161–4.
59. Golden WE, Lavender RC, Metzer WS. Acute postoperative confusion and hallucinations in Parkinson's disease. Ann Intern Med. 1989;111:218–22.

60. Goetz CG. Hallucinations in Parkinson's disease: the clinical syndrome. Adv Neurol. 1999;80:419–23.
61. Gallagher DA, Schrag A. Psychosis, apathy, depression and anxiety in Parkinson's disease. Neurobiol Dis. 2012;46(3):581–9.
62. Factor SA, Molho ES, Podskalny GD, Brown D. Parkinson's disease: drug-induced psychiatric states. Adv Neurol. 1995;65:115–38.
63. Papapetropoulos S, Mash DC. Psychotic symptoms in Parkinson's disease. From description to etiology. J Neurol. 2005;252:753–64.
64. Goetz CG, Leurgans S, Pappert EJ, Raman R, Stemer AB. Prospective longitudinal assessment of hallucinations in Parkinson's disease. Neurology. 2001;57:2078–82.
65. Goetz CG, Wuu J, Curgian L, Leurgans S. Age-related influences on the clinical characteristics of new-onset hallucinations in Parkinson's disease patients. Mov Disord. 2006;21:267–70.
66. Stuebner E, Vichayanrat E, Low DA, Mathias CJ, Isenmann S, Haensch CA. Twenty-four hour non-invasive ambulatory blood pressure and heart rate monitoring in Parkinson's disease. Front Neurol. 2013;4:49.
67. Achary MSN, Govindappa ST, Basu P, Kumarswamy SD, Ramanathan R, Muthane UB. Phenomenology and factors causing psychosis in Parkinson's disease. Mov Disord. 2012;27:S280.
68. Bailbe M, Karolewicz S, Neau JP, Dumas P, Gil R, Association des neurologues du Poitou-Charentes. Hallucinations, delusions, and nocturnal events in 152 Parkinson's patients: a regional survey. Rev Neurol (Paris). 2002;158(2):203–10.
69. Schrag A, Ben-Shlomo Y, Quinn N. How common are complications of Parkinson's disease? J Neurol. 2002;249(4):419–23.
70. Paleacu D, Schechtman E, Inzelberg R. Association between family history of dementia and hallucinations in Parkinson disease. Neurology. 2005;64:1712–5.
71. Terzaghi M, Sinforiani E, Zucchella C, Zambrelli E, Pasotti C, Rustioni V, Manni R. Cognitive performance in REM sleep behaviour disorder: a possible early marker of neurodegenerative disease? Sleep Med. 2008;9(4):343–51.
72. Williams DR, Warren JD, Lees AJ. Using the presence of visual hallucinations to differentiate Parkinson's disease from atypical parkinsonism. J Neurol Neurosurg Psychiatry. 2008;79(6):652–5.
73. Fénelon G, Soulas T, Zenasni F, Cleret de Langavant L. The changing face of Parkinson's disease-associated psychosis: a cross-sectional study based on the new NINDS-NIMH criteria. Mov Disord. 2010;25(6):763–6.
74. Sawada H, Oeda T, Umemura A, Tomita S, Hayashi R, Kohsaka M, Nakano H, Yamamoto K. Hallucinations and delusions in patients with Parkinson's disease – evaluation by the Parkinson psychosis questionnaire. Eur J Neurol. 2011;18 Suppl 2:518.
75. Yadav R, Amar BR, Reddy YCJ, Pal PK. Pattern of psychosis in Parkinson's disease. Parkinsonism Relat Disord. 2012;18 Suppl 1:31.
76. Lee AH, Weintraub D. Psychosis in Parkinson's disease without dementia: common and comorbid with other non-motor symptoms. Mov Disord. 2012;27(7):858–63.
77. Moskovitz C, Moses H, Klawans HL. Levodopa-induced psychosis: a kindling phenomenon. Am J Psychiatry. 1978;135:669–75.
78. Wint DP, Okun MS, Fernandez HH. Psychosis in Parkinson's disease. J Geriatr Psychiatry Neurol. 2004;17(3):127–36.
79. Bell DS. The experimental reproduction of amphetamine psychosis. Arch Gen Psychiatry. 1973;29:35–40.
80. Goetz CG, Tanner CM, Klawans HL. Pharmacology of hallucinations induced by long-term drug therapy. Am J Psychiatry. 1982;139(4):494–7.
81. Glenthøj BY, Hemmingsen R. Dopaminergic sensitization: implications for the pathogenesis of schizophrenia. Prog Neuropsychopharmacol Biol Psychiatry. 1997;21:23–46.
82. Wolters EC. Intrinsic and extrinsic psychosis in Parkinson's disease. J Neurol. 2001;248 Suppl 3:III22–7.

83. Sato M, Chen CC, Akiyama K, Otsuki S. Acute exacerbation of paranoid psychotic state after long-term abstinence in patients with previous methamphetamine psychosis. Biol Psychiatry. 1983;18:429–40.
84. Sato M, Numachi Y, Hamamura T. Relapse of paranoid psychotic state in methamphetamine model of schizophrenia. Schizophr Bull. 1992;18:115–22.
85. Melamed E. Neurobehavioral abnormalities in Parkinson's disease. In: Watts RL, Koller WC, editors. Movement disorders. New York: McGraw Hill; 1996.
86. Goetz CG, Pappert EJ, Blasucci LM, Stebbins GT, Ling ZD, Nora MV, Carvey PM. Intravenous levodopa in hallucinating Parkinson's disease patients: high-dose challenge does not precipitate hallucinations. Neurology. 1998;50(2):515–7.
87. Richelson E. Receptor pharmacology of neuroleptics: relation to clinical effects. J Clin Psychiatry. 1999;60 Suppl 10:5–14.
88. Perry E, Walker M, Grace J, Perry R. Acetylcholine in mind: a neurotransmitter correlate of consciousness? Trends Neurosci. 1999;22:273–80.
89. Whitehouse PJ. Clinical and neurochemical consequences of neuronal loss in the nucleus basalis of Meynert in Parkinson's disease and Alzheimer's disease. Adv Neurol. 1987;45:393–7.
90. Nakano I, Hirano A. Parkinson's disease: neuron loss in the nucleus basalis without concomitant Alzheimer's disease. Ann Neurol. 1984;15:415–8.
91. Papapetropoulos S. Drug-induced psychosis in Parkinson disease: phenomenology and correlations among psychosis rating instruments. Clin Neuropharmacol. 2006;29:59.
92. Goetz CG, Fan W, Leurgans S, Bernard B, Stebbins GT. The malignant course of "benign hallucinations" in Parkinson disease. Arch Neurol. 2006;63:713–6.
93. Moustafa AA, Krishna R, Frank MJ, Eissa AM, Hewedi DH. Cognitive correlates of psychosis in patients with Parkinson's disease. Cogn Neuropsychiatr. 2014;19:381–98 [Epub ahead of print].
94. Harding AJ, Broe GA, Halliday GM. Visual hallucinations in Lewy body disease relate to Lewy bodies in the temporal lobe. Brain. 2002;125(2):391–403.
95. Williams DR, Lees AJ. Visual hallucinations in the diagnosis of idiopathic Parkinson's disease: a retrospective autopsy study. Lancet Neurol. 2005;4:605–10.
96. Papapetropoulos S, McCorquodale DS, Gonzalez J, Jean-Gilles L, Mash DC. Cortical and amygdalar Lewy body burden in Parkinson's disease patients with visual hallucinations. Parkinsonism Relat Disord. 2006;122(4):253–6.
97. Larsen JP, Tandberg E. Sleep disorders in patients with Parkinson's disease. CNS Drugs. 2001;15(4):267–75.
98. Pacchetti C, Manni R, Zangaglia R, Mancini F, Marchioni E, Tassorelli C, Terzaghi M, Ossola M, Martignoni E, Moglia A, Nappi G. Relationship between hallucinations, delusions, and rapid eye movement sleep behavior disorder in Parkinson's disease. Mov Disord. 2005;20(11):1439–48.
99. Pappert EJ, Goetz CG, Niederman FG, Raman R, Leurgans S. Hallucinations, sleep fragmentation, and altered dream phenomena in Parkinson's disease. Mov Disord. 1999;14:117–21.
100. Comella CL, Tanner CM, Ristanovic RK. Polysomnographic sleep measures in Parkinson's disease patients with treatment-induced hallucinations. Ann Neurol. 1993;34:710–4.
101. Arnulf I, Konofal E, Merino-Andreu M, Houeto JL, Mesnage V, Welter ML, Lacomblez L, Golmard JL, Derenne JP, Agid Y. Parkinson's disease and sleepiness. An integral part of PD. Neurology. 2002;58:1019–24.
102. Diedrich NJ, Goetz CG, Raman R, Pappert EJ, Leurgans S, Piery V. Poor visual discrimination and visual hallucinations in Parkinson's disease. Clin Neuropharmacol. 1998;21:289–95.
103. Bodis-Wollner I. Visual deficits related to dopamine deficiency in experimental animals and Parkinson's disease patients. Trends Neurosci. 1990;13(7):296–302.
104. Maurage CA, Ruchoux MM, de Vos R, Surguchov A, Destee A. Retinal involvement in dementia with Lewy bodies: a clue to hallucinations? Ann Neurol. 2003;54:542–7.
105. Onofrj M, Bonanni L, Albani G, Mauro A, Bulla D, Thomas A. Visual hallucinations in Parkinson's disease: clues to separate origins. J Neurol Sci. 2006;248:143–50.

106. Kraft E, Winkelmann J, Trenkwalder C, Auer DP. Visual hallucinations: white matter lesions and disease severity in Parkinson's disease. Acta Neurol Scand. 1999;99(6):362–7.
107. Stebbins GT, Goetz CG, Carrillo MC, Bangen KJ, Turner DA, Glover GH, Gabrieli JD. Altered cortical visual processing in PD with hallucinations. Neurology. 2004;63:1409–16.
108. Holroyd S, Wooten GF. Preliminary fMRI evidence of visual system dysfunction in Parkinson's disease patients with visual hallucinations. J Neuropsychiatry Clin Neurosci. 2006;18(3):402–4.
109. Barnes J, Boubert L, Harris J, Lee A, David AS. Reality monitoring and visual hallucinations in Parkinson's disease. Neuropsychologia. 2003;41:565–74.
110. Gallagher DA, Parkkinen L, O'Sullivan SS, Spratt A, Shah A, Davey CC, Bremner FD, Revesz T, Williams DR, Lees AJ, Schrag A. Testing an aetiological model of visual hallucinations in Parkinson's disease. Brain. 2011;134(Pt 11):3299–309.
111. De la Fuente-Fernandez R, Nunez MA, Lopez E. The apolipoprotein E epsilon 4 allele increases the risk of drug-induced hallucinations in Parkinson's disease. Clin Neuropharmacol. 1999;22(4):226–30.
112. Feldman B, Chapman J, Korczyn AD. Apolipoprotein epsilon4 advances appearance of psychosis in patients with Parkinson's disease. Acta Neurol Scand. 2006;113(1):14–7.
113. Goetz CG, Burke PF, Leurgans S, Berry-Kravis E, Blasucci LM, Raman R, Zhou L. Genetic variation analysis in Parkinson disease patients with and without hallucinations: case–control study. Arch Neurol. 2001;58(2):209–13.
114. Camicioli R, Rajput A, Rajput M, Reece C, Payami H, Hao C, Rajput A. Apolipoprotein E epsilon4 and catechol-O-methyltransferase alleles in autopsy-proven Parkinson's disease: relationship to dementia and hallucinations. Mov Disord. 2005;20(8):989–94.
115. Papapetropoulos S, Farrer MJ, Stone JT, Milkovic NM, Ross OA, Calvo L, McQuorquodale D, Mash DC. Phenotypic associations of tau and ApoE in Parkinson's disease. Neurosci Lett. 2007;414(2):141–4.
116. Chen CC, Lee ST, Wu T, Chen CJ, Chen MC, Lu CS. Short-term effects of bilateral subthalamic stimulation for advanced Parkinson's disease. Chang Gung Med J. 2003;26(5):344–51.
117. Herzog J, Volkmann J, Krack P, Kopper F, Pötter M, Lorenz D, Steinbach M, Klebe S, Hamel W, Schrader B, Weinert D, Müller D, Mehdorn HM, Deuschl G. Two-year follow-up of subthalamic deep brain stimulation in Parkinson's disease. Mov Disord. 2003;18(11):1332–7.
118. Castelli L, Perozzo P, Zibetti M, Crivelli B, Morabito U, Lanotte M, Cossa F, Bergamasco B, Lopiano L. Chronic deep brain stimulation of the subthalamic nucleus for Parkinson's disease: effects on cognition, mood, anxiety and personality traits. Eur Neurol. 2006;55(3):136–44.
119. Vesper J, Haak S, Ostertag C, Nikkhah G. Subthalamic. Nucleus deep brain stimulation in elderly patients – analysis of outcome and complications. BMC Neurol. 2007;7:7.
120. Stephenson R, Houghton D, Sundarararjan S, Doty RL, Stern M, Xie SX, Siderowf A. Odor identification deficits are associated with increased risk of neuropsychiatric complications in patients with Parkinson's disease. Mov Disord. 2010;25(13):2099–104.
121. Kitayama M, Wada-Isoe K, Irizawa Y, Nakashima K. Association of visual hallucinations with reduction of MIBG cardiac uptake in Parkinson's disease. J Neurol Sci. 2008;264:22–6.
122. Sawada H, Oeda T, Umemura A, Tomita S, Hayashi R, Kohsaka M, Yamamoto K, Sudoh S, Sugiyama H. Subclinical elevation of plasma C-reactive protein and illusions/hallucinations in subjects with Parkinson's disease: case–control study. PLoS One. 2014;9(1):e85886.
123. Wolters EC, Berendse HW. Management of psychosis in Parkinson's disease. Curr Opin Neurol. 2001;14:499–504.
124. Fernandez HH, Donnelly EM, Friedman JH. Long-term outcome of clozapine use for psychosis in parkinsonian patients. Mov Disord. 2004;19(7):831–3.
125. Fernandez HH, Trieschmann ME, Okun MS. Rebound psychosis: effect of discontinuation of antipsychotics in Parkinson's disease. Mov Disord. 2005;20(1):104–5.
126. Ramirez-Ruiz B, Junque C, Marti MJ, Valldeoriola F, Tolosa E. Cognitive changes in Parkinson's disease patients with visual hallucinations. Dement Geriatr Cogn Disord. 2007;23(5):281–8.
127. Uc EY, Struck LK, Rodnitzky RL, Zimmerman B, Dobson J, Evans WJ. Predictors of weight loss in Parkinson's disease. Mov Disord. 2006;21(7):930–6.

128. Goetz CG, Stebbins GT. Risk factors for nursing home placement in advanced Parkinson's disease. Neurology. 1993;43:2227–9.
129. Kempster PA, O'Sullivan SS, Holton JL, Revesz T, Lees AJ. Relationships between age and late progression of Parkinson's disease: a clinico-pathological study. Brain. 2010;133(Pt 6):1755–62.
130. Goetz CG, Stebbins GT. Mortality and hallucinations in nursing home patients with advanced Parkinson's disease. Neurology. 1995;45:669–71.
131. Hindle JV. The practical management of cognitive impairment and psychosis in the older Parkinson's disease patient. J Neural Transm. 2013;120(4):649–53.
132. NICE guideline CG103, Delirium: diagnosis, prevention and management. http://www.nice.org.uk/guidance/CG103.
133. Hindle JV. Neuropsychiatry. In: Playfer J, Hindle J, editors. Parkinson's disease in the older patient. 2nd ed. Oxford: Radcliffe; 2008.
134. The Parkinson Study Group. Low-dose clozapine for the treatment of drug-induced psychosis in Parkinson's disease. N Engl J Med. 1999;340(10):757–63.
135. Schulte P. Risk of clozapine-associated agranulocytosis and mandatory white blood cell monitoring. Ann Pharmacother. 2006;40(4):683–8.
136. Taylor D, Paton C, Kapur S. The Maudsley prescribing guidelines. 10th ed. London: Informa Healthcare; 2010.
137. Eng ML, Welty TE. Management of hallucinations and psychosis in Parkinson's disease. Am J Geriatr Pharmacother. 2010;8(4):316–30.
138. Bleakley S. Identifying and reducing the risk of antipsychotic drug interactions. Prog Neurol Psychiatry. 2012;16(2):20–4.
139. Shotbolt P, Samuel M, David A. Quetiapine in the treatment of psychosis in Parkinson's disease. Ther Adv Neurol Disord. 2010;3(6):339–50.
140. Huybrechts KF, Schneeweiss S, Gerhard T, Olfson M, Avorn J, Levin R, Lucas JA, Crystal S. Comparative safety of antipsychotic medications in nursing home residents. J Am Geriatr Soc. 2012;60(3):420–9.
141. Huybrechts KF, Gerhard T, Crystal S, Olfson M, Avorn J, Levin R, Lucas JA, Schneeweiss S. Differential risk of death in older residents in nursing homes prescribed specific antipsychotic drugs: population based cohort study. BMJ. 2012;344:e977.
142. Murray M. Role of CYP pharmacogenetics and drug-drug interactions in the efficacy and safety of atypical and other antipsychotic agents. J Pharm Pharmacol. 2006;58(7):871–85.
143. Seppi K, Weintraub D, Coelho M, Perez-Lloret S, Fox SH, Katzenschlager R, Hametner EM, Poewe W, Rascol O, Goetz CG, Sampaio C. The movement disorder society evidence-based medicine review update: treatments for the non-motor symptoms of Parkinson's disease. Mov Disord. 2011;26 Suppl 3:S42–80.
144. Goldman JG, Vaughan CL, Goetz CG. An update expert opinion on management and research strategies in Parkinson's disease psychosis. Expert Opin Pharmacother. 2011;12(13):2009–24.
145. Emre M, Aarsland D, Albanese A, Byrne EJ, Deuschl G, De Deyn PP, Durif F, Kulisevsky J, van Laar T, Lees A, Poewe W, Robillard A, Rosa MM, Wolters E, Quarg P, Tekin S, Lane R. Rivastigmine for dementia associated with Parkinson's disease. N Engl J Med. 2004;351(24):2509–18.
146. Burn D, Emre M, McKeith I, De Deyn PP, Aarsland D, Hsu C, Lane R. Effects of rivastigmine in patients with and without visual hallucinations in dementia associated with Parkinson's disease. Mov Disord. 2006;21(11):1899–907.
147. Cummings J, Isaacson S, Mills R, Williams H, Chi-Burris K, Corbett A, Dhall R, Ballard C. Pimavanserin for patients with Parkinson's disease psychosis: a randomised, placebo-controlled phase 3 trial. Lancet. 2014;383(9916):533–40.
148. Li CT, Tsai SJ, Hwang JP. Pramipexole-induced psychosis in Parkinson's disease. Psychiatry Clin Neurosci. 2008;62(2):245.
149. Habermeyer B, Kneifel S, Lotz-Bläuer I, Müller-Spahn F. Psychosis in a case of schizophrenia and Parkinson's disease. J Neuropsychiatry Clin Neurosci. 2008;20(3):373–5.

Chapter 7 Neuropsychiatric Manifestations in Atypical Parkinsonian Syndromes

Iva Stankovic and Gregor K. Wenning

Introduction

Neuropsychiatric symptoms are common in atypical parkinsonian disorders. Among a range of psychopathology, cognitive impairment is the best described feature in dementia with Lewy bodies (DLB) and progressive supranuclear palsy (PSP), while apraxia has been carefully studied in corticobasal degeneration (CBD). Multiple system atrophy (MSA) has been traditionally considered as a disorder without psychiatric symptoms, despite growing evidence suggesting they may be an integral part of the disease. Different behavioral, psychiatric, and personality disturbances frequently overlap, establishing behavioral symptoms as quite insufficient diagnostic markers especially in the early stages of the disease. Considering the heterogeneous pathological and neurochemical substrates underlying the similar clinical appearance, future work on larger series of post-mortem proven cases is warranted to determine the true prevalence and to better assess neuropsychiatric problems. Sleep problems frequently occur in the premotor phase of synucleinopathies, representing the key issue that may underpin efforts to develop neuroprotective therapy. Despite relatively sufficient data on anti-dementing drugs in DLB, limited evidence exist on their use in other atypical parkinsonisms. Similarly, the efficacy and tolerability of commonly used psychotropic agents is widely unknown, highlighting an urgent need for well designed double-blind placebo-controlled trials to evaluate their effectiveness.

I. Stankovic, MD
Movement Disorders Department, Neurology Clinic, Clinical Center of Serbia, Dr. Subotica 6, Belgrade 11000, Serbia
e-mail: idstanko139@gmail.com

G.K. Wenning, MD, PhD, MSC (✉)
Division of Neurobiology, Department of Neurology, Innsbruck Medical University, Anichstrasse 35, Innsbruck A-6020, Austria
e-mail: gregor.wenning@i-med.ac.at

H. Reichmann (ed.), *Neuropsychiatric Symptoms of Movement Disorders*, Neuropsychiatric Symptoms of Neurological Disease,
DOI 10.1007/978-3-319-09537-0_7

Neuropsychiatric Manifestations in Multiple System Atrophy

Introduction

Multiple system atrophy is characterized by various combinations of parkinsonism, cerebellar ataxia, autonomic failure, urogenital dysfunction, and corticospinal disorders, with the widespread oligodendroglial alpha-synuclein accumulation, as a pathological hallmark of the disease. The differentiation between two main motor subtypes of MSA including parkinsonian variant (MSA-P) and cerebellar variant (MSA-C) is based on the predominantly affected basal ganglia or cerebellar circuits. Although neuropsychiatric features are not reported commonly as in other parkinsonian disorders, the increasing evidence on a wide spectrum of cognitive and psychiatric disturbances, together with well described sleep disorders, led to the increased interest in those symptoms recently. However, consensus diagnostic criteria for MSA consider dementia and hallucinations as nonsupporting features [1], although recent studies estimated dementia prevalence rates of up to 31 % [2, 3] and psychosis rates of up to 9 % [4]. Despite the lack of longitudinal neuropsychiatric assessment in pathologically proven cases, several lines of evidence suggest an interaction of subcortical deafferentation and intrinsic cortical pathology underlying cognitive decline, while more detailed evaluation is needed to better elucidate the origin of psychiatric symptoms in MSA.

Cognitive Impairment

Although global cognitive impairment is not a consistent feature of MSA, a recent study revealed reduced Mini-Mental State Examination (MMSE) scores in 26 % of MSA patients [2]. The mean prevalence of cognitive impairment in MSA is 13 % to 31 % [2, 3], with mild, moderate, and severe impairment in 22 %, 2 %, and 0.5 % of confirmed MSA cases, respectively [5]. Despite comparative studies between MSA-P and MSA-C patients reveal diverse findings [6–8], difficulties in immediate recall in MSA-P and impaired learning and long-term memory in MSA-C compared to controls may reflect different subcortical degeneration patterns, pointing the roles of basal ganglia and cerebellum in cognitive processes. Time interval to reach clinically significant symptoms is estimated to be 7 years [3]. The presence of cognitive impairment in almost 50 % of the patients surviving more than 8 years (7 %) [2] indicates that if the disease would not have such a rapid course, it would be possible to recognize even more demented patients, comparably to high dementia rate in advanced Parkinson's disease (PD) in long-term follow-up studies. In favor of this are 14 % of MSA patients found to be demented in the last year prior to death [3] and exceptional long-term survival cases with mean onset of dementia after 17 years [9]. Aiming to overcome the weakness of the existing consensus criteria classifying dementia as a nonsupporting feature [1], several researchers omitted the dementia criterion of the consensus statement and defined dementia according to the Parkinson's disease dementia (PDD) criteria, Diagnostic and Statistical Manual of Mental Disorders, Fourth Edition-revised criteria, cut-off values of dementia rating scales or employed other clinical MSA criteria which only define "signs of severe dementia" as an exclusion criterion.

Frontal-executive dysfunction is a prominent cognitive disturbance affecting 32 % to 49 % of MSA patients [2, 7, 10]. A diversity of impaired executive processes have been reported in 40 % of MSA-P patients [7], including salient verbal dysfluency [8, 11], impaired speed of thinking, problem solving, attentional set shifting, mental flexibility [8], and abstract reasoning with more perseverative tendencies [8], while reports regarding conceptual thinking and response inhibition are sparse [6, 8, 11]. Abnormal Frontal Assessment Battery (FAB) [7] and longer time needed to complete Trail Making Test (TMT) [6] are accompanied with conflicting reports on Wisconsin Card Sorting Test (WCST) and Stroop performance in similar proportion of MSA-C patients [6, 7, 8]. Verbal fluency is moderately decreased in some [6], but not in all MSA-C cohorts [8], possibly influenced by depression and anxiety. Impairments of attention and working memory in MSA are similar to that observed in PSP [2]; however, intact attention and working memory have also been reported in both MSA-P and MSA-C [6, 7].

Memory decline, noted in 10 % to 66 % MSA patients [2, 7, 10], includes learning [7], recall [2, 7, 10], and less commonly recognition difficulties [2]. Impaired spontaneous immediate recall is reported in 16.4 % MSA-P patients, while learning, delayed recall, recognition, and visual memory [6, 7, 8, 11] are less often impaired. While learning deficit is the most prominent memory dysfunction in MSA-C, variable results have been reported regarding recall [6, 7] and recognition disturbances [6].

MSA patients exhibit some visuospatial and constructional difficulties compared to controls [8, 10], although sometimes inconsistently reported [2, 12]. While MSA-P show impairment in visuospatial abilities [8] presumably due to attention deficits, Kawai and colleagues found visuospatial impairment as the only cognitive difficulty in MSA-C [8], while other results regarding this are not convincing [6]. Language functions seem to be preserved in the majority of MSA patients [10, 13], although have not been studied carefully. Apraxia is present in 8 % to 10 % of both MSA motor subtypes and may be attributed to dysfunction of supplemental motor and premotor areas.

A correlation between pontine, midbrain, and cerebellar atrophy and decline in different cognitive domains as well as global cognition in MSA patients [14], supported by observed cerebellar hypoperfusion associated with visuospatial decline in MSA-C [8] and postmortem widespread degenerative changes in basal ganglia and cerebellar circuits [5] favor the hypothesis of primary subcortical deafferentation of cortical regions. On the other hand, a characteristic pattern of prefrontal, frontal, temporal, and parietal cortical atrophy in MSA-P [15] and MSA-C [16], supported by variety of post-mortem degenerative changes, has been reported. The correlations between prefrontal atrophy and overall memory scores in MSA [6] and between dorsolateral prefrontal hypoperfusion and visuospatial impairment in both motor MSA subtypes and executive dysfunction in

MSA-P [8], supported by frontal hypometabolism in early MSA-C, spreading to other cortical regions in advanced disease [10], contrary to steady cerebellar hypometabolism, argue for primary cortical involvement in the cognitive deficits. Brenneis and colleagues reported a marked progression of brain atrophy in patients with MSA-P including striatum, mesencephalon, thalamus, and cerebellum, but also cortical regions such as the primary sensorimotor cortex, supplementary motor area, lateral premotor cortex, medial and middle frontal gyrus, orbitofrontal cortex, insula, posterior parietal cortex, and hippocampus. While short disease duration was correlated with progression of subcortical atrophy, longer disease duration was correlated with increasing atrophy in the cortical areas and cerebellar hemispheres, thus suggesting that early degeneration of the basal ganglia drives late-onset cortical atrophy [15]. Degeneration of pedunculopontine nucleus (PPN) and dorsolateral tegmental nuclei (DLTN) [17] in accordance with diminished cortical and subcortical acetylcholinesterase activity [18] and increased amyloid burden in some demented MSA cases are likely to be additional contributors to the cognitive decline.

Behavioral and Psychiatric Manifestations

Behavioral and psychiatric changes in MSA include frequent depression, apathy, and anxiety. Approximately 40 % to 85 % MSA patients harbor at least dysthymia or mild depression [7, 19, 20], while 28 % to 50 % are moderately to severely depressed [19, 20]. The comparative studies of the rates of depression in MSA, PSP [2, 21], and PD [7] yield conflicting results. The depressive symptoms most frequently identified by MSA patients are fatigue, dissatisfaction, loss of libido, work inhibition, sadness, and hopelessness [19]. Anxiety occurs in 37 % of MSA patients similarly as in PSP [21] and less frequently compared to PD patients [7]. Although high levels of depression and anxiety are present in both MSA motor subtypes [6–8], MSA-P patients tend to be more depressed compared to more anxious MSA-C patients [6]. The mood disturbances and anxiety influence executive, memory, and visuospatial performance [7], albeit not in all cohorts [2]. Depression is one of the major contributors to the poor life satisfaction in MSA patients. However, the weak correlation between cognitive impairment and quality of life is presumably due to the insufficient recognition of cognitive decline in MSA. MSA patients often appear to be more apathetic with a blunted affect compared to PD patients [7]. Other psychiatric symptoms may be also present in MSA, including anhedonia, panic attacks, aggressiveness, unreasonable fear and delirium, aberrant motor behavior, irritability, and disinhibition [7]. While hallucinations are very infrequent (9 %) [4], presumably due to the younger age, lower total levodopa dose, and structural changes affecting predominantly the brainstem, basal ganglia, and related motor regions, confusion occurs somewhat more commonly (17.2 %) in MSA.

Sleep Disorders

MSA is considered as a synucleinopathy with the most severe sleep-related disorders clearly recognized as a part of the disease. Determinants of sleep disturbances in MSA include longer disease duration, higher motor scores, more disability, and depression. Since the self-awareness about sleep problems is often poor, polysomnography is requisite for REM sleep behavior disorder (RBD) diagnosis and assessment of other associated, potentially fatal sleep disorders. The estimated rate of RBD in MSA of 88 % to 100 % points that the absence of RBD is strongly questionable for MSA diagnosis. The fact that in 30–50 % of the patients RBD symptoms precede the onset of typical clinical signs of MSA for years or decades affirms RBD as a premotor symptom of an evolving neurodegenerative disorder. Interestingly, parkinsonism in MSA significantly improves during RBD compared to wakefulness. However, RBD-related movements are not resulting from the restoration of the dopaminergic loop because postsynaptic dopaminergic receptors are diminished in MSA. While 20 % of patients with RBD report episodes of sleep walking or sleep terror in the childhood, 10 % have positive family history for this disorder [22–24].

Sleep fragmentation is the most frequent sleep complaint reported in 53 % of patients, followed by early waking (33 %) and insomnia (20 %). MSA sleep pattern includes reduced total sleep time, low sleep efficiency, reduction of both rapid eye movements (REM) sleep and slow wave sleep, increased periodic limb movements in sleep (PLMS), and restless leg syndrome (RLS). MSA-C patients are reported to exhibit higher REM sleep latency and apnea/hypopnea index, contrary to MSA-P patients who endorse RLS more commonly. Besides more frequent RBD, MSA patients also perform REM sleep without atonia, higher PLMS index, less total sleep time, and RLS more commonly compared to PD patients [22, 24, 25].

MSA-related breathing disorders include nocturnal stridor, as an exclusive feature of 13 % to 24 % of MSA patients [5, 22, 25], and obstructive sleep apnea (OSA) occurring in 15 % to 37 % of patients. Stridor is associated with reduced survival due to the pharyngeal and laryngeal obstruction possibly leading sudden death during sleep and may precede onset of motor symptoms in 29 % of patients [25].

Treatment Considerations

Pharmacological treatment strategies for neuropsychiatric manifestations in MSA are very limited, which may be due to the underestimation of those symptoms in MSA. There is no interventional study with any of the neuropsychiatric symptoms defined as the primary outcome measure in MSA. Encouraging evidence of antidepressants as anti-inflammatory and synuclein-reducing agents shown to improve motor abilities but not depressive symptoms in transgenic mouse models and MSA patients by modulating serotonergic transmission settled a trace for the future investigation [26].

The treatment of RBD and sleep-related disorders is the same as in DLB. However, before prescribing clonazepam in MSA, ruling out stridor and OSA is needed, since it may worsen apneas. Patients prone to upper airway obstruction may be treated with melatonin. There is some evidence of efficacy of serotonergic therapy in maintaining the glottis opening during sleep.

Conclusion and Future Directions

Neuropsychiatric manifestations in MSA became increasingly perceived in the era of the nonmotor symptoms recognition in other parkinsonian disorders. Executive functions and fluency are the most commonly affected, while attention, memory, and visuospatial domains are less often impaired. Despite relatively sparse reports for the distinction in cognitive patterns of MSA-P and MSA-C patients, available evidence suggest that visuospatial impairment and learning disturbances appear more typically in MSA-C patients, while MSA-P patients seem to exhibit more executive problems and recall deficits improving with cueing. Deafferentation from subcortical structures as an early feature and intrinsic cortical pathology contributing later into the disease jointly underlie cognitive disturbances in MSA. The prospective longitudinal studies on sufficient number of autopsy-proven cases, based on detailed neuropsychology and psychiatry assessment, correlated with imaging evidence is requisite for better understanding of clinical features and pathophysiological underpinnings of neurobehavioral and cognitive changes in MSA. Next step would be to assess the efficacy and tolerability of commonly used medications in other parkinsonian disorders including cholinesterase inhibitors (ChEIs), memantine, antidepressants, and anxiolytics. However, initially, cognitive and psychiatric symptoms should be included as endpoints in future clinical studies in MSA. While careful assessment and treatment of sleep problems should be provided due to potentially fatal outcomes, treatment of comorbid depression in these patients will likely improve their life satisfaction, despite the presence of other debilitating deficits.

Neuropsychiatric Manifestations in Dementia with Lewy Bodies

Introduction

Dementia with Lewy bodies is the second most common neurodegenerative cause of dementia after Alzheimer's disease (AD) with the estimated prevalence of 15 % to 30 % of all dementia cases [27]. The central clinical feature of DLB is cognitive impairment associated with extrapyramidal signs, fluctuating cognition, and well-formed recurrent visual hallucinations arbitrary arising within 12 months from parkinsonism onset. Additionally, RBD is listed as a suggestive feature, while depression, hallucinations in other modalities, and systematized delusions are supportive for DLB diagnosis [28]. DLB and PDD share similar neurochemical and neuropathological background despite distinctive clinical appearance and most likely represent different points in the Lewy body (LB) disease spectrum [29]. Several lines of evidence suggest that cholinergic deficits in selective brain regions along with LB pathology and neuronal loss underlie cognitive and psychiatric features of DLB. Although traditionally considered as a disease of alpha-synuclein aggregates, the concomitant amyloid pathology frequently co-occurs, influencing psychiatric symptoms [28, 30].

Hallucinations and Delusions

Visual hallucinations (VH) are one of the major clinical features of DLB [28], usually occurring in around 70 % of patients, although the rates vary from 25 % to 90 % [31]. VH are well-formed, three-dimensional, vivid, colorful, and mute images of adults, animals, children, or objects, reoccurring in the low stimulating environment typically early in the course of the disease [31, 32]. Auditory hallucinations may be present in 11 % to 45 % of patients [31], while hallucinations in other modalities are less common. The presence or recent history of VH in patients with mild dementia seems to be the strongest predictor of DLB diagnosis with 99 % specificity [33]. While the associations between VH and older age, later disease onset, vulnerability to antiparkinsonian agents, and the severity of dementia are conflicting [34–36], visuospatial and visual information processing impairment invariably predicts psychosis. Genetic analyses failed to find any marker of genetic susceptibility for psychosis in DLB patients so far. Hallucinatory syndrome and psychosis are more frequent in DLB compared to other synucleinopathies, [13, 35] while the comparative studies with AD show opposite results [32, 35]. Clinical correlates of hallucinations in DLB are different from those in PD, suggesting that neurobiological differences between disorders are not merely quantitative. Delusions including paranoid ideation, phantom boarder, Capgras syndrome, and TV characters misidentifications occur somewhat less frequently than VH, affecting 13 % to 75 % of patients [31].

Visual inattention, the main cognitive determinant for VH, combined with fluctuations in consciousness and disturbed perceptual processes are proposed in "perception and attention deficit model" of VH. Existing evidence suggest that it is most likely that VH are related to disruption of cholinergic projections to higher tertiary visual association regions of the temporal cortex [37] which contain abundant LB pathology [38] despite the limited atrophy and local pathological changes [39]. Therefore, extrastriatal visual pathway involved in color and shape recognition is primarily affected. The metabolic and perfusion reductions in the occipital cortex and precuneus improving after donepezil treatment [40] with variable, usually not prominent atrophy [27], implicate that occipital-temporal visual stream abnormalities for object and face recognition are preferably due to reduced occipital cholinergic inputs [37]. Additionally, changes in amygdala [38] fail to modulate visual processing according to cognition and emotion, while dysfunctions of dorsal visual steam and anterior cingulate cortex and its limbic inputs [34] are responsible for changes in spatial vision and motion perception [37]. While there are the contradictory findings regarding the influence of hypodopaminergic state, the increased activity of the serotonergic system is associated with VH [41]. The association of distinguishable cerebral networks with different psychotic symptoms in DLB along with damage of frontal regions [37] suggests that delusions may be neurobiologically distinct from VH.

Behavioral and Psychiatric Manifestations

Behavioral changes debut characteristically early in DLB sometimes many years prior presenting cognitive decline or parkinsonism. Behavioral and psychiatric problems affect majority of patients and weakly correlate with cognitive decline [31]. Depression and anxiety are recognized as risk factors for DLB, occurring more frequently than in AD [31, 42] and PDD patients [35] and on the similar rate as in PD and MSA patients [13]. Despite variable depression prevalence reported, 14 % to 33 % of patients exhibit major depressive disorder [31]. Among initially depressed patients, 73 % suffer persistent symptoms, while 23 % develop depression incidentally [43]. The profile of depression in DLB includes low mood, diminished future outlook, and increased worry more frequently than decreased concentration, apathy, or the lack of energy. At least half of DLB patients report anxiety which can be related to frightening hallucinations experience. Anxiety is associated with depression and higher disability in everyday life functioning, but not with agitation and cognitive performance; however, cognitive impairment substantially increases the odds for anxiety [42]. The association between depression and anxiety symptoms and frontal hypometabolism [40] highlights the frontal lobe involvement in neuropsychiatric symptoms in DLB.

The personality changes in DLB include diminished emotional responsiveness, relinquishing hobbies, growing apathy, purposeless hyperactivity [32], disinhibition [13, 36], agitation, irritability, aberrant motor behavior, anhedonia, and loss of energy, while inappropriate hilarity and sexual misdemeanor do not occur [32, 36]. Somatoform disorders occur in up to 19 % of DLB patients showing different motor and nonmotor patterns of hysteria, bizarre somatic delusions, catatonic posture stereotypes, and negativism, often characterized by psychotic elements [44]. Quality of life determinants in DLB patients include neuropsychiatric disturbances, independency in activities of daily living, delusions, and apathy [45]. Although caregiver burden improves after the initiation of ChEIs, it returns to the baseline level after long-term treatment [46].

Cognitive Impairment

The cognitive profile of substantial attention, executive, and visuospatial dysfunction with relatively preserved memory and naming is characteristic for DLB patients and highly distinguishable from that of AD patients representing dominant memory and naming difficulties [28]. DLB and PDD share the overall similar cognitive decline, which is more pronounced compared to PD and MSA [13]. DLB can pass through non-amnestic or amnestic mild cognitive impairment (MCI) stage evolving into LB disease after approximately 2.6 years [47]. The cumulative proportion of patients who proceed from non-amnestic MCI to DLB is 45 % in the 4-year and 59 % in the 10-year follow-up. Patients with attention-executive or visuospatial MCI are 10 times more likely to develop DLB than AD, suggesting that the non-amnestic MCI may predict underlying LB pathology [47].

A disproportionately salient visuospatial decline particularly concerning the visual distractibility irrespective of the environmental intrusions is the neuropsychological hallmark of the disease in 74 % of patients [33]. The visuospatial decline is more profound compared to PDD and AD [29] implicating its differential diagnostic value. While the early emphasis on presence of visuospatial impairment substantially improves the diagnostic sensitivity, its absence emerges as the best negative predictor for the diagnosis [33]. Therefore, a brief assessment using the Clock Drawing Test or the Pentagon Copying Test may be of the greatest value in the correct and early detection of DLB patients. A prognostic implication of visuospatial dysfunction is reflected through its strong association with the rapid rate of global cognitive decline and VH [30].

The dominance of general and widespread attentional breakdown, another important neuropsychological feature of DLB, becomes more apparent when greater task demands are given, especially when additional recruitment of attention is needed for the executive or visuospatial processes [48]. Although inattention has been reported as an important distinguishing feature from AD and PDD patients [49], such observations are sometimes inconsistent.

Executive dysfunction, reported in as many as 75 % of DLB patients [50], is nearly always more pronounced as compared to AD, while reports concerning verbal dysfluency have been more opposed. Frontal executive dysfunction in DLB is on the lower rate compared to PDD [29]. There is a distinction between both the letter and category fluency compromised in DLB and prominent category dysfluency in AD [51]. Positive applause sign has been noted in as many as 60 % of patients [52]. Importantly, executive performance in DLB may be influenced by impaired visuospatial skills in tasks with visually given stimuli [51].

Learning and recognition decline are frequent in DLB [13, 49]. Although often present, recall deficits are not as salient as in AD, albeit not in all studies [49]. Recall deficits likely result from pervasive attentional deficit preventing initial encoding, contrary to AD where encoding is severely diminished. Further, semantic memory impairment overlaps with visuospatial and executive deficits, providing poor performance on the picture meaning tasks [51]. The overall memory scores are similar to PDD and worse compared to PSP patients [29]. Despite language impairment is not one of the core cognitive features of DLB [49], it may be present in the form of confabulations, speech incoherence, and increased environmental verbal intrusions. Naming is similarly [49] or less frequently impaired compared to that in AD [30]. No praxis deficits have been observed in DLB patients [52].

The imaging and histopathology evidence of the neuronal loss in midbrain, hypothalamus, and basal forebrain supported by the reduced cortical acetylcholinesterase (ChAT) activity [53] and altered cholinergic receptors [34], suggest the principal role of the disruption of ascending cholinergic pathways from nucleus basalis of Meynert (nbM), DLTN, and PPN in cognitive and psychiatric manifestations in DLB [17, 27]. Severe neocortical cholinergic denervation [53] and extensive cortical ChAT decline beginning in early-stage disease favor the cholinergic origin of dementia. A relative sparing of temporoparietal cortex, hippocampus, and amygdala serve as potential explanation for preserved episodic memory in DLB [27, 39]. Nevertheless, there are controversial reports regarding the relationship between cognitive performance and neocortical LB and ChAT activity and the influence of AD pathology on the rate of cognitive decline [30].

Cognitive and Behavioral Fluctuations

Fluctuations represent brief episodes of increased confusion and cognitive impairment, interruptions of consciousness, diminished arousal, prolonged sleep, daytime drowsiness, disorganized speech, or staring into space for long periods [32]. Although fluctuations are noted in 46 % of patients [27], their occurrence and severity may be difficult to capture since they range from minutes to days [32]. Attentional deficits underlie and alternate in parallel with cognitive fluctuations in intervals from seconds to hours. Bradshaw and colleagues suggest that second-to-second variations reflect basic, continuous, subclinical level of attentional dysregulation provoked by ascending cholinergic depletion, while more robust, clinically significant individual episodes, influenced by situational condition or task demands, are likely triggered by impaired cortical influence on attention processing [48]. Neurochemical evidence suggest that amplification of nicotinic receptors in thalamus, temporal cortex, and hippocampus [54] and muscarinic M4 receptors in the anterior cingulate cortex [34] together with the loss thalamic inputs from PPN and DLTN [17] influences small variations in neurotransmission causing the instability of mechanisms underlying disturbances of consciousness in DLB. Despite the hypothesized distinct relationship between the damage of the cholinergic system and attention and consciousness disturbances, the neuropathological and neurochemical evidence do not support this causality [17], pointing that magnitude of cholinergic transmission depends on the complex interplay with other neurotransmitter systems.

Sleep Disorders

RBD usually precedes the onset of cognitive decline or parkinsonism for 10 or more years and together with MCI represents a prodromal phase of LB disease [47], improving the overall diagnostic accuracy when incorporated in the diagnostic clinical criteria [28]. Nightmares without atonia and excessive daytime sleepiness (EDS) may also portend other clinical signs [47]. The early metabolic changes in the occipital lobe and characteristic early EEG abnormalities in patients with RBD subsequently evolving into DLB suggest an opportunity for the neuroprotective measures in the preclinical disease phase.

REM-related phenomena occur in 50 % to 87 % of more likely younger male patients with the earlier onset of visual hallucinations and parkinsonism relative to dementia onset and shorter dementia duration while the associations between RBD and dementia severity are diverse [36, 55, 56]. Histopathologically, patients who exhibit RBD have lower AD pathology burden in the hippocampus and amygdala, while reports regarding the predominance of limbic vs. neocortical LB type are adversative [55, 56]. While the "bottom-up" progression through Braak staging has been proposed in DLB with RBD, DLB patients without RBD presumably have early corticolimbic Lewy-related pathology with the "top-down" progression, although autopsy-based study assessing this issue is missing [55]. RBD may be related to alpha-synuclein-mediated degenerative changes of sleep-regulating nuclei in the pontine tegmentum and basal forebrain. However, imaging and postmortem findings of neuronal loss in PPN and DLTN without apparent relationship to RBD symptoms suggest its modulatory effect, rather than the central role [17]. Additionally, gray matter loss in cerebellum and hippocampal gyrus represents characteristic structural change in synucleinopathies with RBD.

A little data exist on other common sleep disorders in DLB. RBD is often complicated with the increase in the PLMS, associated with the decrease in the dopaminergic activity. The rate of EDS is at least similar compared to that in PD and more frequent compared to AD. Recurrent dream enactment behavior, sleep-disordered breathing, reduced sleep efficiency, arousal episodes, dysrhythmic breathing, sleep talking, insomnia, and overall impaired sleep structure have been reported relatively frequently, while RLS has not been described in DLB patients [57].

Treatment Considerations

Drugs enhancing central cholinergic function offer a rationally based therapeutic approach targeting mainly cognitive and hallucinatory syndromes. ChEIs are the widely accepted first-line treatment with good efficacy and tolerability, acceptable adversative events (AE), and proven maintenance of the effect after long-term administration [46]. All the interventional trials with ChEIs have shown the improvement neuropsychiatric symptoms, while effects on cognitive performance are not always promising [58]. Additionally, an extensive reduction in amyloid deposition in patients treated with ChEIs suggests a significant impact upon this key disease substrate.

Clinically important improvements with rivastigmine include diminished hallucinations, delusions, apathy, anxiety, agitation, indifference, sleep disorders, and aberrant motor behavior, while the efficacy in enhancing cognitive functions is limited and variably reported [59], except for attention-related cognitive deficits. The donepezil dose of 10 mg daily is recommended for improving cognitive and psychiatric manifestations, and reducing the caregiver burden [60]. There is so far no compelling evidence that any one ChEI is better than the other in treating DLB. The worsening of parkinsonism and cardiac dysrhythmia remains the major concerns during the use of ChEIs [46], although nausea, vomiting, and anorexia are observed relatively frequently (31.5 %) [46, 59]. Prolonging the intervals between dose increases has been shown to be associated with improved tolerability for this class of drugs. The issue of whether to switch or stay on the first prescribed ChEI in case of intolerance or absence of a clinically apparent effect still depends on clinician's subjectivity, since it has not been systematically investigated.

However, 24 % to 35 % of patients have psychosis resistant to ChEIs [59]. Treatment of DLB-related psychosis is based on reducing environmental risk factors, avoiding medicamental polypragmasia and drugs with anticholinergic effect. The particularly disturbing and resistant hallucinations need to be treated with quetiapine, clozapine, or olanzapine, since the evidence of their effectiveness are mostly supportive. Given the narrow therapeutic window of quetiapine and significant side effects of clozapine, careful monitoring should be considered. The neuroleptics and atypical antipsychotics should be avoided, due to the potent antidopaminergic effects frequently precipitating the malignant neuroleptic syndrome in 27 % to 53 % of DLB patients [61]. Both improvement and worsening of hallucinations were noted with memantine use with only a small benefit in cognition. Memantine has been proven as efficient in overall sleeping and nighttime behavior improvement, but not in the treatment of EDS [62].

The low efficacy of antidepressants in cognitively impaired patients with the high risk of adverse events together with treatment-related parahippocampal thinning suggests the need to reevaluate treatment approaches for depression and the role of antidepressants in patients with DLB. Since the density of serotonin 1A receptors is increased in temporal cortex, adjuvant serotonergic antagonist may improve treatment of depression in dementia [63]. Despite there have been no systematic studies on the management of depression, selective serotonin reuptake inhibitors and serotonin-norepinephrine reuptake inhibitors are preferred, while tricyclic antidepressants and those with anticholinergic properties should generally be avoided [28]. Electroconvulsive therapy and transcranial magnetic stimulations are reported as effective and safe therapeutic tools for drug therapy-resistant depression in DLB.

Except one small double-blind, placebo-controlled melatonin trial [64], no other study of similar design has been reported for other drug treatment for RBD. The first-line therapy for RBD is clonazepam commonly effective at doses of 0.25 to –0.5 mg/night, but doses above 1 mg nightly are necessary in some patients. Melatonin in doses ranging from 3 to 15 mg/night and ramelteon, melatonin receptors agonist, can be effective either as monotherapy or in conjunction with clonazepam when either melatonin or clonazepam alone is ineffective. Other drugs reported to improve RBD include memantine, pramipexole, donepezil, levodopa, carbamazepine, triazolam, clozapine, and quetiapine. RBD can be precipitated or aggravated by certain classes of medications, particularly the new generation of antidepressant drugs including mirtazapine and venlafaxine or excessive consumption of caffeine or chocolate.

Conclusion and Future Directions

Among disorders presenting with parkinsonism, DLB is widely regarded as a neuropsychiatric illness according to current clinical criteria [28]. The specific fluctuating cognitive and behavioral pattern allows its differentiation from other dementing syndromes. Visuospatial and attentional deficits are the neuropsychological hallmark of the disease. The executive disturbances are very frequent, influencing performance in other cognitive domains while memory is often mildly affected with relatively preserved recall. Neuropsychological testing therefore has a valuable role in differentiation among demented patients, especially in the early disease when non-amnestic MCI may predict underlying LB disease. Peculiar early VH occurring simultaneously with onset of parkinsonism can help to distinguish DLB from PDD. Sleep-related problems may precede the onset of dementia, and the combination of those symptoms should facilitate the diagnosis of DLB. Depression together with the range of other psychiatric manifestations is very common in DLB and should be early appreciated and appropriately treated affording the opportunity to lessen caregiver burden and improve patient and caregiver outcomes. A growing body of evidence suggests that neuropsychiatric manifestations in DLB originate from widespread cholinergic denervation, although additional influence of LB and AD-like pathology needs to be considered.

The issue of accurate clinical identification of DLB patients is increasingly important not only in the light of functional disability, prognosis, and caregiver burden, but for choosing the appropriate treatment strategy considering a good efficacy and tolerability of ChEIs and avoiding classic neuroleptics. Considering the limited cognitive improvement, ChEIs nonresponders could be good candidates for future trials with new medications. Despite six randomized controlled trials in DLB [58], future trials with different classes of medications, mainly antidepressants and antipsychotics, are needed. Finally, reduced dopamine transporter binding and substantia nigra hypoechogenicity in patients with idiopathic RBD who are about to develop neurodegenerative disorder within 5 years represent valuable markers for screening eligible patients to be enrolled in future trials of disease-modifying or neuroprotective therapy [65].

Neuropsychiatric Manifestations in Progressive Supranuclear Palsy

Introduction

The classical form of progressive supranuclear palsy, Steele-Richardson-Olszewski syndrome (PSP-RS), is a tauopathy presenting with supranuclear vertical gaze palsy, axial rigidity, postural instability, and symmetric akinetic-rigid syndrome poorly responsive to levodopa. Even from the initial clinical descriptions, PSP-RS is recognized as a prototypical "subcortical dementia." PSP-parkinsonism (PSP-P) is a more benign PSP subtype with asymmetric parkinsonian features, non-axial dystonia, at least initial levodopa responsivity, and pathologically less severe and a subtly different tau accumulation [66]. Considering the significant clinical overlaps among tauopathies and different phenotypic presentations within PSP, it is not surprising that at least 20 % to 30 % of patients remain undiagnosed during life [66, 67]. The core frontal lobe symptomatology in PSP results from both the disruption of subcortico-frontal inputs and internal frontal cortical pathology, with the minor contribution from cholinergic deafferentation and possibly co-occurring AD-like changes.

Cognitive Impairment

The prototypical "subcortical dementia" is characterized by impaired executive functioning, diminished attention, and psychomotor slowing. While some degree of cognitive impairment is present in up to 85 % of PSP patients [2, 68], 34 % of patients score below 25 on MMSE [2]. Cognitive impairment commonly, although not consistently, remains unrelated to the duration of illness [2, 68, 69], while the results are conflicting regarding the predictive value of an early dementia on shortened survival. The longitudinal studies of the disease progression reveal diverse findings, from the lack of progression of cognitive impairment over the years to more than twice as double increase in its prevalence between the first 2 years and the advanced disease stage [69]. Dementia occurs in 62 % of PSP-RS patients who reach the clinical milestone for dementia earlier, compared to 28 % demented PSP-P patients [3].

Frontal executive dysfunction, exhibited by 55 % to 88 % of patients, comprises a range of impaired abilities [2, 68], classically manifested by decreased verbal fluency [2, 70], more perseverative errors on TMT and WCST, and impaired control over attention, planning, set shifting, reasoning, and execution of sequential actions [2, 11, 68, 71]. Verbal fluency has been most profoundly affected [2] with the reverse pattern of more declined lexical compared to semantic fluency from that seen in AD. Executive dysfunction markedly influences performance in all cognitive domains. An increased rate of frontal lobe signs from 46 % to 58 % in median

2.2 years period, contrary to more pronounced decline in other symptoms, contrasts the associations between fontal decline and increased rates of midbrain and frontal cortical atrophy over time [14]. Whether executive functions deteriorate in parallel or independently from behavioral functioning also remains unclear [68, 72, 73].

Applause sign is a frequent motor perseveration in 70 % to 90 % of patients [52]. Impaired scores on verbal fluency and inhibitory control tests can predict worse outcome on applause sign task, which originates from insufficient planning and inability to stop once relieved automatic activities due to the basal ganglia and frontal lesions [74]. Despite earlier reports on its ability to clinically distinguish PSP from PD and behavioral variant of frontotemporal dementia (bvFTD), it should not be used as a diagnostic value, as suggested recently, due to its insufficient specificity.

An increasing frontal atrophy has been associated with growing number of errors on the WCST and decline in Paced Auditory Serial Addition Test and FAB performance in a longitudinal study [14]. More precisely, decline on Stroop and Weigl executive tests are shown to be associated with the hypoperfusion in the posterior part of midcingulate cortex [75], while disrupted fronto-occipital connections are found in patients with severe dysexecutive syndrome. The marked contribution of the brainstem and subcortical structures damage to the cognitive dysfunction is shown through the strong association between a decline in the FAB score and increased rates of midbrain atrophy [14]. Moreover, the significant correlation between poor executive and overall cognitive performance with frontal and cerebellar atrophy suggests the additional role of dysfunctional frontocerebellar circuits [14]. Thalamic pathology disrupting thalamocortical connections is also related to cognitive decline in PSP.

Memory decay pattern of impaired free recall and mild deficits in recognition and learning which improve after cuing, presumably derived from inefficient retrieval strategies due to executive dysfunction, is typical for subcortical dementia. This pattern is robustly contrasting one seen in cortical dementia such as AD. However, analyzing performance in a large group of PSP patients, Gerstenecker and colleagues found low average or only mild impairment in a range of memory functions [68]. In general, memory decline, observed in 17 % to 63 % of patients [2, 68], is milder compared to PDD, DLB, and AD [29] and more severe compared to MSA [2]. However, no difference between PSP, PD, and controls has been observed in terms of short-term memory, delayed recall, and recognition proving its benignity [68, 70]. Structurally normal hippocampal volume in PSP is in keeping with neuropsychological findings [76]. PSP endorse some visuospatial problems (8 % – 24 %) [2, 68], which rather reflect an overall cognitive decline [12].

The rates of logopenia have been variably reported, from more than a quarter to almost all PSP patients affected [70, 73]. Logopenia and anomia both correlate with the disease severity, with the latter being very infrequent in the early disease stages, compared to the evolved disease when 17 % of patients become anomic [70]. Although in the earlier reports, naming was observed as normal despite severe dysfluency, which is known as "verbal adynamia" or "dynamic aphasia," it may be impaired together with comprehension in 19 % of patients [68].

Traditional consideration of PSP-RS patients as prone to develop more significant cognitive impairment compared to PSP-P patients has been demonstrated in the study by O'Sullivan and colleagues [3]. Despite PSP-RS patients have been reported to endorse more neuropsychiatric problems, lower conceptualization subscore on FAB, and dissociative caregivers and patients reports on the degree of apathy, the results of another cohort showed comparable rates of general cognitive decline, frontal dysfunction, and apathy compared to PSP-P patients [77]. Impaired transcallosal inhibition, a sign of altered callosal integrity, correlating with cognitive dysfunction in PSP-RS, but not in PSP-P, probably reflects more severe cognitive decline in the former group.

Ideomotor apraxia in PSP is characterized by impaired transitive movements with more sequencing errors, likely originating from dysfunction of the anterior frontal cortical areas and striatum [78]. The variable rates of other forms of apraxia, including 10 % of patients with the eyelid opening apraxia [73] and 86 % of patients with verbal apraxia on Frontal Behavioral Inventory [70], are consistently less frequent compared to CDB.

Behavioral and Psychiatric Manifestations

Behavioral changes in PSP sometimes remain in the shadow of the motor, oculomotor, and cognitive symptoms. Personality changes, present in 77 % of patients, are usually not as severe and bizarre as occur in bvFTD. However, 20 % of commonly younger patients with PSP have predominant behavioral and cognitive presentation, which often results in establishing the incorrect diagnosis of bvFTD. They do not differentiate in survival compared to other PSP patients, highlighting that frontal symptoms are not predictors of survival. Almost half of the variance of frontal behavioral scores has been explained by disease severity suggesting, although not without exceptions [79], that behavioral and cognitive changes occur in parallel with the motor impairment [70].

Apathy is the most pervasive and almost universal behavioral disturbance, reported in 35 % to 92 % of PSP patients [70, 71, 73, 79, 80], of whom 43 % to 66 % are moderately to severely apathetic [70, 80]. Other negative symptoms including lacking spontaneity, indifference, inflexibility, loss of insight, and disorganization may be also dominant [11, 72, 73] and are far more prevalent compared to positively disinhibited behavior [11]. The rate of diminished motivation in PSP is lower compared to that in bvFTD but significantly higher compared to PD [11, 72] and corticobasal syndrome [73]. Apathy is unrelated to other neuropsychiatric symptoms [80], while variably related to executive functioning [71, 80] and the disease duration, suggesting that disruption of different frontal subcortical circuits independently contributes neuropsychiatric and cognitive symptoms in PSP [71]. The dissociation between apathy and motor impairment further suggests it is not dopamine dependent [73].

Among positive frontal symptoms, disinhibition and agitation affect around one third of the patients [29, 71, 80], while poor judgment is somewhat more frequent (67 %) [11] and aberrant motor behavior less frequent (<14 %) [80]. Inappropriate crying and laughter are assigned to emotional lability [80], likely as a part of pseudobulbar affect. Often combined increased anxiety (18 % – 37 %), nervousness and irritability (33 %) are present in a significant proportion of patients, although not in all the cohorts [21, 71, 80]. Anxiety may also arise along with the agitation and impaired attention [71].

Depression is relatively variably reported in PSP patients [21, 29, 71, 80, 81], affecting up to two thirds of patients, of whom 16 % to 19 % have moderate to severe depressive symptoms [80]. Patients who are diagnosed with PSP more likely develop depression within the next year and are more often depressed if remain cognitively unimpaired [2]. Depression is more common in PSP than in MSA [21] and PD [72]. Despite apathy and depression are both often reported, they seem to be unrelated [71], sharing only 1 % of the variance and it is believed that they represent distinct processes [80]. Life quality is strongly related with cognitive disability and depression, while frontal lobe symptoms including apathy are reported as more burdensome by caregivers than by patients [80].

Various forms of antisocial behavior including physical assault (30 %), hypersexuality (30 %), neglect of the traffic rules (30 %), public urination (10 %), and obsessive compulsive behavior (24 %) are relatively common in PSP patients [81]. Hallucinations (5–13 %) and delusions (5 %), uncooperativeness, resentment, belligerence, and irresponsibility are rarely present [71, 80–82]. Stereotypic behavior and alterations in eating habits are significantly less common compared to bvFTD patients [81].

Among personality changes, PSP patients exhibit poorer lie and sarcasm comprehension [83, 84]. Deficits in the recognition of the basic negative emotions are supposed to be either linked to the ventral frontal cortex atrophy [85] or alternatively to more widespread brain lesions. However, impaired ability to comprehend verbalized opinions and intentions contrasting preserved comprehension of more explicit visually given perspectives of talking points to focal deficits of social cognition [84]. Diminished social dominance, loss of interpersonal warmth, and extraversion are quite frequent. Executive dysfunction seems to be insufficient to account for the social cognitive deficits, although foci of frontal atrophy are linked to the integration of socially relevant stimuli and interpretation of their social meaning [83].

More frequent disinhibition compared to less hallucination, delusion, and depression represent the typical differences between PSP and PD-specific neuropsychiatric profiles [72], while more apathy and less irritability is distinguishing from AD [71] and CBS [73]. Both the severity and frequency of positive symptoms in PSP are significantly less common compared to that of bvFTD, which accounts for the biggest difference between the disorders.

A broad body of evidence suggests that degeneration in both subcortical and cortical sites correlates with the severity of behavioral symptoms. Significant negative correlations were observed between frontal behavioral functions and frontal gray matter atrophy, precisely the atrophy of posterior lateral frontal lobes and inferior fronto-occipital fasciculus due to frontal changes, supported by other imaging evidence of atrophy along with higher neurofibrillary tangles density in frontal regions [79, 80, 86]. The very high rate of apathy suggests the core dysfunction of medial frontal and orbitofrontal regions, proven to correlate with behavioral disturbances [85]. Neuroradiological and histopathological reports of a more marked involvement of the frontal lobes, more precisely orbitofrontal circuit [85] in PSP than in PD extend findings of more severe behavioral symptoms in PSP patients [80], suggesting a greater involvement of intrinsic structural changes within the frontal cortex. Depression is associated with the hypometabolism in dorsolateral prefrontal cortex, while obsessive compulsive behavior may be related to the dysfunction of fronto-caudate-thalamus-cerebellum circuit. On the other hand, disruption of cortical inputs secondary to subcortical pathology [72] is supported by the association between midbrain atrophy and behavioral symptoms [85] and between apathy and putaminal gray matter loss in severely affected patients [79].

Lesions in midbrain and basal forebrain cholinergic nuclei may contribute behavioral and cognitive disturbances. The greatest vulnerability of cholinergic neurons in DLTN compared to milder cholinesterase activity reduction in nbM and PPN may be characteristic for PSP. Preferential loss of thalamic cholinergic innervation along with the reduction in thalamic ChAT activity for 24 %, compared to mildly reduced cortical cholinergic activity points towards the minimal influence of the thalamocortical denervation on behavioral and cognitive symptoms, which is in the line with insufficient efficacy of ChEIs in PSP [71, 87].

Sleep Disorders

PSP patients exhibit poor quality of sleep in terms of reduced sleep efficiency, PLMS, sleep-disordered breathing, RBD, and RLS. Acting out dreams has occurred rarely in 13 % and frequently in 7 % of patients in one study [82]. Additionally, unspecified sleep changes after the disease onset have been reported in as much as 63 % of patients [82]. OSA and vocal cord paralysis have been described on isolated cases with PSP. PSP patients seem less aware of their sleep problems, hence direct questions should be provided in order to access features of disrupted sleep.

Treatment Considerations

Despite some evidence of the beneficial effect of short-acting ChEIs-like physostigmine on memory and visuospatial features, donepezil does not improve cognitive functioning and has possible detrimental effects on motor functions in PSP [88] and therefore cannot be currently recommended for treatment in PSP patients. Decrease in FAB score associated with treatment with coenzyme Q10 in a daily dose of 5 mg/kg body weight, along with mild clinical amelioration, improving energy metabolism, and good tolerability provides an encouraging evidence of its potential neuroprotective effect [89]. Zolpidem, a GABA agonist of the benzodiazepine receptor, has been shown to ameliorate aggressiveness and agitation in a PSP patient, possibly enhancing reduced neurotransmission of GABA in striatum and globus pallidus.

Conclusion and Future Directions

Cognitive decline and psychiatric manifestations in PSP characteristically disclose frontal lobe impairment with pronounced executive dysfunction strongly influencing functioning in other cognitive domains and salient frontal behavioral signs, with apathy and other negative symptoms predominating over the hyperfrontal behavior. Nevertheless, clinical appearance is highly variable, not only quantitatively from one to another patient [80], but also qualitatively presenting with a range of impairments in mood, personality, and social functioning. The dominant subcortical pattern of impaired cognition allows differentiation from AD, while behavioral changes, despite many overlaps, are distinctive from bvFTD, mainly in terms of their severity. Sleep disorders are not exclusively related to synuclein aggregation disorders, but may also be a part of the clinical spectrum of tauopathies. It becomes clear that RBD is not related to a specific pathological mechanism but rather to localizational distribution of tau pathology in regions like brainstem nuclei critically involved in RBD pathophysiology. Sleep problems are poorly investigated in PSP and polysomnography studies in post-mortem confirmed cases could give answers about the influence of tau pathology on the sleep pattern. Since APOE is a risk factor for the co-occurrence of AD-type pathology, the issue of its contribution to cognitive and behavioral symptoms needs to be elucidated in future studies.

Despite the wide appreciation of PSP as disorder of pronounced dementia and psychiatric features and some evidence of possibly distinctive frontal pattern with the lack of self-perception in PSP-RS group, the comparative study of PSP-RS and PSP-P patients assessing cognitive and behavioral presentation complemented with the structural and functional imaging should be promising for sufficient differentiation between PSP subtypes. Treatment options for neuropsychiatric and cognitive problems in PSP including ChEIs are very limited, highlighting the lack of placebo-controlled trials with cognitive and psychiatric symptoms as outcome measures. Therefore, an effort should be directed towards understanding pathophysiological mechanism of neuropsychiatric symptoms in PSP aiming to develop sufficient treatment strategies and neuroprotective therapy.

Neuropsychiatric Manifestations in Corticobasal Syndrome

Introduction

The classical clinical description of corticobasal degeneration includes unilateral arm rigidity, bradykinesia and fixed dystonic posture poorly responsive to levodopa, associated with apraxia, alien limb and cortical sensory loss. Histopathologically, CBD is tauopathy with dominant unilateral parietal and frontal lobar atrophy. Broad evidence suggest that the clinical presentation of CBD may be highly variable. Dominant behavioral changes may mimic frontotemporal lobar degeneration; isolated dysphasia can mislead towards the diagnosis of primary progressive aphasia; vertical gaze palsy and recurrent falls may lead to a diagnosis of PSP-RS, while predominant cognitive dysfunction without marked extrapyramidal symptomatology may masquerade as AD. Marked cognitive impairment, behavioral, and language symptoms, solely presented or accompanied with motor and other cortical signs once referred as exclusion criteria for the diagnosis of CBD, now represent the distinct phenotypic variants of the disease [90]. Considering widely overlapping clinical symptoms with other neurodegenerative disorders presentations, an umbrella term corticobasal syndrome (CBS) has been introduced for discrete clinical presentation corresponding to postmortem diagnosis in up to half of the cases [67, 91].

Apraxia

Asymmetric apraxia, defined as an inability to perform purposeful skilled movements, is a neurobehavioral hallmark of CBD and one of the best predictors for the diagnosis when initially present in 45 % of patients [90]. Ideomotor apraxia is the most common form affecting 75 % of patients [91]. Despite the fairly preserved everyday activities with the apraxic hand, patients with ideomotor apraxia exhibit different degrees of impairment on specific tasks known as "automatic-voluntary dissociation." Limb-kinetic apraxia is an associated feature in some patients, while ideational apraxia arises usually later into the disease. Alien limb phenomenon develops within 1–2 years after the symptom onset on apraxic hand in half of the patients [91] and has been considered to arise due to the lack of the inhibitory control of inferior frontal gyrus over involuntary motor responses. Orobuccofacial apraxia , eyelid opening apraxia, dressing apraxia, and apraxia of speech have been less frequently reported in CBD patients.

Currently accepted framework for understanding apraxia is based on impairment on two main components involved in praxis: the conceptual-representational system, which provides an abstract representation of the action, and the production-execution component, integrating sensorimotor presentation of the action and motor processes needed for its organization and execution. Therefore, the production of skilled movements requires translation of movement representation into specific pattern in motor cortex while disruption on any of those sites may lead to apraxia. The role of frontal and parietal regions including the superior parietal lobule and supplemental motor area in praxis system integration devoted to storage of learned skilled movements and sensorimotor transformations has been confirmed in the positron emission tomography and voxel-based morphometry studies. Diffusion tensor imaging analysis further revealed disrupted fibers between frontal and parietal lobes, within parietal lobe, hand cortical areas, and corpus callosum. Visual information, basal ganglia, and sensory impairment may also contribute to ideomotor apraxia. CBD patients perform worse on production tasks at early disease, while conceptual and representational tasks become more affected as the disease progresses [92]. Given the progressive nature of the disease, it is possible that affection of both hemispheres into the illness accounts for execution deficits in both patients with dominant and nondominant hemisphere affection.

Behavioral and Psychiatric Manifestations

Behavioral and personality changes in CBD patients including apathy or inertion, disinhibition, repetitive behavior, inattention, and hyperorality which, associated with executive dysfunction, can resemble the core symptoms sufficient to meet the criteria for possible bvFTD [93]. Other signs of inadequate social behavior encompass increased agitation, aggressiveness, impulsiveness, hypersexuality, excessive spending, inappropriate laughter, antisocial, bizarre, and obsessive compulsive behaviors [94, 95]. Negative frontal symptoms such as apathy, aspontaneity, and loss of insight seem to be more prevalent compared to "hyperfrontal" syndrome [73]. Frontal lobe behavior may be present at onset in 29 % to 46 % of CBD patients [90, 91] and in up to 60 % of patients during the course of the illness [90, 91, 96, 97]. Patients who present with striking personality changes may become demented later and/or may develop motor signs of CBD, while some of them solely present with behavioral symptoms [97]. Since increased utilization behavior is related to the release of parietal lobe activities, it is possible that dysfunction of this region is related to normal utilization process in CBD [98]. The gray matter loss in frontal, orbitofrontal, dorsomedial, and dorsolateral prefrontal areas and striatum are reported in patients that would be classified as frontal behavioral-spatial syndrome [90]. VH and sleep problems are rare in CBD [82, 99].

Usually subtle depression has been observed in 20 % to 30 % of CBD patients at onset, compared to up to 73 % of patients who can be depressed at some point during the disease [90, 91, 94, 99, 100]. Preserved insight in some patients is associated with frequent complaints about depressive mood [94]. Compared to AD [100] and PSP [99], CBD patients endorse more depressive symptoms. Based on evidence of disruption in fronto-subcortical circuits involved in mediating emotional functions in PD and CBD patients, the same pattern of depression in both disorders has been indicated [99]. Apathy, irritability, and rare disinhibition (7 %) [94] are parts of the same syndrome associated with frontal lobe release signs rather than independent behavioral domains in CBD patients [99]. Apathy seems to be burdensome, particularly if co-occurring with disinhibition, while dementia is a milder contributor [101].

Cognitive Impairment

Cognitive impairment in CBD ranges from mild impairment to severe dementia. The cognitive decline may be the initial symptom in 36 % of patients [91], while up to 70 % of patients show signs of dementia during the disease [90, 91]. Patients initially presenting with cognitive symptoms usually have lower overall cognitive performance compared to patients with initial motor presentation [96]. Cognitive deterioration over time has been noted in many domains and is greatest in CBD compared to PD and PSP patients [102].

Language syndromes such as nonfluent aphasia are present in up to half of the CBD patients and represent one of the hallmarks of the disease [90, 91, 96]. Progressive aphasia may be an initial symptom in a group of CBD patients who subsequently develop motor symptoms and vice versa, aphasia syndrome may arise during the disease course after onset of extrapyramidal or other cortical symptoms, with no later differences between groups [96].

Originally mild dysphasia with word-finding difficulties shows tendency of changing towards transcortical motor aphasia over time. Additionally, effortful speech is present in around half of the patients at onset, suggesting that motor impairment together with speech apraxia and aprosodic speech contribute overall language disturbance [94]. Predominantly receptive aphasic disturbances are not characteristic for CBD patients at least at onset. However, in the end-stage disease, 57 % of patients present comprehension impairment, mostly in understanding complex sentences, that may be related to sensory aphasia, but more likely ideomotor apraxia or executive dysfunction [94]. Agraphia may be present in 30 % to 40 % of patients, due to language, comprehension, executive, motor disturbances, or less often apraxia (20 %) [94]. Impaired oral and written spelling contribute writing impairment even in non-aphasic patients. The relationship between the side of motor onset and hemisphere atrophy with language syndromes is unclear. Although it is generally assumed that left hemisphere atrophy is related to aphasia, it seems not to be a rule in CBD patients. Similar aphasia scores in patients with left- and right-sided onset [96] are supported by imaging evidence of mostly symmetrical parietal atrophy in pathologically proven CBD cases [97].

Neuropsychologically, patients with CBD show tendency to generate a small number of low-frequency rather than high-frequency words, similarly to PSP patients, which may be explained by affection of cortical areas responsible for lexical retrieval and phonological processing during word generation, such as pars triangularis of the inferior frontal gyrus and the dorsolateral prefrontal cortex [102]. Contrary to clear-cut phonological and semantic fluency impairment, results regarding naming are diverse. Normal naming function has been observed in majority of CBD patients, while mildly affected naming improves with provision of phonemic clues in some cases [94, 100]. Both fluency and naming are reported to be worse in patients presenting with cognitive symptoms compared to those with classical motor presentation [96]. Comprehension related to single words is preserved initially and impairment is suggested to be to a certain extent due to executive problems [94], apart from dysphasia. All the language functions significantly deteriorate over time, regardless of the time of the symptom onset in the disease course [96]. Increased severity of dementia can be associated with language decline, and since most CBD patients show gradual language decline, it seems to be the most useful method to quantitatively assess cognitive deterioration. Additionally, neuropsychological testing becomes impossible in many patients in later disease stages due to aphasia, and language assessment remains the only function useful for tracking the disease progression in late-stage disease [94].

Frontal-executive dysfunction associated with frontal behavioral symptoms is common throughout the disease [94, 97, 98]. Murray and colleagues reported dysexecutive syndrome in all 15 autopsy-proven CBD patients emphasizing its high frequency in one of the largest post-mortem confirmed case studies assessing cognitive functioning [94]. Impaired planning and mental search (60–70 %), followed by perseverations (40 %) and inattention (7 %) [94] may be selectively affected also in mildly demented patients [100]. Applause sign is reported as positive in nearly 40 % of CDB patients, similarly as in DLB [52]. Patients with CBD exhibit more severe executive dysfunction compared to AD patients [100], while poor performance of WCST and lexical fluency compared to relatively preserved semantic fluency resembles executive dysfunction in PSP [98]. Markedly reduced fluency probably originates from medial frontal lobe, left temporal lobe, and basal ganglia dysfunction [100] suggesting the role of both frontal-subcortical circuits and temporal regions in dysfluency in CBD. Imaging evidence suggest that dysexecutive syndrome in CBD originates from bilateral perirolandic cortex and striatal atrophy showing fronto-subcortical pattern [97, 98], while attention deficits presumably originate from medial frontal lobes, basal ganglia, and locus coeruleus dysfunction [100].

In the context of broad cognitive difficulties, memory seems to be relatively spared even late into the disease [94]. While some studies have shown normal memory functions [98, 100], others have reported a decline in memory scores [96]. The performance on immediate and long-delay free recall and false positives at recognition subtests is similar to that of PSP and much better than that of AD patients matched for the severity of dementia [98], attributed to the poor usage of strategies of retrieval and encoding rather than pure memory impairment related to medial temporal lobes. However, 78 % of patients with CBS-AD phenotype have short-term memory loss [97]. Semantic memory is preserved or mildly impaired in CBD patients even late into the disease. However, a slight decline over time in word-picture matching has been recognized.

Up to half of CBD patients endorse visuospatial and visuoconstructional difficulties [94, 98], and impairment in this domain is one of diagnostic criteria for frontal-behavioral-spatial syndrome [90]. Typically, spatial location deficits are more severe compared to object-related deficits [12]. Although the role of diminished visual scanning in poor performance is apparent, it has been suggested that spatial ability is more affected than perceptual due to more pronounced damage of dorsal than ventral occipitoparietal cortex. Focal visual syndromes, such as Balint syndrome, visuomotor apraxia, visual gnosia, or hemianopsia, although rare, may be a presenting or major feature of CBD [94]. They may be so profound that patients have problems how to understand or draw simple objects, read, drive, use coins, and focus their eyes. Neuropathologic correlates of visuospatial dysfunction in those cases account for atypical occipital lobe pathology indicating the distinct CBD-posterior cortical atrophy phenotype. These patients may also demonstrate total Gerstmann syndrome or isolated acalculia, agraphia, and problems with identifying body parts that precede or are more prominent in comparison to other motor, cognitive, or behavioral symptoms. Visuospatial functions usually correlate with global cognitive decline and seem to be more affected compared to PD and MSA patients, while evidence is variable for CBD vs. PSP patients [12, 102]. Over time, they decline significantly [94] compared to PD and PSP [102], but no clear correlation with disease duration and disease severity has been obtained [12].

Conclusion and Future Directions

Neuropsychiatric symptoms are an important part of the clinical spectrum of CBD. Behavioral changes, mostly linked to frontal disequilibrium, are present more frequently in a form of "hypofrontal" syndrome. Personality changes are sometimes odd or unusual mimicking those in bvFTD, while depression is present in many patients resembling other subcortical dementia syndromes. Severe language dysfunction even in non-aphasic patients together with decline in visuospatial and executive functions represents a backbone of the cognitive disorder in CBD. Aphasia is a hallmark of the disease which allows a distinction from other parkinsonian disorders, while mostly intact memory together with motor impairment allows the distinction from AD. To date, there is no evidence for the treatment of dementia in CBD.

Future research in the field of CBD requires larger cohorts of pathologically confirmed CBD cases. CBD is a rare disorder and the largest studies to date encompass not more than thirty autopsy-proven cases. Depending on the predominant clinical presentation, patients initially present to movement disorder or dementia clinics accounting for the referral bias. Finally, most of the existing studies with pathologically confirmed cases are retrospective. Future studies assessing neuropsychiatric disturbances in the light of neuroanatomical underpinnings and treatment options are warranted.

References

1. Gilman S, Wenning GK, Low PA, Brooks DJ, Mathias CJ, Trojanowski JQ, et al. Second consensus statement on the diagnosis of multiple system atrophy. Neurology. 2008;71:670–6.
2. Brown RG, Lacomblez L, Landwehrmeyer BG, Bak T, Uttner I, Dubois B, et al. Cognitive impairment in patients with multiple system atrophy and progressive supranuclear palsy. Brain. 2010;133:2382–93.

3. O'Sullivan SS, Massey LA, Williams DR, Silveira-Moriyama L, Kempster PA, Holton JL, et al. Clinical outcomes of progressive supranuclear palsy and multiple system atrophy. Brain. 2008;131:1362–72.
4. Williams DR, Lees AJ. Visual hallucinations in the diagnosis of idiopathic Parkinson's disease: a retrospective autopsy study. Lancet Neurol. 2005;4:605–10.
5. Wenning GK, Tison F, Ben Shlomo Y, Daniel E, Quinn NP. Multiple system atrophy: a review of 203 pathologically proven cases. Mov Disord. 1997;12:133–47.
6. Chang CC, Chang YY, Chang WN, Lee YC, Wang YL, Lui CC, et al. Cognitive deficits in multiple system atrophy correlate with frontal atrophy and disease duration. Eur J Neurol. 2009;16:1144–50.
7. Siri C, Duerr S, Canesi M, Delazer M, Esselink R, Bloem BR, et al. A cross-sectional multicenter study of cognitive and behavioural features in multiple system atrophy patients of the parkinsonian and cerebellar type. J Neural Transm. 2013;120:613–8.
8. Kawai Y, Suenaga M, Takeda A, Ito M, Watanabe H, Tanaka F, et al. Cognitive impairments in multiple system atrophy: MSA-C vs MSA-P. Neurology. 2008;70:1390–6.
9. Petrovic IN, Ling H, Asi Y, Ahmed Z, Kukkle PL, Hazrati LN, et al. Multiple system atrophy-parkinsonism with slow progression and prolonged survival: a diagnostic catch. Mov Disord. 2012;27:1186–90.
10. Lyoo CH, Jeong Y, Ryu YH, Lee SY, Song TJ, Lee JH, et al. Effects of disease duration on the clinical features and brain glucose metabolism in patients with mixed type multiple system atrophy. Brain. 2008;131:438–46.
11. Pillon B, Gouider-Khouja N, Deweer B, Vidailhet M, Malapani C, Dubois B, et al. Neuropsychological pattern of striatonigral degeneration: comparison with Parkinson's disease and progressive supranuclear palsy. J Neurol Neurosurg Psychiatry. 1995;58:174–9.
12. Bak TH, Caine D, Hearn VC, Hodges JR. Visuospatial functions in atypical parkinsonian syndromes. J Neurol Neurosurg Psychiatry. 2006;77:454–6.
13. Kao AW, Racine CA, Quitania LA, Kramer JH, Christine CW, Miller BL. Cognitive and neuropsychiatric profile of the synucleinopathies: Parkinson's disease, dementia with Lewy bodies and multiple system atrophy. Alzheimer Dis Assoc Disord. 2009;23:365–70.
14. Paviour DC, Price SL, Jahanshahi M, Lees AJ, Fox NC. Longitudinal MRI in progressive supranuclear palsy and multiple system atrophy: rates and regions of atrophy. Brain. 2006;129:1040–9.
15. Brenneis C, Egger K, Scherfler C, Seppi K, Schocke M, Poewe W, et al. Progression of brain atrophy in multiple system atrophy. A longitudinal VBM study. J Neurol. 2007;254:191–6.
16. Brenneis C, Boesch SM, Egger KE, Seppi K, Scherfler C, Schocke M, et al. Cortical atrophy in the cerebellar variant of multiple system atrophy: a voxel-based morphometry study. Mov Disord. 2006;21:159–65.
17. Schmeichel AM, Buchhalter LC, Low PA, Parisi JE, Boeve BW, Sandroni P, et al. Mesopontine cholinergic neuron involvement in Lewy body dementia and multiple system atrophy. Neurology. 2008;70:368–73.
18. Mazere J, Meissner WG, Sibon I, Lamare F, Tison F, Allard M, et al. [(123)I]-IBVM SPECT imaging of cholinergic systems in multiple system atrophy: a specific alteration of the ponto-thalamic cholinergic pathways (Ch5-Ch6). Neuroimage Clin. 2013;8:212–7.
19. Gill CE, Khurana RK, Hibler RJ. Occurrence of depressive symptoms in Shy-Drager Syndrome. Clin Auton Res. 1999;9:1–4.
20. Benrud-Larson LM, Sandroni P, Schrag A, Low PA. Depressive symptoms and life satisfaction in patients with multiple system atrophy. Mov Disord. 2005;20:951–7.
21. Schrag A, Sheikh S, Quinn NP, Lees AJ, Selai C, Mathias C, et al. A comparison of depression, anxiety, and health status in patients with progressive supranuclear palsy and multiple system atrophy. Mov Disord. 2010;25:1077–81.
22. Ghorayeb I, Yekhlef F, Chrysostome V, Balestre E, Bioulac B, Tison F. Sleep disorders and their determinants in multiple system atrophy. J Neurol Neurosurg Psychiatry. 2002;72:798–800.

23. Jecmenica-Lukic M, Poewe W, Tolosa E, Wenning GK. Premotor signs and symptoms of multiple system atrophy. Lancet Neurol. 2012;11:361–8.
24. Cochen De Cock V, Debs R, Oudiette D, Leu S, Radji F, Tiberge M, et al. The improvement of movement and speech during rapid eye movement sleep behaviour disorder in multiple system atrophy. Brain. 2011;134:856–62.
25. Moreno-Lopez C, Santamaria J, Salamero M, Del Sorbo F, Albanese A, Pellecchia MT, et al. Excessive daytime sleepiness in multiple system atrophy (SLEEMSA study). Arch Neurol. 2011;68:223–30.
26. Ubhi K, Inglis C, Mante M, Patrick C, Adame A, Spencer B, et al. Fluoxetine ameliorates behavioral and neuropathological deficits in a transgenic model mouse of α-synucleinopathy. Exp Neurol. 2012;234:405–16.
27. Whitwell JL, Weigand SD, Shiung MM, Boeve BF, Ferman TJ, Smith GE, et al. Focal atrophy in dementia with Lewy bodies on MRI: a distinct pattern from Alzheimer's disease. Brain. 2007;13:708–19.
28. McKeith IG, Dickson DW, Lowe J, Emre M, O'Brien JT, Feldman H, et al. Diagnosis and management of dementia with Lewy bodies: third report of the DLB consortium. Neurology. 2005;65:1863–72.
29. Aarsland D, Litvan I, Salmon D, Galasko D, Wentzel-Larsen T, Larsen JP. Performance on the dementia rating scale in Parkinson's disease with dementia and dementia with Lewy bodies: comparison with progressive supranuclear palsy and Alzheimer's disease. J Neurol Neurosurg Psychiatry. 2003;74:1215–20.
30. Hamilton JM, Salmon DP, Galasko D, Raman R, Emond J, Hansen LA, et al. Visuospatial deficits predict rate of cognitive decline in autopsy-verified dementia with Lewy bodies. Neuropsychology. 2008;22:729–37.
31. Ballard C, Holmes C, McKeith I, Neill D, O'Brien J, Cairns N, et al. Psychiatric morbidity in dementia with Lewy Bodies: a prospective clinical and neuropathological comparative study with Alzheimer's disease. Am J Psychiatry. 1999;156:1039–45.
32. Galvin JE, Malcom H, Johnson D, Morris JC. Personality traits distinguishing dementia with Lewy bodies from Alzheimer disease. Neurology. 2007;68:1895–01.
33. Tiraboschi P, Salmon DP, Hansen LA, Hofstetter RC, Thal LJ, Corey-Bloom J. What best differentiates Lewy body from Alzheimer's disease in early-stage dementia? Brain. 2006;129:729–35.
34. Teaktong T, Piggott MA, McKeith IG, Perry RH, Ballard CG, Perry EK. Muscarinic M2 and M4 receptors in anterior cingulate cortex: relation to neuropsychiatric symptoms in dementia with Lewy bodies. Behav Brain Res. 2005;161:299–05.
35. Johnson DK, Watts AS, Chapin BA, Anderson R, Burns JM. Neuropsychiatric profiles in dementia. Alzheimer Dis Assoc Disord. 2011;25:326–32.
36. Caputo M, Monastero R, Mariani E, Santucci A, Mangialasche F, Camarda R, et al. Neuropsychiatric symptoms in 921 elderly subjects with dementia: a comparison between vascular and neurodegenerative types. Acta Psychiatr Scand. 2008;117:455–64.
37. Nagahama Y, Okina T, Suzuki N, Matsuda M. Neural correlates of psychotic symptoms in dementia with Lewy bodies. Brain. 2010;133:557–67.
38. Harding AJ, Broe GA, Halliday GM. Visual hallucinations in Lewy body disease relate to Lewy bodies in the temporal lobe. Brain. 2002;125:391–03.
39. Burton EJ, McKeith IG, David J, Burn DJ, Williams ED, O'Brien JT. Cerebral atrophy in Parkinson's disease with and without dementia: a comparison with Alzheimer's disease, dementia with Lewy bodies and controls. Brain. 2004;127:791–800.
40. Kobayashi K, Sumiya H, Nakano H, Akiyama N, Urata K, Koshino Y. Detection of Lewy body disease in patients with late-onset depression, anxiety and psychotic disorder with myocardial meta-iodobenzylguanidine scintigraphy. Int J Geriatr Psychiatry. 2010;25:55–65.
41. Perry EK, Marshall E, Kerwin J, Smith CJ, Jabeen S, Cheng AV, et al. Evidence of a monoaminergic–cholinergic imbalance related to visual hallucinations in Lewy body dementia. J Neurochem. 1990;55:1454–6.

42. Hynninen MJ, Breitve MH, Rongve A, Aarsland D, Nordhus IH. The frequency and correlates of anxiety in patients with first-time diagnosed mild dementia. Int Psychoger. 2012;24:1771–8.
43. Fritze F, Ehrt U, Hortobagyi T, Ballard C, Aarsland D. Depressive symptoms in Alzheimer's disease and Lewy body dementia: a one-year follow-up study. Dement Geriatr Cogn Disord. 2011;32:143–9.
44. Onofrj M, Thomas A, Tiraboschi P, Wenning G, Gambi F, Sepede G, et al. Updates on Somatoform disorders (SFMD) in Parkinson's disease and dementia with Lewy bodies and discussion of phenomenology. J Neurol Sci. 2011;310:166–71.
45. Boström F, Jönsson L, Minthon L, Londos E. Patients with dementia with Lewy bodies have more impaired quality of life than patients with Alzheimer disease. Alzheimer Dis Assoc Disord. 2007;21:150–4.
46. Ikeda M, Mori E, Kosaka K, Iseki E, Hashimoto M, Matsukawa N, et al. Donepezil-DLB Study Investigators. Long-term safety and efficacy of donepezil in patients with dementia with Lewy bodies: results from a 52-week, open-label, multicenter extension study. Dement Geriatr Cogn Disord. 2013;36:229–41.
47. Ferman TJ, Smith GE, Kantarci K, Boeve BF, Pankratz VS, Dickson DW. Nonamnestic mild cognitive impairment progresses to dementia with Lewy bodies. Neurology. 2013;81:2032–8.
48. Bradshaw JM, Saling M, Anderson V, Hopwood M, Brodtmann A. Higher cortical deficits influence attentional processing in dementia with Lewy bodies, relative to patients with dementia of the Alzheimer's type and controls. J Neurol Neurosurg Psychiatry. 2006;77:1129–35.
49. Park KW, Kim HS, Cheon SM, Cha JK, Kim SH, Kima JW. Dementia with Lewy bodies versus Alzheimer's disease and Parkinson's disease dementia: a comparison of cognitive profiles. J Clin Neurol. 2011;7:19–24.
50. Johns EK, Phillips NA, Belleville S, Goupil D, Babins L, Kelner N, et al. Executive functions in frontotemporal dementia and Lewy body dementia. Neuropsychology. 2009;23:765–77.
51. Lambon Ralph MA, Powell J, Howard D, Whitworth AB, Garrard P, Hodges JR. Semantic memory is impaired in both dementia with Lewy bodies and dementia of Alzheimer's type: a comparative neuropsychological study and literature review. J Neurol Neurosurg Psychiatry. 2001;70:149–56.
52. Isella V, Rucci F, Traficante D, Mapelli C, Ferri F, Appollonio IM. The applause sign in cortical and cortical-subcortical dementia. J Neurol. 2013;260:1099–103.
53. Perry EK, Irving D, Kerwin JM, McKeith IG, Thompson P, Collerton D, et al. Cholinergic transmitter and neurotrophic activities in Lewy body dementia: similarity to Parkinson's and distinction from Alzheimer disease. Alzheimer Dis Assoc Disord. 1993;7:69–79.
54. Pimlott SL, Piggott M, Ballard C, McKeith I, Perry R, Kometa S, et al. Thalamic nicotinic receptors implicated in disturbed consciousness in dementia with Lewy bodies. Neurobiol Dis. 2006;21:50–6.
55. Dugger BN, Boeve BF, Murray ME, Parisi JE, Fujishiro H, Dickson DW, et al. Rapid eye movement sleep behavior disorder and subtypes in autopsy-confirmed dementia with Lewy bodies. Mov Disord. 2012;27:72–8.
56. Murray ME, Ferman TJ, Boeve BF, Przybelski SA, Lesnick TG, Liesinger AM, et al. MRI and pathology of REM sleep behavior disorder in dementia with Lewy bodies. Neurology. 2013;81:1681–9.
57. Pao WC, Boeve BF, Ferman TJ, Lin SC, Smith GE, Knopman DS, et al. Polysomnographic findings in dementia with Lewy bodies. Neurologist. 2013;19:1–6.
58. Aarsland D, Ballard C, Rongve Broadstock AM, Svenningsson P. Clinical trials of dementia with Lewy bodies and Parkinson's disease dementia. Curr Neurol Neurosci Rep. 2012;12:492–501.

59. McKeith I, Del Ser T, Spano PF, Emre M, Wesnes K, Anand R, et al. Efficacy of rivastigmine in dementia with Lewy bodies: a randomised, double-blind, placebo-controlled international study. Lancet. 2000;356:2031–6.
60. Mori E, Ikeda M, Kosaka K; Donepezil-DLB Study Investigators. Donepezil for dementia with Lewy bodies: a randomized, placebo-controlled trial. Ann Neurol. 2012;72:41–52.
61. Aarsland D, Perry R, Larsen JP, McKeith IG, O'Brien JT, Perry EK, et al. Neuroleptic sensitivity in Parkinson's disease and parkinsonian dementias. J Clin Psychiatry. 2005;66:633–7.
62. Emre M, Tsolaki M, Bonuccelli U, Destée A, Tolosa E, Kutzelnigg A; 11018 Study Investigators. Memantine for patients with Parkinson's disease dementia or dementia with Lewy bodies: a randomised, double-blind, placebo-controlled trial. Lancet Neurol. 2010;9:969–77.
63. Sharp SI, Ballard CG, Ziabreva I, Piggott MA, Perry RH, Perry EK, et al. Cortical serotonin 1A receptor levels are associated with depression in patients with dementia with Lewy bodies and Parkinson's disease dementia. Dement Geriatr Cogn Disord. 2008;26:330–8.
64. Kunz D, Mahlberg R. A two-part, double-blind, placebo-controlled trial of exogenous melatonin in REM sleep behaviour disorder. J Sleep Res. 2010;19:591–6.
65. Iranzo A, Tolosa E, Gelpi E, Molinuevo JL, Valldeoriola F, Serradell M, et al. Neurodegenerative disease status and post-mortem pathology in idiopathic rapid-eye-movement sleep behaviour disorder: an observational cohort study. Lancet Neurol. 2013;12:443–53.
66. Williams DR, de Silva R, Paviour DC, Pittman A, Watt HC, Kilford L. Characteristics of two distinct clinical phenotypes in pathologically proven progressive supranuclear palsy: Richardson's syndrome and PSP-parkinsonism. Brain. 2005;128:1247–58.
67. Hughes AJ, Daniel SE, Ben-Shlomo Y, Lees AJ. The accuracy of diagnosis of parkinsonian syndromes in a specialist movement disorder service. Brain. 2002;125:861–70.
68. Gerstenecker A, Mast B, Duff K, Ferman TJ, Litvan I, ENGENE-PSP Study Group. Executive dysfunction is the primary cognitive impairment in progressive supranuclear palsy. Arc Clin Neuropsychol. 2013;28:104–13.
69. Ghosh BCP, Carpenter RH, Rowe JB. A longitudinal study of motor, oculomotor and cognitive function in progressive supranuclear palsy. PLoS One. 2013;8(9):e74486.
70. Cordato NJ, Halliday GM, Caine D, Morris JGL. Comparison of motor, cognitive, and behavioral features in progressive supranuclear palsy and Parkinson's disease. Mov Disord. 2006;21:632–8.
71. Litvan I, Mega MS, Cummings JL, Fairbanks L. Neuropsychiatric aspects of progressive supranuclear palsy. Neurology. 1996;47:1184–9.
72. Aarsland D, Litvan I, Larsen JP. Neuropsychiatric symptoms of patients with progressive supranuclear palsy and Parkinson's disease. J Neuropsychiatry Clin Neurosci. 2001;13:42–9.
73. Borroni B, Alberici A, Agosti C, Cosseddu M, Padovani A. Pattern of behavioral disturbances in corticobasal degeneration syndrome and progressive supranuclear palsy. Int Psychogeriatr. 2009;21:463–8.
74. Somme J, Gómez-Esteban JC, Tijero B, Berganzo K, Lezcano E, Zarranz JJ. The applause sign and neuropsychological profile in progressive supranuclear palsy and Parkinson's disease. Clin Neurol Neurosurg. 2013;115:1230–3.
75. Chiu WZ, Papma JM, de Koning I, Donker KL, Seelaar H, Reijs AE, et al. Midcingulate involvement in progressive supranuclear palsy and tau positive frontotemporal dementia. J Neurol Neurosurg Psychiatry. 2012;83:910–5.
76. Cordato NJ, Duggins AJ, Halliday GM, Morris JG, Pantelis C. Clinical deficits correlate with regional cerebral atrophy in progressive supranuclear palsy. Brain. 2005;128:1259–66.
77. Srulijes K, Mallien G, Bauer S, Dietzel E, Groger A, Ebersbach G, et al. In vivo comparison of Richardson's syndrome and progressive supranuclear palsy-parkinsonism. J Neural Transm. 2011;118:1191–7.
78. Pharr V, Uttl B, Stark M, Litvan I, Fantie B, Grafman J. Comparison of apraxia in corticobasal degeneration and progressive supranuclear palsy. Neurology. 2001;56:957–63.

79. Josephs KA, Whitwell JL, Eggers SC, Senjem ML, Jack CR Jr. Gray matter correlates of behavioral severity in progressive supranuclear palsy. Mov Disord. 2011;26:493–8.
80. Gerstenecker A, Duff K, Mast B, Litvan I; ENGENE-PSPStudy Group. Behavioral abnormalities in progressive supranuclear palsy. Psychiatry Res. 2013;210:1205–10.
81. Yatabe Y, Hashimoto M, Kaneda K, Honda K, Ogawa Y, Yuuki S, et al. Neuropsychiatric symptoms of progressive supranuclear palsy in a dementia clinic. Psychogeriatrics. 2011;11:54–9.
82. Diederich NJ, Leurgans S, Fan W, Chmura TA, Goetz CG. Visual hallucinations and symptoms of REM sleep behavior disorder in Parkinsonian tauopathies. Int J Geriatr Psychiatry. 2008;23:598–603.
83. Ghosh BCP, Calder AJ, Peers PV, Lawrence AD, Acosta-Cabronero J, Pereira JM, et al. Social cognitive deficits and their neural correlates in progressive supranuclear palsy. Brain. 2012;135:2089–102.
84. Shany-Ur T, Poorzand P, Grossman SN, Growdon ME, Jang JY, Robin S, Ketelle RS, et al. Comprehension of insincere communication in neurodegenerative disease: lies, sarcasm, and theory of mind. Cortex. 2012;48:132–41.
85. Cordato NJ, Pantelis C, Halliday GM, Velakoulis D, Wood SJ, Stuart GW, et al. Frontal atrophy correlates with behavioural changes in progressive supranuclear palsy. Brain. 2002;125:789–800.
86. Brenneis C, Seppi K, Schocke M, Benke T, Wenning GK, Poewe W. Voxel based morphometry reveals a distinct pattern of frontal atrophy in progressive supranuclear palsy. J Neurol Neurosurg Psychiatry. 2004;75:246–9.
87. Hirano S, Shinotoh H, Shimada H, Aotsuka A, Tanaka N, Ota T, et al. Cholinergic imaging in corticobasal syndrome, progressive supranuclear palsy and frontotemporal dementia. Brain. 2010;133:2058–68.
88. Litvan I, Phipps M, Pharr V, Hallett M, Grafman J, Salazar A. Randomized placebo-controlled trial of donepezil in patients with progressive supranuclear palsy. Neurology. 2001;57:467–73.
89. Stamelou M, Reuss A, Pilatus U, Magerkurth J, Niklowitz P, Eggert KM, et al. Short-term effects of coenzyme Q10 in progressive supranuclear palsy: a randomized, placebo-controlled trial. Mov Disord. 2008;23:942–9.
90. Armstrong MJ, Litvan I, Lang AE, Bak TH, Bhatia KP, Borroni B, et al. Criteria for the diagnosis of corticobasal degeneration. Neurology. 2013;80:496–503.
91. Wenning GK, Litvan I, Jankovic J, Granata R, Mangone CA, McKee A, et al. Natural history and survival of 14 patients with corticobasal degeneration confirmed at postmortem examination. J Neurol Neurosurg Psychiatry. 1998;64:184–9.
92. Goldmann Gross R, Grossman M. Update on apraxia. Curr Neurol Neurosci Rep. 2008;8:490–6.
93. Rascovsky K, Hodges JR, Knopman D, Mendez MF, Kramer JH, Neuhaus J, et al. Sensitivity of revised diagnostic criteria for the behavioural variant of frontotemporal dementia. Brain. 2011;134:2456–77.
94. Murray R, Neumann M, Forman MS, Farmer J, Massimo L, Rice A, et al. Cognitive and motor assessment in autopsy-proven corticobasal degeneration. Neurology. 2007;68:1274–83.
95. Ling H, O'Sullivan SS, Holton JL, Revesz T, Massey LA, Williams DR, Paviour DC, Lees AJ. Does corticobasal degeneration exist? A clinicopathological re-evaluation. Brain. 2010;133:2045–57.
96. Kertesz A, Martinez-Lage P, Davidson W, Munoz DG. The corticobasal degeneration syndrome overlaps progressive aphasia and frontotemporal dementia. Neurology. 2000;55:1368–75.
97. Lee SE, Rabinovici GD, Mayo MC, Wilson SM, Seeley WW, Stephen J, et al. Clinicopathological correlations in corticobasal degeneration. Ann Neurol. 2011;70:327–40.
98. Pillon B, Blin J, Vidailhet M, Deweer B, Sirigu A, Dubois B, et al. The neuropsychological pattern of corticobasal degeneration: comparison with progressive supranuclear palsy and Alzheimer's disease. Neurology. 1995;45:1477–83.

99. Litvan I, Cummings JL, Mega M. Neuropsychiatric features of corticobasal degeneration. J Neurol Neurosurg Psychiatry. 1998;65:717–21.
100. Massman PJ, Kreiter KT, Jankovic J, Doody RS. Neuropsychological functioning in cortical-basal ganglionic degeneration: differentiation from Alzheimer's disease. Neurology. 1996;46:720–6.
101. Armstrong N, Schupf N, Grafman J, Huey ED. Caregiver burden in frontotemporal degeneration and corticobasal syndrome. Dement Geriatr Cogn Disord. 2013;36:310–8.
102. Rittman T, Ghosh BC, McColgan P, Breen DP, Evans J, Williams-Gray CH, et al. The Addenbrooke's cognitive examination for the differential diagnosis and longitudinal assessment of patients with parkinsonian disorders. J Neurol Neurosurg Psychiatry. 2013;84:544–51.

Chapter 8
Neuropsychiatric Disturbances in Dystonia

Paolo Amami, Lucrezia Islam, Dirk Dressler, and Alberto Albanese

Abbreviations

BoNT	Botulinum neurotoxin
DRD	Dopa-responsive dystonia
M-D	Myoclonus-dystonia
NBIA	Neurodegeneration with brain iron accumulation
OCD	Obsessive-compulsive disorder
PKAN	Pantothenate kinase-associated neurodegeneration
PLAN	PLA2G6-mutation-associated neurodegeneration

P. Amami, PsyD
Department of Psychology, Milano-Bicocca University, via Celoria, 11, Milan 20133, Italy

Movement Disorders Unit, IRCCS Istituto Neurologico Carlo Besta, via Celoria, 11, Milan 20133, Italy
e-mail: paolo.amami@istituto-besta.it

L. Islam, MD
Department of Psychiatry, University of Milan Medical School, Ospedale San Paolo, Via Antonio Di Rudini 8, Milan 20131, Italy
e-mail: lucrezia.islam@unimi.it

D. Dressler, MD, PhD
Movement Disorders Section, Department of Neurology, Hanover Medical School, Carl-Neuberg-Str. 1, Hannover D-30625, Germany
e-mail: ressler.dirk@mh-hannover.de

A. Albanese, MD (✉)
Department of Neurology, Catholic University, via Celoria, 11, Milan 20133, Italy

Movement Disorders Unit, IRCCS Istituto Neurologico Carlo Besta, via Celoria, 11, Milan 20133, Italy
e-mail: alberto.albanese@unicatt.it

H. Reichmann (ed.), *Neuropsychiatric Symptoms of Movement Disorders*,
Neuropsychiatric Symptoms of Neurological Disease,
DOI 10.1007/978-3-319-09537-0_8

RDP	Rapid onset dystonia parkinsonism
SCID	Structural clinical interview for DSM
Y-BOCS	Yale-Brown obsessive-compulsive scale

Introduction

Dystonia is a hyperkinetic movement disorder that has been recognized quite recently. It is characterized by sustained or intermittent muscle contractions causing abnormal, often repetitive, movements, postures, or both. Dystonic movements are typically patterned and twisting and may be tremulous. Dystonia is often initiated or worsened by voluntary action and overflow muscle activation [1]. Dystonic syndromes are classified along two axes based on motor features. Axis I defines the clinical characteristics using five descriptors: age at onset, body distribution, temporal pattern, coexistence of other movement disorders, or other neurological manifestations. Based on the first axis, two main groups of dystonia syndromes can be recognized: isolated and combined. Axis II provides an etiological classification depicting nervous system anatomy and distinguishing inherited from acquired forms [1] (Table 8.1).

Since its first description by Oppenheim in 1911, dystonia has been retained as a pure motor disorder. In recent years, non-motor features have been increasingly

Table 8.1 Classification of dystonia [1]

Axis I. Clinical characteristics	
Clinical characteristics of dystonia	
Age at onset	Infancy (birth to 2 years)
	Childhood (3–12 years)
	Adolescence (13–20 years)
	Early adulthood (21–40 years)
	Late adulthood (>40 years)
Body distribution	Focal
	Segmental
	Multifocal
	Generalized (with or without leg involvement)
	Hemidystonia
Temporal pattern	Disease course
	Static
	Progressive
	Variability
	Persistent
	Action specific
	Diurnal
	Paroxysmal

Table 8.1 (continued)

Associated features	
Isolated dystonia or combined with another movement disorder	Isolated dystonia
	Combined dystonia
Occurrence of other neurological or systemic manifestations	List of co-occurring neurological manifestations
Axis II. Etiology	
Nervous system pathology	Evidence of degeneration
	Evidence of structural (often static) lesions
	No evidence of degeneration or structural lesion
Inherited or acquired	Inherited
	Autosomal dominant
	Autosomal recessive
	X-linked recessive
	Mitochondrial
	Acquired
	Perinatal brain injury
	Infection
	Drug
	Toxic
	Vascular
	Neoplastic
	Brain injury
	Psychogenic
	Idiopathic
	Sporadic
	Familial

recognized and neuropsychiatric abnormalities are a relevant part of the non-motor phenomenology [2, 3]. Many studies have assessed the occurrence of psychiatric symptoms in dystonia syndromes. Current evidence suggests that psychiatric symptoms occur at an increased rate in dystonia patients compared to the general population, with differences in the type and severity of symptoms depending on the specific syndrome [2–4]. The most frequent reported disturbances include depression, anxiety, and obsessive-compulsive disorder (OCD).

A relatively small number of studies on cognition have been published, and this topic is still evolving. Overall, subtle cognitive deficits were found in executive and visuospatial domains, while dementia has been observed only in dystonia syndrome associated with neurodegeneration [2, 3]. An open question pertains to the origin of neuropsychiatric symptoms, whether they are a primary feature of dystonia or the consequence of harboring a disabling motor disease.

We review here the occurrence of psychiatric and cognitive features in different forms of dystonia using the current classification scheme. We specifically deal with isolated dystonias, which represent the most common prototypical form, and with selected types of combined dystonias.

Isolated Dystonia Syndromes

Isolated dystonia is characterized by occurrence of features of dystonia with no other neurological sign except for tremor [1]. This term encompasses many forms previously described as "pure" or "primary" dystonias [5]. The clinical spectrum covers different ages at onset and a variety of affected body parts. The most common forms include cervical dystonia, limb dystonia, blepharospasm, oromandibular dystonia, and laryngeal dystonia [6]. The extension of body involvement is interrelated with age of onset. Early-onset isolated dystonia is a progressive disorder that often begins in a limb and subsequently progresses generalizing to other limbs and the trunk. Isolated late-onset dystonia is often focal and usually involves the craniocervical muscles or one arm; generalization is unusual. Isolated dystonia syndromes are mainly idiopathic or genetic, more rarely acquired [6]. DYT1 dystonia is due to autosomal dominant mutation of the TOR1A gene [7]. This is an often young-onset disease with a typical phenotype characterized by progressive dystonia that, when it does not lead to fixed postural deformities, is associated with a relatively high level of functioning [8]. DYT1 accounts up to 50 % of early-onset isolated dystonia syndromes in non-Jews [9]. A second hereditary form of isolated dystonia is linked to mutations in the THAP1 gene (DYT6) [10]. This is an autosomal dominant disease with adolescent or adult onset, characterized by craniocervical or focal dystonia affecting the upper limbs [11]. Two other inherited isolated forms have been identified: DYT13 [12] and DYT21 [13].

Psychiatric Profile

Early studies have implicated psychological factors in the origin of isolated dystonia. A century ago, isolated dystonia was considered a hysterical syndrome expressing an unresolved psychological conflict. In 1977, Bindman and Tibbetts presented ten patients with focal hand dystonia and "obsessional personalities" describing three types of writer's cramp: writer's cramp arising from a conflict in obsessional subjects, writer's cramp beginning as social phobia in less obsessional subjects, and hysterical dysgraphia [14].

The hypothesis of a psychodynamic origin of dystonia was dismissed, but psychopathology remained a significant topic for the negative consequences on patients' quality of life [15]. Evidence suggests that in isolated dystonia, comorbid psychiatric disturbances occur with a higher than expected rate [3, 4]. Table 8.2 reviews the studies on psychopathologies in isolated dystonia. The prevalence of lifetime or current psychiatric disorders has been estimated to range between 30 and 50 % [3, 4]. Major depression has been reported in about 30 % of patients, being the most common diagnosis, anxiety disorders in about 25 %, including social phobia in 20 %, panic disorder in 10 %, and OCD in 6.8–19.7 % [3]. In a large study, 86 patients with isolated dystonia were compared with a general population sample of

Table 8.2 Studies on psychiatric features of isolated dystonias [16–35]

Author, year	Study type	Sample size	Assessment	Main findings
Broocks, 1998 [17]	Case-control	13 BSP, 13 HSP	SCID, SCL-90, HOCI	Patients in the blepharospasm group had significantly more obsessive-compulsive symptoms than the patients with hemifacial spasm
Wenzel, 1998 [18]	Case series	44 CD	SCID-I	High lifetime prevalence of psychiatric disorders (66 %), including panic disorder (30 %), major depressive disorder (25 %), substance abuse (13.6 %), and OCD (6.8 %). In 43 % of patients psychiatric disorder began before dystonia onset
Gündel, 2001 [19]	Case-control	116 CD, 483 general population	SCID-I, SCL-90, SPS, SIAS	Higher lifetime prevalence of anxiety (50 %), in particular social phobia (41 %), and mood disorders (16 %) was found in dystonic patients
Cavallaro, 2002 [20]	Case-control	76 focal dystonia, 129 general population	Clinical psychiatric examination, Y-BOCS	Prevalence of OCD (20 %) and family morbidity risk in dystonic patients were higher than in general population
Moraru, 2002 [21]	Case series	40 CD	BDI, SCL-90, SCID	55 % of patients fulfilled the criteria for at least one lifetime psychiatric disorder. The most frequent psychiatric disorders were anxiety (40 %) and major depressive disorders (37.5 %). In 43 % of patients (42.5 %) psychiatric symptoms began prior to the onset of CD
Müller, 2002 [22]	Case series with treatment	131 CD, 89 BSP	BDI	At baseline 47 % of CD and 37 % of BSP patients had depression. After BoNT treatment, BDI improved by a mean of 17 % in CD

(continued)

Table 8.2 (continued)

Author, year	Study type	Sample size	Assessment	Main findings
Gündel, 2003 [23]	Case-control	48 CD, 48 alopecia areata	SCID-I, SCL-90, SPS	The prevalence of psychiatric disorders was higher in CD (77 %) compared to patients with alopecia areata (42 %). 69 % of CD patients fulfilled the criteria for current anxiety disorders and 19 % for mood disorders
Heiman, 2004 [24]	Case-control	96 symptomatic DYT1, 60 non-symptomatic DYT1, 65 noncarriers	CIDI	Increased risk for recurrent major depressive disorder in both symptomatic and non-symptomatic carriers compared with noncarriers. DYT1 patients had earlier age at onset of recurrent major depression than noncarriers
Gündel, 2007 [25]	Case-control	48 LD, 27 vocal fold paralysis	SCID-I, SCL-90	Higher prevalence of current psychiatric disorders in LD subjects (42 %) compared to vocal fold paralysis patients (19 %). LD patients have more severe voice impairment and longer disease duration compared to vocal fold paralysis patients
Heiman, 2007 [26]	Case-control	96 symptomatic DYT1, 60 non-symptomatic DYT1, 65 noncarriers	CIDI, MOCI	OCD/OCS are not increased in DYT1 mutation carriers compared with noncarriers, nor is OCD associated with manifesting DYT1 dystonia
Ochudlo, 2007 [27]	Case series with treatment	33 BSP	MADRAS	Treatment with BoNT is accompanied by a reduction in depressive symptoms
Bugalho, 2008 [28]	Case-control	45 dystonic patients (15 BSP, 15 CD, 15 WC), 27 HS	SCL-90, Y-BOCS	Dystonic patients had higher intensity of OCS when compared to HS

Lewis, 2008 [29]	Case series	329 focal and generalized dystonia	BDI, BCS, RSES	30 % reported moderate to severe depression; disfigurement, negative body concept, low self-esteem, and quality of life were important contributors to depression
Lencer, 2009 [16]	Case-control	86 focal dystonia, 3943 general population	SCID-I and II, NEO-FFI	Compared with the population based sample, dystonic patients had increased risk for any psychiatric disorder. Highest chances were found for social phobia, agoraphobia, panic disorder, OCD, alcohol abuse, and drug dependence. Dystonic patients had increased rates for OCD and avoidant personality disorders
Fabbrini, 2010 [30]	Case-control	89 dystonic patients (34 CD, 28 BSP, 16 LD, 11 AD), 26 HSP, 62 HC	SCID-, HAM-A, BDI, Y-BOCS	Higher prevalence of depressive disorders was found in CD and BPS patients than in healthy controls. In 69 % of dystonic patients who had psychiatric disorders, these started before onset of dystonia
Barahona-Corrêa, 2011 [31]	Cross-sectional	45 focal dystonia, 46 controls (HSP, cervical spondyloarthropathy, or carpal tunnel syndrome), 30 HS	MINI, SCL-90, Y-BOCS	Dystonic patients had higher OCS score compared to both control groups. Major depression and generalized anxiety are the most frequent psychiatric diagnoses in dystonic patients
Dias, 2011 [32]	Case-control	30 focal dystonia and 30 PD	MINI, Y-BOCS, BDI, HAM-A, LS	PD patients had higher rates of major depression and generalized anxiety disorder, while patients with dystonia had an increased severity of OCS
Duane, 2011 [33]	Case series	117 CD	MMPI	50 % had evidence of depression, 32 % evidence of anxiety, and 32 % evidence of obsessiveness

(continued)

Table 8.2 (continued)

Author, year	Study type	Sample size	Assessment	Main findings
Mula, 2012 [34]	Cross-sectional	19 focal dystonia, 18 HSP, 23 HS	SCID-I, HADS, SCL-90, SCI-OBS-SR, Y-BOCS	The prevalence of OCD was significantly higher in both dystonic and HSP patients than in HS. Dystonic patients and HSP patients differed regarding the thematic contents of obsessions and compulsions
Lehn, 2014 [35]	Cross-sectional	103 focal dystonia, 78 HSP, 93 HS	Y-BOCS, BAI, BDI	Dystonic patients had higher scores of OCS, anxiety, and depression compared to HSP and HS

AD arm dystonia, *BAI* Beck anxiety inventory, *BCS* body concept scale, *BDI* Beck depression inventory, *BoNT* botulinum neurotoxin, *BSP* blepharospasm, *CD* cervical dystonia, *CIDI* composite international diagnostic interview, *HADS* hospital anxiety depression scale, *HAM-A* Hamilton rating scale for anxiety, *HOCI* Hamburg obsession/compulsion inventory, *HS* healthy subjects, *HSP* hemifacial spasm, *LD* laryngeal dystonia, *LS* Liebowitz social anxiety scale, *MADRAS* Montgomery-Asberg depression rating scale, *MINI* mini-international neuropsychiatric inventory, *MMPI* Minnesota multiphasic personality inventory, *MOCI* Maudsley obsessive-compulsive inventory, *NEO-FFI* 5 factor inventory, *OBS-SR* obsessive-compulsive spectrum self-report, *OCD* obsessive-compulsive disorder, *OCS* obsessive-compulsive symptoms, *PD* Parkinson's disease, *RSES* Rosenberg's self-esteem scale, *SCID* structured clinical interview schedule, *SCI-OBS-SR* structured clinical interview for obsessive-compulsive spectrum self-report, *SCL-90* symptoms checklist 90 item, *SIAS* social interactions anxiety scale, *SPS* social phobia scale, *Y-BOCS* Yale-Brown obsessive-compulsive scale, *WC* writer's cramp

3,943 subjects using a detailed psychiatric assessment [16]. Patients had an increased frequency for many psychiatric disorders compared to the general population, and some patients showed two or more coexisting conditions. The highest prevalence was found for major depression, anxiety disorders, alcohol abuse, and drug dependence. Most of the psychiatric disorders appeared before the onset of dystonia.

In a recent case-control study, different forms of isolated dystonia were compared for prevalence of psychiatric comorbidity assessed with the Structured Clinical Interview for Diagnostic and Statistical Manual of Mental Disorders (SCID) [30]. Overall, 53 % of patients with isolated dystonia had a diagnosis of psychiatric disorders compared to 24 % of healthy control subjects. The prevalence of depressive disorders in cervical dystonia (26 %) and blepharospasm (39 %) was higher than in healthy control (5 %), while the frequency of anxiety disorders, OCD, or adjustment disorder approached that of healthy subjects. No difference was found in the frequency of any specific psychiatric disorder in patients with laryngeal dystonia or limb dystonia and healthy controls. In 35 of 51 patients with psychiatric disorders, these started before the onset of dystonia.

It is debated whether psychiatric disorders represent a consequence of having a disabling and stigmatizing disease or they are instead a primary clinical feature of dystonia. Psychiatric symptoms, particularly depression and anxiety, may be sensitive to physical disability and social stigma. In a study on the impact of botulinum neurotoxin (BoNT) treatment on depressive symptoms, 33 patients with blepharospasm were analyzed [27]. Twenty exhibited depressive symptoms prior to treatment, with 11 patients displaying mild depressive symptoms, 6 patients with moderate depressive symptoms, and 3 patients with severe depressive symptoms. Depressive symptoms decreased on average by 56 % after treatment [27]. In keeping with this, it has been observed that successful treatment with BoNT improves depressive symptoms in a number of isolated dystonia types [22, 36]. These findings support the view that depression may partly be a consequence of the motor impairment and that it can be ameliorated by improving disability and reduce visibility of the movement disorder. The hypothesis that psychiatric symptoms of dystonia can be reactive to motor impairment has been further tested in studies using subjects with a similar motor impairment and no central nervous system involvement as controls. In a recent study, 89 patients with various types of isolated dystonia were compared to 62 healthy subjects and 26 patients with hemifacial spasm regarding the frequency of some psychiatric disturbances [30]. Depression was more frequent in subjects with cervical dystonia and blepharospasm [30].

Social stigma has been considered as a factor that contributes to psychiatric disturbances in dystonia. A study exploring the role of social stigma compared 48 subjects with alopecia areata, a skin condition causing significant hair loss, and 48 patients with cervical dystonia matched for age, gender, and body image dissatisfaction [23]. In subjects with cervical dystonia, a significantly higher psychiatric comorbidity was found compared to subjects with alopecia areata, despite the fact that the latter can be at least as socially embarrassing. This consisted mainly in anxiety and depressive disorders. This finding suggests that psychiatric symptoms may also be a primary expression of dystonia and not necessarily an aftermath of disfigurement.

Special attention has been given to OCD, which occurs with an especially high frequency in isolated dystonia, although the studies addressing this topic have provided inconsistent results. One study compared 13 patients with blepharospasm with 13 patients with hemifacial spasm [17]. In this study, patients with blepharospasm had significantly more obsessive-compulsive symptoms than patients with hemifacial spasm. Another study assessed the prevalence and severity of OCD in 30 patients with isolated dystonia and 30 matched controls with Parkinson's disease [32]. A higher prevalence of OCD was found in dystonia patients, whereas Parkinson's disease patients exhibited greater rates of major depression and generalized anxiety disorder. While some studies reported greater OCD severity in patients with isolated dystonia, others were unable to replicate this finding [37, 38]. Another study assessed 12 patients with writer's cramp by means of the Yale-Brown obsessive-compulsive scale (Y-BOCS) using two control groups: 12 patients with diseases of peripheral origin (7 patients with carpal tunnel syndrome, 3 with cervical spondylotic radiculopathy, 1 with chronic inflammatory demyelinating polyneuropathy, 1 with myasthenia gravis) and 12 age- and gender-matched healthy controls employed as clerks or secretaries [39]. The additional control group was included to test the hypothesis that OCD may be a consequence of functional impairment. Mean Y-BOCS scores were 5.8 for the writer's cramp group, 1 for the disease control group, and 1 for the healthy control group, respectively. The fact that patients with writer's cramp scored higher than patients with functional impairment of peripheral origin supported the hypothesis that basal ganglia dysfunction is involved in both writer's cramp and OCD [39].

Studies of monogenetic isolated dystonias have shed further light on the relationship between motor and psychiatric phenomenology. In a study attempting to determine if affective symptoms might be a manifestation of the DYT1 mutation, 96 manifesting mutation carriers, 60 non-manifesting mutation carriers, and 65 noncarriers were compared [24]. All subjects underwent complete psychiatric assessment by means of a standardized psychiatric interview. The risk for recurrent major depressive disorder was increased in both non-manifesting carriers and manifesting carriers compared to noncarriers. Mutation carriers also had earlier age at onset of recurrent major depressive disorder than noncarriers. The severity of motor signs was not associated with the likelihood of recurrent depression. The analysis of non-manifesting subjects (i.e., non-manifesting carriers compared to noncarriers) showed that non-manifesting carriers were over four times more likely than noncarriers to exhibit recurrent major depressive disorder. These findings support the hypothesis that recurrent major depression is a phenotypic expression of the DYT1 mutation. In another study, the hypothesis that OCD might be a clinical expression of the DYT1 gene was tested [26]. DYT1 manifesting and non-manifesting carriers and noncarriers underwent a structured clinical interview. Three manifesting carriers (3 %), one non-manifesting carriers (2 %), and three noncarriers (5 %) met criteria for current OCD. Similarly, the prevalence of a lifetime history of OCD did not differ between the three groups. Based on this evidence OCD is not part of clinical expression of DYT1 mutation [26].

Cognitive Profile

Earlier studies either found no cognitive dysfunction [40, 41] or found that dystonia patients score better than controls on measures of general intelligence [42]. Therefore, isolated dystonia patients were described as "intelligent" and "the brightest in family" [41–43]. Such presumed higher intelligence of patients with isolated dystonia was subsequently questioned [44]. Current evidence suggests that no major cognitive impairment occurs in isolated dystonia patients. Some studies show that selective executive or visuospatial deficits may be present, but it is unclear how functionally relevant such deficits are. Many studies that compared patients with isolated dystonia and healthy subjects on several cognitive domains found no differences on long-term verbal and visual memory [28, 45–48], short-term memory [46–49], learning [45, 50], attention [46, 49, 50], executive functions [28, 45–48, 50], or language [49]. Other observations reported lower performance of isolated dystonia patients on categorization and set-shifting [28], extra-dimensional set-shifting [49], verbal memory with retroactive interference [51], use of allocentric cue in visual memory [52], and mental manipulation of personal and extra-personal space [53]. Table 8.3 reviews the studies on cognition in isolated dystonia.

Only one study has characterized the cognitive phenotype in DYT1 [51]. This assessed manifesting patients harboring DYT1 mutation and non-manifesting carriers matched for age, gender, mother tongue, and education on an extensive neuropsychological battery. No differences were found between non-manifesting carriers and control, while manifesting DYT1 patients showed increased verbal memory difficulties when exposed to retroactive interference. No other cognitive domains were found impaired [51].

Several shortcomings of the current literature reduce the capacity to test hypotheses regarding the role of cognitive dysfunction in isolated dystonia. The quality of most of the studies is limited by small size and sample heterogeneity. Some potentially meaningful variables including age, premorbid intellectual ability, age of disease onset, duration of the disease, body distribution of dystonic symptoms, or genotype are not usually considered. Furthermore, use of "pencil and paper" neuropsychological tests instead of computerized versions probably reduced sensibility and increased examiner-related errors. Overall, the more consistent evidence is for deficits of executive and visuospatial functions.

The observation of cognitive deficits in isolated dystonia has raised the question of whether such dysfunctions are primary, or the consequences of potential confounding factors. One possible issue relates to the effect of medications used to treat dystonia, especially anticholinergic agent or benzodiazepines. In one study, isolated focal dystonia patients were evaluated with an extensive neuropsychological battery before and after treatment with anticholinergic medication [45]. Before treatment, no differences were found between patients and control subjects regarding intelligence, memory, executive, and visuospatial functions. With anticholinergic medication, dystonic patients showed lower performance on verbal memory and speed of information processing [45]. A second potential mechanism leading to lower

Table 8.3 Studies on cognitive impairment in isolated dystonia [45–54]

Author, year	Study type	Sample size	Assessment	Main findings
Taylor, 1991 [45]	case-control with treatment	12 focal dystonia, 25 HS	WAIS, WMS (logical passages and visual reproduction), DRT, TT, BSRT, CALT, BC, item 99, SCWT, WFT, WCST	At baseline there were no differences between patients and HS. After treatment with trihexyphenidyl, patients showed lower performances on processing speed and immediate and delayed explicit memory
Leplow, 1994 [54]	Case-control	18 CD, 18 HS	SV, RWT, BPT, RMRT, JLO, DL, SD	Patients showed marked deficits in extra-personal orientation and atypical displacement errors to the right when requested to set the subjective vertical
Hinse, 1996 [53]	Case-control	15 CD, 15 HC	JVV, JLO, RWT, POT, RMRT, RMDS	Patients performed significantly worse on spatial tasks requiring mental manipulation of personal space
Jahanshahi, 2003 [50]	Case-control	10 isolated dystonia, 12 HS	WFT, WCST, SCWT, MDT, SORNS, RNG, VVCAL, PVSAT, DT	Dystonic patients showed lower performance in WFT and DT compared to HS
Scott, 2003 [49]	Case series	14 isolated dystonia	CANTAB (intra/extra-dimensional set-shifting, reaction time, spatial working memory, spatial span, stockings of Cambridge, rapid visual information processing test), RSPM, SDMT, SCWT, TMT, WFT, BNT, JLO, SCOLP (speed of comprehension), RMT, AMIPB (story recall), WAIS (digit span), CF	Patients failed at the extra-dimensional set-shifting phase of the intra/extra-dimensional set- shifting subtest of the CANTAB
Ploner, 2005 [52]	Case-control	16 CD, 16 HS	SMT (egocentric short-term spatial memory, egocentric long-term spatial memory, allocentric short-term spatial memory, allocentric long-term spatial memory)	The absolute performances on SMT of patients and HS were similar; however, while HS used egocentric or allocentric spatial representations, patients used only a allocentric strategy

Balas, 2006 [51]	Case-control	20 symptomatic DYT1, 20 non-symptomatic DYT1, 28 noncarriers	RSPM, RAVLT, RCF, WFT, TMT, SCWT, CANTAB (intra/extra dimensional set-shifting, stockings of Cambridge, spatial working memory, spatial span forward and reverse), WAIS (digit span, similarities, symbol search), JLO	Symptomatic DYT1s performed worse on verbal learning due to a greater retroactive memory interference and better on semantic verbal fluency test
Allam, 2007 [46]	case-control with BoNT treatment	9 BSP, 9 HS	RAVLT, SAT, WMS (digit forward and reversed), SCWT, WAIS (digit symbol)	At baseline BSP patients had lower score on test of sustained attention. After BoNT treatment there were no differences between BSP patients and HS
Alemàn, 2009 [47]	Case-control	20 BSP, 17 HS	FDT, RSPM, LT, WMS (list of words, spatial location) WCST, oral TMT, DR, TD	Dystonic patients performed lower than HS on motor programming, visual working memory, and tactile recognition
Romano, 2011 [48]	Case-control	45 CCD, 37 HS	n-Back, TMT, WCST, WMS	Dystonic patients had lower performance on working memory, set-shifting, visual short-term memory, processing speed, and set-shifting

AMIPB adult memory and information processing battery, *BC* block counting, *BNT* Boston naming test, *BoNT* botulinum neurotoxin, *BPT* body placing test, *BSP* blepharospasm, *BSRT* Buschke selective reminding test, *BVRT* Benton visual retention test, *CALT* conditional associative learning test, *CANTAB* Cambridge neuropsychological test automated battery, *CCD* craniocervical dystonia, *CD* cervical dystonia, *CF* medical college of Georgia complex figures, *DL* dot localizations, *DR* digital recognition, *DRT* delayed recognition span test, *DT* dual task, *FDT* five digits test, *HS* healthy controls, *JLO* judgment of line orientation, *JVV* judgment of the visual vertical, *LT* Luria's task, *MDT* missing digit test, *POT* personal orientation test, *PVSAT* paced visual serial addition test, *RAVLT* Rey auditory verbal learning test, *RCF* Rey complex figure, *RMDS* road map of direction sense, *RMRT* Ratcliff's mental reorientation test, *RMT* recognition memory test, *RNG* random number generation, *RSPM* Raven's standard progressive matrices, *RWT* route-walking test, *SAT* Toulouse-Pieron sustained attention test, *SCOLP* speed and capacity of language processing test, *SCWT* Stroop color-word test, *SD* spontaneous drawing, *SDMT* symbol digit modalities test, *SMT* spatial memory task, *SORNS* self-ordered random number sequences, *SV* subjective vertical, *TD* tactile denomination, *TMT* trial making test, *TT* tower of Toronto, *VVCAL* visual-visual conditions associative learning, *WAIS* Wechsler adult intelligence scale, *WC* writer's cramp, *WCST* Wisconsin card sorting test, *WFT* words fluency test, *WMS* Wechsler memory scale performance on cognitive test depends on disability related to dystonia. This has been highlighted in one study assessing cognitive performance of isolated dystonic patients before and after treatment with BoNT [46]. At baseline, despite well-preserved general intellectual skills, patients showed a deficit of sustained attention compared to control. After BoNT treatment, there was an increase of sustained attention scores and the differences with control group were no more significant [46]. These data support the idea that attention dysfunction in isolated dystonia may be in part secondary to the disrupting effects of motor symptoms. Treatment with BoNT alleviating motor symptoms may consequently improve sustained attention. Furthermore, executive functions were showed to improve also in a group of generalized dystonia patients after deep brain stimulation of the globus pallidus internus [55]. A further confounding factor is the possible occurrence of psychiatric disorders. Concurrent mood disorders may lead to impairment in executive function. It has been reported that pseudodementia may occur in patients with untreated low mood [56] and that patients with OCD can have executive function deficits [57, 58]. Recent studies that controlled for these possible confounding variables suggest that executive and visuospatial deficits are primary symptoms of isolated dystonia. A case-control study on blepharospasm patients found impairment of complex movements planning, motor dexterity, visuospatial working memory, and tactile object recognition [47]. These executive and visuospatial deficits remained significant also after correction for age, duration of disease, severity of blepharospasm, and degree of depression. Furthermore, a recent study involving cranial dystonic patients showed that cognitive dysfunction persisted even after controlling for pharmacological treatment and the effect of motor symptoms [48]. Executive functions, verbal and visual memory, were assessed in isolated dystonic patients and healthy subjects matched for age, gender, socioeconomic status, and premorbid intellectual functioning. None of the subjects were depressed, none of the patients took dopaminergic or anticholinergic drugs, and all patients were assessed 4 or 5 weeks after treatment with BoNT, when treatment provides the peak of effect. Dystonic patients showed lower performance compared to healthy subjects in tasks assessing working memory, processing speed, visual motor ability, and short-term memory. The authors retained that these deficits were not the consequence of motor phenomenology of dystonia but might rather reflect cortical and subcortical changes that characterized the pathophysiology of the disease [48].

Combined Dystonias

Combined syndromes are characterized by the association of dystonia with other movement disorder, i.e., myoclonus or parkinsonism [1]. The phenomenological expression is wide and dystonia may not be necessarily the prominent motor sign. Most of dystonia syndromes previously defined as "plus" or "heredodegenerative" are now covered by this heading. Various dominant, recessive, or X-linked inherited genes are being identified in combined dystonia [59]. Recent evidence has suggested that neuropsychiatric symptoms may be part of the phenotypical spectrum of combined syndromes. However, definitive conclusions are difficult to draw, as few studies are available. Here, we review the neuropsychiatric features of the most common combined dystonia syndromes.

Dopa-Responsive Dystonia

Dopa-responsive dystonia (DRD), also named Segawa disease [60], is a rare treatable form of dystonia. The clinical spectrum is variable and related to age of disease onset. DRD commonly starts in childhood with lower limb involvement and gait difficulties. The disease commonly progresses to generalized dystonia and retains diurnal fluctuations of symptoms, concurrent or subsequent development of parkinsonism, and a dramatic response to levodopa medication [60, 61]. The adult-onset forms have different signs at presentation, i.e., dystonic or resting tremor or mild akinetic-rigid parkinsonism, and are characterized by various types of focal dystonias [61]. In about 50 % of the affected subjects, DRD is caused by dominantly inherited mutations of the GCH1 gene (DYT5a) [62]. A minority of patients show autosomal recessive inheritance involving mutations of TH (DYT5b) [63] or SPR genes [64]. Patients with DRD were initially described as free from mental or psychological abnormalities [61]. However, recent reports observed the occurrence of non-motor features including neuropsychiatric disturbances.

Psychiatric Profile

Case reports [65–67] and family studies [68–71] have shown that psychiatric symptoms, including depression, anxiety, and OCD, can be part of DRD phenomenology. In a retrospective study of 34 GCH1 mutation carriers, high prevalence of recurrent episodes of depressive disorders, including either nonreactive mood swings or major depression, was noted [68]. A recent meta-analysis of 70 DRD patients reported high rate of depression (34 %), anxiety (19 %), and OCD (9 %) [72]. In contrast with these findings, one case-control study highlighted that the risk for psychiatric symptoms is not increased in DRD patients [73]. In this study, 23 levodopa-treated GCH1 mutation carriers from 13 different families and 26 healthy age-matched controls were assessed for depression and anxiety with standardized rating scales, and no differences between the two groups were found [73]. The issue whether the DRD phenotypes includes psychiatric abnormalities has to be considered still unsettled. All the studies variably suffer from shortcomings, including lack of a control group, small sample size, lack of standardized assessment, or bias in sample selection.

Cognitive Profile

Evidence on cognition in DRD is limited. Cognitive domains have been commonly considered in the normal range, and only few patients were reported with cognitive decline [74, 75]. Among 34 GCH1 carriers, difficulties in sustained attention were detected in four patients and verbal memory deficits in three [68]. Only one study examined global intellectual functioning in DRD patients based on a standardized measure [71]. In this study, 14 carriers of CGH1 gene mutation (seven subjects younger than 18 years of age and seven adults) from two families were investigated using the Wechsler intelligence scales. The results revealed that six out of seven adults and three out of seven children had intellectual functioning at a borderline level to mild mental retardation [71]. Although these results are preliminary, the data might suggest that cognitive impairment is associated with CGH1-related DRD, at least in some families. Case-control studies with standardized cognitive assessment are needed to characterized cognitive features in the DRD population.

Myoclonus-Dystonia

Myoclonus-dystonia (M-D) is characterized by alcohol-responsive myoclonus accompanied by dystonia in approximately two-thirds of patients [76]. The jerks mainly occur in the upper limbs, trunk, and neck, whereas cervical dystonia and writer's cramp are the most frequent dystonia types [76, 77]. The onset is typically in the young age, usually in the first or the second decade of life. Mutations of SGCE gene (DYT11) represent the most common cause of M-D with estimated rate at near 50 % in familial cases and 13 % in sporadic cases [78–80]. SGCE mutations are inherited in autosomal dominant fashion with a reduced penetrance due to maternal imprinting. Although there is controversy across studies, in the past few decades evidence has emerged that psychiatric symptoms and cognitive impairments may be part of the clinical spectrum of M-D.

Psychiatric Profile

Psychiatric features including OCD, alcohol misuse, anxiety, depression, and psychosis have been noted in M-D families [77, 81–86]. However, few controlled studies were carried out and no consensus has been reached on the types of psychiatric comorbidity. It is also unknown whether psychiatric symptoms are a primary expression of M-D phenomenology or a consequence of having a chronic disease since the childhood. The majority of controlled studies compared manifesting SGCE mutation carriers against non-manifesting carriers and healthy controls. The available evidence suggests that higher prevalence of psychiatric disorders, especially OCD and alcohol misuse, characterized manifesting mutation carriers compared to non-manifesting carriers and healthy control [87–90]. OCD has been retained a direct expression of SCGE gene mutation, while alcohol misuse has been considered secondary to attempts of self-medication [88, 90].

A recent study compared a group of M-D mutation carriers with a control group matched for severity of motor disability [89]. In this study, a group of 27 DYT 11 patients were compared to 45 subjects with alcohol-responsive tremor matched for disease duration, gender, and alcohol use. Compared to control subjects, DYT11 patients were eight times more likely to have OCD and five times more likely to have alcohol dependence and generalized anxiety disorder [89]. In addition, no association was noted between psychiatric disorders and motor severity, suggesting that the psychopathology may be independent from motor disability. However, the association between SGCE gene mutation and psychiatric symptoms is not confirmed by all observations. In a case-control study, 27 DYT11 mutation carriers (14 manifesting and 13 non-manifesting) and 42 control subjects from one large M-D family were studied [91]. Manifesting mutation carriers showed a high prevalence of depression, anxiety, and panic attacks, while the commonly reported association with OCD or alcohol misuse was not confirmed by this study [91]. The scores of depression and anxiety scales correlated with the severity of motor signs and the non-manifesting carriers did not differ from controls. Foncke and colleagues concluded that the high prevalence of psychiatric symptoms was the consequence of having a disabling disease [91]. Recently, a case-control study compared M-D patients with and without SGCE gene mutation [92]. M-D patients with SGCE mutation had higher prevalence of anxiety disorders compared to M-D patients without mutation, while both groups had higher frequency of depression compared to healthy control [92]. Interestingly, also in this study no association between DYT11 and OCD was observed. The authors suggested that the occurrence of anxiety disorders may be a direct expression of harboring a SGCE mutation, while the occurrence of depression may be a consequence of being affected by a disabling disorder.

Cognitive Profile

Earlier single-case observations in affected families reported inconsistent result [93–95]. Two recent studies from the same Dutch research group have investigated in detail the topic of cognitive profile in M-D, but the inconsistencies still remain. In the abovementioned series by Foncke and colleagues [91], the DYT11 patients performed equal to SGCE asymptomatic carriers and familial noncarriers on several cognitive measurements. The neuropsychological assessment involved attention and processing speed, executive function, and language. In the study by van Tricht and colleagues [92], a relation between DYT11 and the occurrence of executive dysfunction including set shifting, set maintenance, and working memory was described. On the contrary, patients without SCGE mutation showed only a subtle deficit on semantic fluency. No relation between defective cognitive performances and motor impairment or medication was found, suggesting that executive dysfunction may be a primary symptom of M-D linked to DYT11 [92]. Because of the limited sample size, the conclusions drawn are provisional and further studies have to be performed to elucidate the topic of cognitive profile in M-D.

Rapid-Onset Dystonia-Parkinsonism

Rapid-onset dystonia-parkinsonism (RDP) is a rare autosomal dominant movement disorder with reduced penetrance caused by a variety of missense mutations in the ATP1A3 gene (DYT12) [96]. The onset is between the teens and the twenties; symptoms develop abruptly, in hours or weeks, frequently after a mental or physical stressor [97]. The phenotypic expression is variable and characterized by dystonia, signs of parkinsonism, dysarthria, and dysphagia [97].

Psychiatric Profile

The evidence on psychopathologies in RDP is limited and only anecdotal. Depression and anxiety symptoms, including social phobia, were reported in some patients carrying ATP1A3 gene mutations, but standardized evaluations are unavailable [97, 98]. In keeping with this, in a family study three siblings carrying an ATP1A3 gene mutation were examined by means of structured psychiatric interview [99]. The psychiatric evaluation demonstrated mood alterations and anxiety in all. Two siblings received a diagnosis of panic disorder and bipolar disorder as well as OCD and substance abuse disorder. The third sibling reached diagnostic threshold for dysthymia and had a prior diagnosis of psychosis, occurring before the motor onset. Case-control studies with standardized assessment of psychiatric symptoms are needed to highlight the psychiatric phenotype of RDP patients.

Cognitive Profile

Few studies have inquired on cognitive features of patients with RDP and current evidence shows that cognitive impairment is not unusual in these patients pointing out a possible relation between ATP1A3 gene and cognition [97, 99, 100]. The three siblings of the previous study by Barbano and colleagues [99] were assessed also on tests of verbal and nonverbal memory and executive functions. Their performances were under the normative value for tests of verbal fluency and set shifting, suggesting that executive dysfunction may occur in RDP. In keeping with this observation, the only detailed study on cognitive performance confirms that cognitive impairment may be part of RDP phenomenology. Cook and colleagues [100] compared memory, attention, and executive functions of 29 ATP1A3 mutation carriers and 29 familial noncarriers control. The patient group performed worse than controls on tests of verbal and nonverbal memory, set shifting, and attention. These differences remained significant also after controlling for processing speed, depression, psychosis, and substance abuse. The prevalence of cognitive deficit was higher in ATP1A3 carriers, especially for attention and executive functions, although it should be noted that impaired performance was not equally observed among RDP patients for any measure. The motor symptoms may have some influence on these results, as a significant negative correlation between the severity of motor status and the scores of test based on processing speed and motor response was found [100]. It is noteworthy that many RDP patients had learning difficulties during school that was not related to impaired motor functioning. Therefore, in some cases, cognitive impairment or intellectual difficulties could be a premorbid feature of RDP [100].

Neurodegenerations with Brain Iron Accumulation

Neurodegenerations with brain iron accumulation (NBIA) encompasses a heterogeneous group of disorders characterized by excessive regional brain iron deposition, particularly within some basal ganglia nuclei. The clinical spectrum is wide, as NBIA can manifest at variable age, ranging from early childhood to late adulthood, with various combinations of movement disorders, seizures, pyramidal signs, visual disturbances, and neuropsychiatric symptoms [101, 102]. The core NBIA syndromes are: pantothenate kinase-associated neurodegeneration (PKAN) [103] and PLA2G6-mutation-associated neurodegeneration (PLAN) [104]. Recent advances in genetic have recognized further genes causing NBIAs [105].

NBIAs, particularly the formerly called Hallervorden-Spatz syndrome, have been traditionally associated with low intellectual level [106]. However, also due to the rarity of these conditions, the studies on neuropsychiatric features are limited to single-case reports or families. There is overall insufficient knowledge on the neuropsychiatric symptoms and their course.

PKAN

PKAN, originally described as Hallervorden-Spatz syndrome, is an autosomal recessive disorder caused by mutations in the PANK2 gene, accounting for near half cases of NBIA [107]. The classic presentation is characterized by early age of onset, occurring before age 6 in almost of the cases, with gait or postural difficulty [108, 109]. The course is progressive and the phenotype encompasses either pyramidal or extrapyramidal features with prominent dystonia, especially with oromandibular involvement. Oculomotor abnormalities are also common. Adult-onset patients show atypical phenotype with less severe motor signs and neuropsychiatric involvement.

Psychiatric symptoms are common in the adult form and can often antedate the motor onset. Psychiatric onset, including emotional lability, personality change, aggression, impulsivity, OCD, and depression, has been described [110, 111]. Motor and vocal tics and obsessions, suggestive of Tourette syndrome, have also been reported [112].

A limited number of studies were carried out on cognitive profile of PKAN. Cognitive deficits may occur in typical and atypical variants, and dementia has been described in adult-onset patients [109]. Problems with executive functioning, attention, visual and verbal memory, or judgment have been reported in PKAN [113–115]. The degree of cognitive dysfunction varies between subjects, from selective executive deficits [116] to mild cognitive impairment [117] and dementia [109, 115]. Notwithstanding, there are observations reporting no cognitive dysfunction in PKAN patients [118, 119].

In a study investigating intellectual functioning in PKAN, 16 subjects were assessed [120]. Their global intellectual functioning was quite variable, from high average to well below average. Age of disease onset correlated with measures of intellectual functioning, adaptive functioning, and disease severity.

PLAN

PLAN is also an autosomal recessive NBIA caused by mutations in the PLA2G6 gene [104]. Similarly to PKAN, the phenotypic expression varies according to age of onset. The most common form has young age of onset, progressive motor and mental retardation, cerebellar ataxia, trunk hypotonia, pyramidal signs, and visual disturbances caused by optic atrophy. The atypical forms onset later and are characterized by dystonia-parkinsonism, pyramidal signs, eye movement abnormalities, cognitive decline, and psychiatric symptoms.

Single-case and case series reported that neuropsychiatric symptoms, including emotional lability, compulsions, hyperactivity, reduced attention span, and behavioral disturbances, become prominent as disease progresses [107]. A recent 8-year longitudinal study analyzed a series of 24 subjects from 25 unrelated families [121]. At disease onset mood or behavioral changes occurred in 9 % of subjects and cognitive impairment in 4.6 %; after 8 years, 95 % of the patients showed psychiatric disorders and 91.4 % had cognitive decline.

Pathophysiology

Knowledge on neuropsychiatric features of dystonia syndromes is at its infancy. Evidence suggests that at least some psychiatric or cognitive features may share common neurobiological pathways with dystonia, whereas others may be coincidental findings or may be a reaction to motor signs.

The pathophysiology of dystonia is complex and currently poorly understood. Probably, it involves dysfunctions of several central nervous system circuits underpinning control of voluntary movements [122, 123]. Earlier neuropathological studies in acquired dystonias suggest that basal ganglia lesions can produce the movement disorder, but also the thalamus, brainstem, parietal lobe, and cerebellar lesions were considered causative [124, 125]. The basal ganglia involvement in dystonia has been further supported by imaging studies in sporadic and hereditary cases. Studies using voxel-based morphometry have shown increased volume in the putamen, thalamus, sensorimotor cortex, and cerebellum in sporadic dystonia [126, 127] and in DYT1 manifesting- and non-manifesting carriers [128]. Diffusion tensor imaging shows increased fractional anisotropy in the fiber tracts connecting the basal ganglia, cortex, and cerebellum [129].

The basal ganglia have been traditionally recognized as a main part of the complex network regulating movements, but in the last 20 years, basal ganglia non-motor functions have been increasingly recognized. A first account on the pathophysiology of motor and non-motor features was provided by the Alexander-DeLong model of cortico-striato-thalamo-cortical loops [130]. These loops involve projections from specific cortical areas to separate regions within subcortical nuclei that recurrently are connected to the same areas of cortex through specific thalamic relay nuclei [131]. While in this initial model the loops were retained largely segregated, currently it has been shown that transfer of information can occur between these circuits [132]. Therefore, the functional organization of basal ganglia is conditioned largely by their connections with specific cerebral cortex regions. Basal ganglia have connection with dorsolateral prefrontal cortex and lateral orbitofrontal cortex, i.e., the associative loop, and with the medial orbitofrontal cortex, the anterior cingulate, the agranular insular cortex, the amygdala, and the hippocampus, i.e. the limbic loop.

The basal ganglia functional subdivision follows a dorsal-ventral gradient whereby the dorsolateral region of the striatum is engaged in sensorimotor functions, the dorsomedial striatum in associative functions, and the ventral striatum in motivational and emotional function. Therefore, disorders affecting the basal ganglia tend to present with a combination of motor and non-motor symptoms, arising from the specific anatomo-functional organization of these loops [133]. Abnormalities at this level have been related to pathophysiology of depression [134] and OCD [135]. Focal infarction of the basal ganglia can cause dystonia associated with new-onset OCD and depression [136]. Furthermore, in recent years deep brain stimulation of some basal ganglia nuclei has been increasingly used for the treatment of psychiatric conditions including Gilles de la Tourette syndrome, OCD, refractory depression, and addiction [137]. Based on their connections with prefrontal and parietal cortex, the basal ganglia also influence cognitive functions, especially in the executive and visuospatial domains. An amount of evidence sustains the role of basal ganglia in reinforcement learning [138], cognitive control [138], category learning [139], sequential decision-making [140], and working memory [141]. Cognitive impairment and dementia were shown in many pathologies involving basal ganglia including Parkinson's disease, Huntington disease, and progressive supranuclear palsy [133].

Dysfunction in fronto-striatal circuitry may provide a neurobiological explanation for the higher incidence of neuropsychiatric features in isolated and combined dystonias. Further studies of inherited dystonia syndromes will allow generating new hypotheses on the role of specific molecules in the origin of neuropsychiatric symptoms in dystonia.

Implications for Treatment

Unfortunately, no double-blind trials have specifically addressed how to treat neuropsychiatric abnormalities associated with dystonia. Psychiatric treatment should address the underlying psychopathologic conditions, but the coexistence of dystonia and neuropsychiatric disorders has multiple implications. Firstly, if neuropsychiatric symptoms are reactive to motor impairment, the treatment of motor condition may result in improvement of psychiatric symptoms. Some studies reported improvement of psychiatric symptoms in dystonia patients after treatment with BoNT [22, 27, 50]. A second issue pertains to the possible worsening of dystonia after prescription of some psychiatric medications. Special caution should be used when administering antipsychotics, given that anti-dopaminergic drugs are known to worsen and even cause dystonia or tardive dyskinesia [142, 143]. Similarly, selective serotonin reuptake inhibitors may induce worsening of dystonia [144].

Prior to the current era, dystonia was considered a psychogenic condition and treated with psychotherapy to alleviate motor symptomatology. Current knowledge has reversed such view: dystonia is a motor condition with the possible association of psychiatric features. However, psychotherapy in dystonia can be useful for the treatment of psychiatric symptoms. Cognitive-behavioral psychotherapy has shown evidence-based effectiveness in treating depression [145], anxious disorders [146], and OCD [147]. Randomized clinical trials are needed to assess the effectiveness of psychotherapy in dystonia syndromes.

References

1. Albanese A, Bhatia K, Bressman SB, Delong MR, Fahn S, Fung VSC, et al. Phenomenology and classification of dystonia: a consensus update. Mov Disord. 2013;28:863–73.
2. Kuyper DJ, Parra V, Aerts S, Okun MS, Kluger BM. Nonmotor manifestations of dystonia: a systematic review. Mov Disord. 2011;26:1206–17.
3. Stamelou M, Edwards MJ, Hallett M, Bhatia KP. The non-motor syndrome of primary dystonia: clinical and pathophysiological implications. Brain. 2012;135:1668–81.
4. Zurowski M, McDonald WM, Fox S, Marsh L. Psychiatric comorbidities in dystonia: emerging concepts. Mov Disord. 2013;28:914–20.
5. Albanese A, Asmus F, Bhatia KP, Elia AE, Elibol B, Filippini G, et al. EFNS guidelines on diagnosis and treatment of primary dystonias. Eur J Neurol. 2011;18:5–18.
6. Phukan J, Albanese A, Gasser T, Warner T. Primary dystonia and dystonia-plus syndromes: clinical characteristics, diagnosis, and pathogenesis. Lancet Neurol. 2011;10:1074–85.
7. Kramer PL, De Leon D, Ozelius L, Risch N, Bressman SB, Brin MF, et al. Dystonia gene in Ashkenazi Jewish population is located on chromosome 9q32-34. Ann Neurol. 1990;27:114–20.

8. Bressman SB, Raymond D, Wendt K, Saunders-Pullman R, De Leon D, Fahn S, et al. Diagnostic criteria for dystonia in DYT1 families. Neurology. 2002;59:1780–2.
9. Jamora RDG, Tan E-K, Liu C-P, Kathirvel P, Burgunder J-M, Tan LCS. DYT1 mutations amongst adult primary dystonia patients in Singapore with review of literature comparing East and West. J Neurol Sci. 2006;247:35–7.
10. Fuchs T, Gavarini S, Saunders-Pullman R, Raymond D, Ehrlich ME, Bressman SB, et al. Mutations in the THAP1 gene are responsible for DYT6 primary torsion dystonia. Nat Genet. 2009;41:286–8.
11. Almasy L, Bressman SB, Raymond D, Kramer PL, Greene PE, Heiman GA, et al. Idiopathic torsion dystonia linked to chromosome 8 in two Mennonite families. Ann Neurol. 1997;42:670–3.
12. Valente EM, Bentivoglio AR, Cassetta E, Dixon PH, Davis MB, Ferraris A, et al. DYT13, a novel primary torsion dystonia locus, maps to chromosome 1p36.13–36.32 in an Italian family with cranial-cervical or upper limb onset. Ann Neurol. 2001;49:362–6.
13. Norgren N, Mattson E, Forsgren L, Holmberg M. A high-penetrance form of late-onset torsion dystonia maps to a novel locus (DYT21) on chromosome 2q14.3-q21.3. Neurogenetics. 2011;12:137–43.
14. Bindman E, Tibbetts RW. Writer's cramp–a rational approach to treatment? Br J Psychiatry. 1977;131:143–8.
15. Ben-Shlomo Y, Camfield L, Warner T. What are the determinants of quality of life in people with cervical dystonia? J Neurol Neurosurg Psychiatry. 2002;72:608–14.
16. Lencer R, Steinlechner S, Stahlberg J, Rehling H, Orth M, Baeumer T, et al. Primary focal dystonia: evidence for distinct neuropsychiatric and personality profiles. J Neurol Neurosurg Psychiatry. 2009;80:1176–9.
17. Broocks A, Thiel A, Angerstein D, Dressler D. Higher prevalence of obsessive-compulsive symptoms in patients with blepharospasm than in patients with hemifacial spasm. Am J Psychiatry. 1998;155:555–7.
18. Wenzel T, Schnider P, Wimmer A, Steinhoff N, Moraru E, Auff E. Psychiatric comorbidity in patients with spasmodic torticollis. J Psychosom Res. 1998;44:687–90.
19. Gündel H, Wolf A, Xidara V, Busch R, Ceballos-Baumann AO. Social phobia in spasmodic torticollis. J Neurol Neurosurg Psychiatry. 2001;71:499–504.
20. Cavallaro R, Galardi G, Cavallini MC, Henin M, Amodio S, Bellodi L, et al. Obsessive compulsive disorder among idiopathic focal dystonia patients: an epidemiological and family study. Biol Psychiatry. 2002;52:356–61.
21. Moraru E, Schnider P, Wimmer A, Wenzel T, Birner P, Griengl H, et al. Relation between depression and anxiety in dystonic patients: implications for clinical management. Depress Anxiety. 2002;16:100–3.
22. Müller J, Kemmler G, Wissel J, Schneider A, Voller B, Grossmann J, et al. The impact of blepharospasm and cervical dystonia on health-related quality of life and depression. J Neurol. 2002;249:842–6.
23. Gündel H, Wolf A, Xidara V, Busch R, Ladwig KH, Jacobi F, et al. High psychiatric comorbidity in spasmodic torticollis: a controlled study. J Nerv Ment Dis. 2003;191:465–73.
24. Heiman GA, Ottman R, Saunders-Pullman RJ, Ozelius LJ, Risch NJ, Bressman SB. Increased risk for recurrent major depression in DYT1 dystonia mutation carriers. Neurology. 2004;63:631–7.
25. Gündel H, Busch R, Ceballos-Baumann A, Seifert E. Psychiatric comorbidity in patients with spasmodic dysphonia: a controlled study. J Neurol Neurosurg Psychiatry. 2007;78:1398–400.
26. Heiman GA, Ottman R, Saunders-Pullman RJ, Ozelius LJ, Risch NJ, Bressman SB. Obsessive-compulsive disorder is not a clinical manifestation of the DYT1 dystonia gene. Am J Med Genet B Neuropsychiatr Genet. 2007;144B:361–4.
27. Ochudlo S, Bryniarski P, Opala G. Botulinum toxin improves the quality of life and reduces the intensification of depressive symptoms in patients with blepharospasm. Parkinsonism Relat Disord. 2007;13:505–8.

28. Bugalho P, Corrêa B, Guimarães J, Xavier M. Set-shifting and behavioral dysfunction in primary focal dystonia. Mov Disord. 2008;23:200–6.
29. Lewis L, Butler A, Jahanshahi M. Depression in focal, segmental and generalized dystonia. J Neurol. 2008;255:1750–5.
30. Fabbrini G, Berardelli I, Moretti G, Pasquini M, Bloise M, Colosimo C, et al. Psychiatric disorders in adult-onset focal dystonia: a case-control study. Mov Disord. 2010;25:459–65.
31. Barahona-Corrêa B, Bugalho P, Guimarães J, Xavier M. Obsessive-compulsive symptoms in primary focal dystonia: a controlled study. Mov Disord. 2011;26:2274–8.
32. Dias FM, Kummer A, Doyle FC, Harsányi E, Cardoso F, Fontenelle LF, et al. Psychiatric disorders in primary focal dystonia and in Parkinson's disease. Neuropsychiatr Dis Treat. 2011;7:111–6.
33. Duane DD, Bakken EC. Additional clinical observations on psychiatric disorders in adult-onset focal dystonia: a case control study. Mov Disord. 2011;26:1572.
34. Mula M, Strigaro G, Marotta AE, Ruggerone S, Tribolo A, Monaco R, et al. Obsessive-compulsive-spectrum symptoms in patients with focal dystonia, hemifacial spasm, and healthy subjects. J Neuropsychiatry Clin Neurosci. 2012;24:81–6.
35. Lehn A, Mellick G, Boyle R. Psychiatric disorders in idiopathic-isolated focal dystonia. J Neurol. 2014;261:668–74.
36. Jahanshahi M, Marsden CD. Psychological functioning before and after treatment of torticollis with botulinum toxin. J Neurol Neurosurg Psychiatry. 1992;55:229–31.
37. Munhoz RP, Teive HAG, Della Coletta MV, Germiniani FMB, Iwamoto FM, Camargo CHF, et al. Frequency of obsessive and compulsive symptoms in patients with blepharospasm and hemifacial spasm. Arq Neuropsiquiatr. 2005;63:213–6.
38. Fontenelle LF, Pacheco PG, Nascimento PM, de Freitas AR, Rosso AL, Teixeira AL, et al. Obsessive-compulsive symptoms among patients with blepharospasm and hemifacial spasm. Gen Hosp Psychiatry. 2011;33:476–81.
39. Kubota Y, Murai T, Okada T, Hayashi A, Toichi M, Sakihama M, et al. Obsessive-compulsive characteristics in patients with writer's cramp. J Neurol Neurosurg Psychiatry. 2001;71:413–4.
40. Marsden CD, Harrison MJ. Idiopathic torsion dystonia (dystonia musculorum deformans). A review of forty-two patients. Brain. 1974;97:793–810.
41. Riklan M, Cullinan T, Cooper IS. Psychological studies in dystonia musculorum deformans. Adv Neurol. 1976;14:189–200.
42. Eldridge R, Edgar A, Brody J, Cooper IS, Riklan M. Increased intelligence in recessively inherited torsion dystonia (dystonia musculorum deformans). Neurology. 1970;20:410.
43. Eldridge R. The torsion dystonias: literature review and genetic and clinical studies. Neurology. 1970;20:1–78.
44. Nakashima K, Shimoda M, Sato K, Nanba E, Igo M, Takahashi K. Hereditary non-progressive torsion dystonia with intellectual disturbance. Intern Med. 1995;34:843–6.
45. Taylor AE, Lang AE, Saint-Cyr JA, Riley DE, Ranawaya R. Cognitive processes in idiopathic dystonia treated with high-dose anticholinergic therapy: implications for treatment strategies. Clin Neuropharmacol. 1991;14:62–77.
46. Allam N, Frank JE, Pereira C, Tomaz C. Sustained attention in cranial dystonia patients treated with botulinum toxin. Acta Neurol Scand. 2007;116:196–200.
47. Alemán GG, de Erausquin GA, Micheli F. Cognitive disturbances in primary blepharospasm. Mov Disord. 2009;24:2112–20.
48. Romano R, Bertolino A, Gigante A, Martino D, Livrea P, Defazio G. Impaired cognitive functions in adult-onset primary cranial cervical dystonia. Parkinsonism Relat Disord. 2014;20(2):162–5.
49. Scott RB, Gregory R, Wilson J, Banks S, Turner A, Parkin S, et al. Executive cognitive deficits in primary dystonia. Mov Disord. 2003;18:539–50.
50. Jahanshahi M, Rowe J, Fuller R. Cognitive executive function in dystonia. Mov Disord. 2003;18:1470–81.

51. Balas M, Peretz C, Badarny S, Scott RB, Giladi N. Neuropsychological profile of DYT1 dystonia. Mov Disord. 2006;21:2073–7.
52. Ploner CJ, Stenz U, Fassdorf K, Arnold G. Egocentric and allocentric spatial memory in idiopathic cervical dystonia. Neurology. 2005;64:1733–8.
53. Hinse P, Leplow B, Humbert T, Lamparter U, Junge A, Emskötter T. Impairment of visuospatial function in idiopathic spasmodic torticollis. J Neurol. 1996;243:29–33.
54. Leplow B, Stübinger C. Visuospatial functions in patients with spasmodic torticollis. Percept Mot Skills. 1994;78:1363–75.
55. Pillon B, Ardouin C, Dujardin K, Vittini P, Pelissolo A, Cottencin O, et al. Preservation of cognitive function in dystonia treated by pallidal stimulation. Neurology. 2006;66:1556–8.
56. Dobie DJ. Depression, dementia, and pseudodementia. Semin Clin Neuropsychiatry. 2002;7:170–86.
57. Bari A, Robbins TW. Inhibition and impulsivity: behavioral and neural basis of response control. Prog Neurobiol. 2013;108:44–79.
58. Menzies L, Chamberlain SR, Laird AR, Thelen SM, Sahakian BJ, Bullmore ET. Integrating evidence from neuroimaging and neuropsychological studies of obsessive-compulsive disorder: the orbitofronto-striatal model revisited. Neurosci Biobehav Rev. 2008;32:525–49.
59. Charlesworth G, Bhatia KP, Wood NW. The genetics of dystonia: new twists in an old tale. Brain. 2013;136:2017–37.
60. Segawa M, Hosaka A, Miyagawa F, Nomura Y, Imai H. Hereditary progressive dystonia with marked diurnal fluctuation. Adv Neurol. 1976;14:215–33.
61. Segawa M, Nomura Y, Nishiyama N. Autosomal dominant guanosine triphosphate cyclohydrolase I deficiency (Segawa disease). Ann Neurol. 2003;54 Suppl 6:S32–45.
62. Ichinose H, Ohye T, Takahashi E, Seki N, Hori T, Segawa M, et al. Hereditary progressive dystonia with marked diurnal fluctuation caused by mutations in the GTP cyclohydrolase I gene. Nat Genet. 1994;8:236–42.
63. Bräutigam C, Wevers RA, Jansen RJ, Smeitink JA, de Rijk-van Andel JF, Gabreëls FJ, et al. Biochemical hallmarks of tyrosine hydroxylase deficiency. Clin Chem. 1998;44:1897–904.
64. Bonafé L, Thöny B, Penzien JM, Czarnecki B, Blau N. Mutations in the sepiapterin reductase gene cause a novel tetrahydrobiopterin-dependent monoamine-neurotransmitter deficiency without hyperphenylalaninemia. Am J Hum Genet. 2001;69:269–77.
65. Costeff H, Gadoth N, Mendelson L, Harel S, Lavie P. Fluctuating dystonia responsive to levodopa. Arch Dis Child. 1987;62:801–4.
66. Mathen D, Marsden CD, Bhatia KP. SSRI-induced reversal of levodopa benefit in two patients with dopa-responsive dystonia. Mov Disord. 1999;14:874–6.
67. Venna N, Sims KB, Grant PE. Case records of the Massachusetts General Hospital. Case 26-2006. A 19-year-old woman with difficulty walking. N Engl J Med. 2006;355:831–9.
68. Trender-Gerhard I, Sweeney MG, Schwingenschuh P, Mir P, Edwards MJ, Gerhard A, et al. Autosomal-dominant GTPCH1-deficient DRD: clinical characteristics and long-term outcome of 34 patients. J Neurol Neurosurg Psychiatry. 2009;80:839–45.
69. Hahn H, Trant MR, Brownstein MJ, Harper RA, Milstien S, Butler IJ. Neurologic and psychiatric manifestations in a family with a mutation in exon 2 of the guanosine triphosphate-cyclohydrolase gene. Arch Neurol. 2001;58:749–55.
70. Van Hove JLK, Steyaert J, Matthijs G, Legius E, Theys P, Wevers R, et al. Expanded motor and psychiatric phenotype in autosomal dominant Segawa syndrome due to GTP cyclohydrolase deficiency. J Neurol Neurosurg Psychiatry. 2006;77:18–23.
71. López-Laso E, Sánchez-Raya A, Moriana JA, Martínez-Gual E, Camino-León R, Mateos-González ME, et al. Neuropsychiatric symptoms and intelligence quotient in autosomal dominant Segawa disease. J Neurol. 2011;258:2155–62.
72. Tadic V, Kasten M, Brüggemann N, Stiller S, Hagenah J, Klein C. Dopa-responsive dystonia revisited: diagnostic delay, residual signs, and nonmotor signs. Arch Neurol. 2012;69:1–5.
73. Brüggemann N, Stiller S, Tadic V, Kasten M, Münchau A, Graf J, et al. Non-motor phenotype of dopa-responsive dystonia and quality of life assessment. Parkinsonism Relat Disord. 2014;20(4):428–31.

74. Nagata E, Kosakai A, Tanaka K, Segawa M, Fujioka H, Shintaku H, et al. Dopa-responsive dystonia (Segawa disease) -like disease accompanied by mental retardation: a case report. Mov Disord. 2007;22:1202–3.
75. Nitschke M, Steinberger D, Heberlein I, Otto V, Müller U, Vieregge P. Dopa responsive dystonia with Turner's syndrome: clinical, genetic, and neuropsychological studies in a family with a new mutation in the GTP-cyclohydrolase I gene. J Neurol Neurosurg Psychiatry. 1998;64:806–8.
76. Asmus F, Zimprich A, Tezenas Du Montcel S, Kabus C, Deuschl G, Kupsch A, et al. Myoclonus-dystonia syndrome: epsilon-sarcoglycan mutations and phenotype. Ann Neurol. 2002;52:489–92.
77. Asmus F, Gasser T. Dystonia-plus syndromes. Eur J Neurol. 2010;17 Suppl 1:37–45.
78. Zimprich A, Grabowski M, Asmus F, Naumann M, Berg D, Bertram M, et al. Mutations in the gene encoding epsilon-sarcoglycan cause myoclonus-dystonia syndrome. Nat Genet. 2001;29:66–9.
79. Grünewald A, Djarmati A, Lohmann-Hedrich K, Farrell K, Zeller JA, Allert N, et al. Myoclonus-dystonia: significance of large SGCE deletions. Hum Mutat. 2008;29:331–2.
80. Ritz K, Gerrits MCF, Foncke EMJ, van Ruissen F, van der Linden C, Vergouwen MDI, et al. Myoclonus-dystonia: clinical and genetic evaluation of a large cohort. J Neurol Neurosurg Psychiatry. 2009;80:653–8.
81. Misbahuddin A, Placzek M, Lennox G, Taanman JW, Warner TT. Myoclonus-dystonia syndrome with severe depression is caused by an exon-skipping mutation in the epsilon-sarcoglycan gene. Mov Disord. 2007;22:1173–5.
82. Dale RC, Nasti JJ, Peters GB. Familial 7q21.3 microdeletion involving epsilon-sarcoglycan causing myoclonus dystonia, cognitive impairment, and psychosis. Mov Disord. 2011;26:1774–5.
83. Gasser T. Inherited myoclonus-dystonia syndrome. Adv Neurol. 1998;78:325–34.
84. Nygaard TG, Raymond D, Chen C, Nishino I, Greene PE, Jennings D, et al. Localization of a gene for myoclonus-dystonia to chromosome 7q21-q31. Ann Neurol. 1999;46:794–8.
85. Klein C, Schilling K, Saunders-Pullman RJ, Garrels J, Breakefield XO, Brin MF, et al. A major locus for myoclonus-dystonia maps to chromosome 7q in eight families. Am J Hum Genet. 2000;67:1314–9.
86. Kyllerman M, Forsgren L, Sanner G, Holmgren G, Wahlström J, Drugge U. Alcohol-responsive myoclonic dystonia in a large family: dominant inheritance and phenotypic variation. Mov Disord. 1990;5:270–9.
87. Peall KJ, Waite AJ, Blake DJ, Owen MJ, Morris HR. Psychiatric disorders, myoclonus dystonia, and the epsilon-sarcoglycan gene: a systematic review. Mov Disord. 2011;26:1939–42.
88. Hess CW, Raymond D, Aguiar PDC, Frucht S, Shriberg J, Heiman GA, et al. Myoclonus-dystonia, obsessive-compulsive disorder, and alcohol dependence in SGCE mutation carriers. Neurology. 2007;68:522–4.
89. Peall KJ, Smith DJ, Kurian MA, Wardle M, Waite AJ, Hedderly T, et al. SGCE mutations cause psychiatric disorders: clinical and genetic characterization. Brain. 2013;136:294–303.
90. Saunders-Pullman R, Shriberg J, Heiman G, Raymond D, Wendt K, Kramer P, et al. Myoclonus dystonia: possible association with obsessive-compulsive disorder and alcohol dependence. Neurology. 2002;58:242–5.
91. Foncke EMJ, Cath D, Zwinderman K, Smit J, Schmand B, Tijssen M. Is psychopathology part of the phenotypic spectrum of myoclonus-dystonia?: a study of a large Dutch M-D family. Cogn Behav Neurol. 2009;22:127–33.
92. Van Tricht MJ, Dreissen YEM, Cath D, Dijk JM, Contarino MF, van der Salm SM, et al. Cognition and psychopathology in myoclonus-dystonia. J Neurol Neurosurg Psychiatry. 2012;83:814–20.
93. Maréchal L, Raux G, Dumanchin C, Lefebvre G, Deslandre E, Girard C, et al. Severe myoclonus-dystonia syndrome associated with a novel epsilon-sarcoglycan gene truncating mutation. Am J Med Genet B Neuropsychiatr Genet. 2003;119B:114–7.

94. Doheny DO, Brin MF, Morrison CE, Smith CJ, Walker RH, Abbasi S, et al. Phenotypic features of myoclonus-dystonia in three kindreds. Neurology. 2002;59:1187–96.
95. Doheny D, Danisi F, Smith C, Morrison C, Velickovic M, De Leon D, et al. Clinical findings of a myoclonus-dystonia family with two distinct mutations. Neurology. 2002;59:1244–6.
96. De Carvalho AP, Sweadner KJ, Penniston JT, Zaremba J, Liu L, Caton M, et al. Mutations in the Na+/K+ -ATPase alpha3 gene ATP1A3 are associated with rapid-onset dystonia parkinsonism. Neuron. 2004;43:169–75.
97. Brashear A, Dobyns WB, de Carvalho AP, Borg M, Frijns CJM, Gollamudi S, et al. The phenotypic spectrum of rapid-onset dystonia-parkinsonism (RDP) and mutations in the ATP1A3 gene. Brain. 2007;130:828–35.
98. Pittock SJ, Joyce C, O'Keane V, Hugle B, Hardiman O, Brett F, et al. Rapid-onset dystonia-parkinsonism: a clinical and genetic analysis of a new kindred. Neurology. 2000;55:991–5.
99. Barbano RL, Hill DF, Snively BM, Light LS, Boggs N, McCall WV, et al. New triggers and non-motor findings in a family with rapid-onset dystonia-parkinsonism. Parkinsonism Relat Disord. 2012;18:737–41.
100. Cook JF, Hill DF, Snively BM, Boggs N, Suerken CK, Haq I, et al. Cognitive impairment in rapid-onset dystonia-parkinsonism. Mov Disord. 2014;00:1–7.
101. Schneider SA, Hardy J, Bhatia KP. Syndromes of neurodegeneration with brain iron accumulation (NBIA): an update on clinical presentations, histological and genetic underpinnings, and treatment considerations. Mov Disord. 2012;27:42–53.
102. Dusek P, Schneider SA. Neurodegeneration with brain iron accumulation. Curr Opin Neurol. 2012;25:499–506.
103. Zhou B, Westaway SK, Levinson B, Johnson MA, Gitschier J, Hayflick SJ. A novel pantothenate kinase gene (PANK2) is defective in Hallervorden-Spatz syndrome. Nat Genet. 2001;28:345–9.
104. Paisan-Ruiz C, Bhatia KP, Li A, Hernandez D, Davis M, Wood NW, et al. Characterization of PLA2G6 as a locus for dystonia-parkinsonism. Ann Neurol. 2009;65:19–23.
105. Gregory A, Hayflick SJ. Genetics of neurodegeneration with brain iron accumulation. Curr Neurol Neurosci Rep. 2011;11:254–61.
106. Dooling EC, Schoene WC, Richardson EP. Hallervorden-Spatz syndrome. Arch Neurol. 1974;30:70–83.
107. Gregory A, Polster BJ, Hayflick SJ. Clinical and genetic delineation of neurodegeneration with brain iron accumulation. J Med Genet. 2009;46:73–80.
108. Thomas M, Hayflick SJ, Jankovic J. Clinical heterogeneity of neurodegeneration with brain iron accumulation (Hallervorden-Spatz syndrome) and pantothenate kinase-associated neurodegeneration. Mov Disord. 2004;19:36–42.
109. Hayflick SJ, Westaway SK, Levinson B, Zhou B, Johnson MA, Ching KHL, et al. Genetic, clinical, and radiographic delineation of Hallervorden-Spatz syndrome. N Engl J Med. 2003;348:33–40.
110. Oner O, Oner P, Deda G, Içağasioğlu D. Psychotic disorder in a case with Hallervorden-Spatz disease. Acta Psychiatr Scand. 2003;108:394–7; discussion 397–8.
111. Del Valle-López P, Pérez-García R, Sanguino-Andrés R, González-Pablos E. Adult onset Hallervorden-Spatz disease with psychotic symptoms. Actas Españolas Psiquiatr. 2005;39:260–2.
112. Pellecchia MT, Valente EM, Cif L, Salvi S, Albanese A, Scarano V, et al. The diverse phenotype and genotype of pantothenate kinase-associated neurodegeneration. Neurology. 2005;64:1810–2.
113. Cossu G, Melis M, Floris G, Hayflick SJ, Spissu A. Hallervorden Spatz syndrome (pantothenate kinase associated neurodegeneration) in two Sardinian brother with homozygous mutation in PANK 2 gene. J Neurol. 2002;249:1599–600.
114. Molinuevo JL, Martí MJ, Blesa R, Tolosa E. Pure akinesia: an unusual phenotype of Hallervorden-Spatz syndrome. Mov Disord. 2003;18:1351–3.

115. Marelli C, Piacentini S, Garavaglia B, Girotti F, Albanese A. Clinical and neuropsychological correlates in two brothers with pantothenate kinase-associated neurodegeneration. Mov Disord. 2005;20:208–12.
116. Doi H, Koyano S, Miyatake S, Matsumoto N, Kameda T, Tomita A, et al. Siblings with the adult-onset slowly progressive type of pantothenate kinase-associated neurodegeneration and a novel mutation, Ile346Ser, in PANK2: clinical features and (99m)Tc-ECD brain perfusion SPECT findings. J Neurol Sci. 2010;290:172–6.
117. Diaz N. Late onset atypical pantothenate-kinase-associated neurodegeneration. Case Rep Neurol Med. 2013;2013:860201.
118. Aggarwal A, Schneider SA, Houlden H, Silverdale M, Paudel R, Paisan-Ruiz C, et al. Indian-subcontinent NBIA: unusual phenotypes, novel PANK2 mutations, and undetermined genetic forms. Mov Disord. 2010;25:1424–31.
119. Yoon WT, Lee WY, Shin H-Y, Lee S-T, Ki C-S. Novel PANK2 gene mutations in korean patient with pantothenate kinase-associated neurodegeneration presenting unilateral dystonic tremor. Mov Disord. 2010;25:245–7.
120. Freeman K, Gregory A, Turner A, Blasco P, Hogarth P, Hayflick S. Intellectual and adaptive behaviour functioning in pantothenate kinase-associated neurodegeneration. J Intellect Disabil Res. 2007;51:417–26.
121. Zhang P, Gao Z, Jiang Y, Wang J, Zhang F, Wang S, et al. Follow-up study of 25 Chinese children with PLA2G6-associated neurodegeneration. Eur J Neurol. 2013;20:322–30.
122. Vidailhet M, Grabli D, Roze E. Pathophysiology of dystonia. Curr Opin Neurol. 2009;22:406–13.
123. Breakefield XO, Blood AJ, Li Y, Hallett M, Hanson PI, Standaert DG. The pathophysiological basis of dystonias. Nat Rev Neurosci. 2008;9:222–34.
124. Pettigrew LC, Jankovic J. Hemidystonia: a report of 22 patients and a review of the literature. J Neurol Neurosurg Psychiatry. 1985;48:650–7.
125. Obeso JA, Giménez-Roldán S. Clinicopathological correlation in symptomatic dystonia. Adv Neurol. 1988;50:113–22.
126. Zoons E, Booij J, Nederveen AJ, Dijk JM, Tijssen MAJ. Structural, functional and molecular imaging of the brain in primary focal dystonia–a review. Neuroimage. 2011;56:1011–20.
127. Pantano P, Totaro P, Fabbrini G, Raz E, Contessa GM, Tona F, et al. A transverse and longitudinal MR imaging voxel-based morphometry study in patients with primary cervical dystonia. AJNR Am J Neuroradiol. 2011;32:81–4.
128. Carbon M, Argyelan M, Eidelberg D. Functional imaging in hereditary dystonia. Eur J Neurol. 2010;17 Suppl 1:58–64.
129. Fabbrini G, Pantano P, Totaro P, Calistri V, Colosimo C, Carmellini M, et al. Diffusion tensor imaging in patients with primary cervical dystonia and in patients with blepharospasm. Eur J Neurol. 2008;15:185–9.
130. Alexander GE, DeLong MR, Strick PL. Parallel organization of functionally segregated circuits linking basal ganglia and cortex. Annu Rev Neurosci. 1986;9:357–81.
131. Parent A, Hazrati LN. Functional anatomy of the basal ganglia. I. The cortico-basal ganglia-thalamo-cortical loop. Brain Res Brain Res Rev. 1995;20:91–127.
132. Arsalidou M, Duerden EG, Taylor MJ. The centre of the brain: topographical model of motor, cognitive, affective, and somatosensory functions of the basal ganglia. Hum Brain Mapp. 2013;34:3031–54.
133. O'Callaghan C, Bertoux M, Hornberger M. Beyond and below the cortex: the contribution of striatal dysfunction to cognition and behaviour in neurodegeneration. J Neurol Neurosurg Psychiatry. 2014;85:371–8.
134. Nestler EJ, Carlezon WA. The mesolimbic dopamine reward circuit in depression. Biol Psychiatry. 2006;59:1151–9.
135. Milad MR, Rauch SL. Obsessive-compulsive disorder: beyond segregated cortico-striatal pathways. Trends Cogn Sci. 2012;16:43–51.

136. Lauterbach EC, Jackson JG, Price ST, Wilson AN, Kirsh AD, Dever GE. Clinical, motor, and biological correlates of depressive disorders after focal subcortical lesions. J Neuropsychiatry Clin Neurosci. 1997;9:259–66.
137. Krack P, Hariz MI, Baunez C, Guridi J, Obeso JA. Deep brain stimulation: from neurology to psychiatry? Trends Neurosci. 2010;33:474–84.
138. Bullock D, Tan CO, John YJ. Computational perspectives on forebrain microcircuits implicated in reinforcement learning, action selection, and cognitive control. Neural Netw. 2009;22:757–65.
139. Shohamy D, Wagner AD. Integrating memories in the human brain: hippocampal-midbrain encoding of overlapping events. Neuron. 2008;60:378–89.
140. Cabeza R, Nyberg L. Neural bases of learning and memory: functional neuroimaging evidence. Curr Opin Neurol. 2000;13:415–21.
141. Dahlin E, Bäckman L, Neely AS, Nyberg L. Training of the executive component of working memory: subcortical areas mediate transfer effects. Restor Neurol Neurosci. 2009;27:405–19.
142. Tarsy D, Baldessarini RJ. Epidemiology of tardive dyskinesia: is risk declining with modern antipsychotics? Mov Disord. 2006;21:589–98.
143. Thiel A, Dressler D, Kistel C, Rüther E. Clozapine treatment of spasmodic torticollis. Neurology. 1994;44:957–8.
144. Gerber PE, Lynd LD. Selective serotonin-reuptake inhibitor-induced movement disorders. Ann Pharmacother. 1998;32:692–8.
145. Hollon SD, Ponniah K. A review of empirically supported psychological therapies for mood disorders in adults. Depress Anxiety. 2010;27:891–932.
146. Otto MW, Smits JAJ, Reese HE. Cognitive-behavioral therapy for the treatment of anxiety disorders. J Clin Psychiatry. 2004;65 Suppl 5:34–41.
147. Gava I, Barbui C, Aguglia E, Carlino D, Churchill R, De Vanna M, et al. Psychological treatments versus treatment as usual for obsessive compulsive disorder (OCD). Cochrane Database Syst Rev. 2007;(2):CD005333.

Chapter 9
Depression in Huntington's Disease

Christiana Ossig and Alexander Storch

Abbreviations

5-HIAA	5-Hydroxyindoleacetic acid
AES	Apathy evaluation scale
BDI-II	Becks depression inventory-II
CAG repeat	Cytosine adenine guanine repeat
CRF	Corticotropin-releasing factor
CSF	Cerebrospinal fluid
Ham-D	Hamilton rating scale for depression
HD	Huntington's disease
LARS	Lille Apathy Rating Scale
MAOI	Monoamine oxidase inhibitor
MARDS	Montgomery-Asberg rating scale
NPI	Neuropsychiatric inventory
SNRI	Selective noradrenergic reuptake inhibitor
SSRI	Selective serotonin reuptake inhibitor
UHDRS	Unified Huntington's Disease RatingSscale
Y-BOCS	Yale-Brown Obsessive-Compulsive symptom scale

C. Ossig, MD (✉) • A. Storch, MD
Division of Neurodegenerative Diseases, Department of Neurology,
Dresden University of Technology, Fetscherstrasse 74, Dresden 01307, Germany
e-mail: christiana.ossig@uniklinikum-dresden.de;
Alexander.Storch@neuro.med.tu-dresden.de

H. Reichmann (ed.), *Neuropsychiatric Symptoms of Movement Disorders*,
Neuropsychiatric Symptoms of Neurological Disease,
DOI 10.1007/978-3-319-09537-0_9

Introduction

Huntington's disease (HD) is a progressive neurodegenerative disorder that affects movement, cognition, and mood, which was first described in detail by the physician George Huntington in 1872 [1]. HD is an autosomal dominant inherited disease with full penetrance caused by an abnormal expansion of CAG tandem repeat of the huntingtin gene located on the short arm of chromosome 4p16.3 encoding an extended tract of glutamines in the huntingtin protein [2]. Thirty-six repeats or more are considered an elongation. An interesting phenomenon, the so-called anticipation, is the observation that a longer CAG repeat leads to earlier disease onset and faster disease course [3–5]. The mean age at onset of motor symptoms is 30–50 years of age, and duration of HD is approximately 15–20 years after disease onset. The diagnosis is based on clinical symptoms in an individual with a parent with proven HD and is nowadays confirmed by genetic testing. There is a wide range of differential diagnosis, which has to be considered such as chorea-acanthocytosis or Dentato-rubro-pallido-luysian atrophy (DRPLA), which are however all also quite rare [6–9]. HD cannot be cured, but several medical and nonmedical therapeutic strategies to address the specific symptoms are available. Eventually, the progression of HD leads to a complete dependency in daily life, resulting in the need of full-time care and finally death, caused most commonly by pneumonia and secondly by suicide.

HD is a rare neuropsychiatric disorder with a prevalence of 5–10/100,000 in the Caucasian population. However, the prevalence depends mainly on the country referred to, e.g., in Japan, a much lower prevalence of about 1/100,000 is described [10]. Besides the motoric symptoms, psychiatric symptoms including psychosis, irritability, anxiety, apathy, and obsessive–compulsive disorder play a major role in HD [11–13].

The clinical course of the HD consists of three major stages: an "at-risk" stage, a preclinical stage, and a clinical stage [14]. Psychiatric disturbances occur in all stages but may also already present in the early stage of the disease or may even precede motor symptoms [15]. Between 33 and 76 % of patients suffer from psychiatric symptoms throughout their lifetime; among those, depression seems to be most frequent with a prevalence of between 33 and 76 % depending on the study [16, 17]. One could speculate that depression seems to be a natural consequence when facing the risk of inheriting the disease and around the time of genetic testing. However, HD gene-positive carriers present a higher prevalence of major depression prior to clinical onset and show increased depression scores and frequency of suicidal thoughts over time compared to genetic negative tested and thus healthy individuals who have a family history of HD implying a disease intrinsic risk for depression in HD [18, 19].

Depression has been part of the nosology of HD from George Huntington's first description of the disease [1]. Depression is characterized by sadness, loss of interest or pleasure, feelings of guilt or low self-worth, disturbed sleep or appetite, feelings of tiredness, and poor concentration (WHO10/2012). As one of the most common psychiatric disorders, depression is also a frequent feature of many diseases involving basal ganglia including HD [20, 21].

Epidemiology

Depressive symptoms are the most frequent psychiatric conditions in HD with reported prevalence of 33–76 % [16]. It is noted that the variations of prevalence is by large due to the use of different assessment methods with most of them not being validated in HD. Depressive mood in particular is reported in 33–69 % of patients depending on the method of assessment (Unified HD rating scale (UHDRS), or neuropsychiatric inventory (NPI)) [22]. Using the formal DSM-IV criteria, 43 % of HD patients show mood disorders with 29 % having major depression and 14 % nonmajor depression [23]. Compared to the general population with a lifetime prevalence of major depression of around 15 %, depression seems to be part and parcel of HD [24]. Current data suggest that the occurrence of depressive symptoms is independent of HD disease stage [25] and can be considered as a premotor symptom, since it often precedes motor symptom onset years or even decades [14, 26]. Interestingly, patients rate depression as one of the most important symptoms of HD just similar to motor or even cognitive aspects with respect to their quality of life [27].

Anxiety is reported in approximately 40 % of patients [22]. One small study assessed the rate of anxiety at the first hospital admission due to the manifestation of motor symptoms, showing a much higher prevalence of 61 % [28], clearly indicating that the time of assessment is of pivotal relevance. Anxiety is not related to disease stage. The prevalence of irritability as a symptom of the depressive symptom complex and characterized by reduced control over temper that may result in verbal or behavioral outbursts varies between 38 and 73 % of HD patients [22]. Prevalence of apathy range from 34 to 76 % of patients [22], with "loss of energy" (88 %), "impaired performance of ADL" (76 %), and "lack of initiative"(76 %) as the most prevalent symptoms of the apathy symptom cluster. Apathy is related to disease stage with higher frequency of apathy in later disease stages. Obsessive and compulsive symptoms occur frequently in HD, and prevalence varies between 10 and 55 % (52 % using the Yale-Brown Obsessive Compulsive symptom scale (Y-BOCS). However, the percentage of patients completely fulfilling the DSM-IV diagnostic criteria for the obsessive-compulsive disorder is low (<10 %).

The suicide attempt rate is exceptionally high in HD and varies between 10 and 30 % of patients [25, 29]. Death due to suicide among HD patients is four times higher than within the healthy population [17, 30]. Suicide occurs more frequently in early symptomatic individuals and also in presymptomatic gene carriers. Around the time of gene testing and the stage when independence diminishes are the most risky periods for suicide.

Clinical Description

Depression is characterized by sadness, loss of interest or pleasure, feelings of guilt or low self-worth, disturbed sleep or appetite, feelings of tiredness, and poor concentration (WHO10/2012). There is no evidence that the clinical presentation of depression in HD is largely different from major depression. Throughout life, a patient suffering from HD passes through different stages of the disease where psychiatric disturbances become evident. The clinical description in this chapter shall focus on these symptoms, especially on depression in HD.

Depression in HD involves—as in major depression—considerable emotional distress, evidenced by tearfulness, sadness, anxiety, agitation, insomnia, anorexia, feelings of worthlessness and hopelessness, and recurrent thoughts of death [31]. A loss of interest and increasing passive behavior are seen as part of the apathy syndrome. Apathy and depression have to be distinguished and play different roles throughout the course of the disease. Apathy is defined as diminished motivation not attributable to a decreased level of consciousness, cognitive impairment, or emotional distress. Apathy and depression cannot be linked to a specific stage of HD. Like depression, apathy is correlated with neurodegeneration, cognitive dysfunction, and functional decline [32]. Merely, the precise relationship between apathy and depression in HD remains unclear. Up to now, therapeutic strategies are the same.

Irritability may also be a presenting sign in the early stage of HD. It may be expressed with great variation from anger and disputes with family members to physical aggression and violence. Up to 50 % of HD patients report anxiety during the "at-risk" stage, often due to uncertainty about the start and the course of the disease. Further psychiatric symptoms in the early stages may be obsessive–compulsive disorder and hypersexuality. During later stages, psychosis may appear and may present like schizophrenia with paranoid and acoustic hallucinations [13].

Even though there is no correlation of depression in HD with cognitive impairment, motor symptoms, or CAG repeat length [33], depression is associated with changes in cognitive abilities involving verbal fluency, visual memory tasks, spatial span tasks, working memory tasks, and executive function [34]. Thus, this potentially treatable condition that may exacerbate cognitive decline needs to be seriously addressed in HD patients.

Pathophysiology of Depression

The pathophysiological mechanisms mediating depression in HD remain largely enigmatic. Although psychological reactions like handling and adjusting to a terminal neurodegenerative disease with progressive disability may initially play a major role in HD, depression is considered mostly a consequence of the pathology of HD. The pathological correlate in HD is atrophy of the caudate nucleus and putamen, which are involved in the frontal subcortical circuits. Thus, dysfunction and hypometabolism of the frontal cortices, including dorsolateral prefrontal cortices, orbitofrontal cortices, and anterior cingulate cortices are linked to depression in HD [35, 36].

Studies of the cerebrospinal fluid (CSF) of HD patients with depression revealed elevated corticotropin-releasing factor (CRF) and reduced 5-*Hydroxyindoleacetic acid* (5-HIAA) levels. Except of these findings in the CSF, HD patients with depressive disorders did not differ otherwise from HD patients without depression. There was even a positive correlation between severity of major depression and CRF concentration in CSF noted [37].

It is known that some treatments for motor dysfunction in HD such as dopamine antagonists might worsen or even induce depressive symptoms in HD. Exemplarily, tetrabenazine, a dopamine receptor antagonist, is widely used to modify motor symptoms like chorea in HD. Tetrabenazine however is linked to increased depression and high rates of suicide in HD [38]. It is thus recommended to regularly assess depressive symptoms after initiation of new treatments, particularly typical antipsychotics and antichoreatic compounds. If depression occurs, dose reduction of these compounds and reassessment of mood symptoms are necessary [38].

Diagnostic and Assessments

Although depressive symptoms are frequent in HD, their diagnosis might be difficult because of the absence of standardized diagnostic procedures and due to the overlap of some depressive symptoms with motor or other somatic conditions such as weight loss, sleep disorders, and inactivity/parkinsonism. However, it is well accepted that the depressive symptoms in HD as in other basal ganglia disorders are largely part of the disease entity (see above), and discrimination between depressive symptoms and their mimics is not helpful in most. Much more important are the identification of depressive symptoms and the determination of depression management—independent of their pathophysiological classification—in conjunction with other psychiatric condition.

The diagnostic problems resulting from the overlap of depressive conditions with other symptoms of the disease might be overcome by using the "inclusion strategy" in combination with formal diagnostic criteria such as the Diagnostic and Statistical Manual of Mental Disorders IV (or the new version: DSM-V) or the International Classification of Diseases (ICD-10), similar as recommended for the diagnosis of depression in Parkinson's disease [39]. The "inclusion strategy" judges all relevant symptoms as "depressive" and includes them into the diagnostic decision, independent of their overlap with other psychiatric or motor symptoms. This strategy might overdiagnose depression in HD but hopefully avoids undertreatment of depressive symptoms in HD.

In a clinical setting, depression (including its severity) can be easily assessed using the Becks Depression Inventory-II (BDI-II), a 21-question multiple-choice self-report inventory. Also, the Hamilton Rating Scale for Depression (Ham-D) consisting of 17 items and the Montgomery-Asberg Rating Scale (MARDS) as a 10-item questionnaire are widely used. Even though the behavioral section of the Unified Huntington's Disease rating Scale (UHDRS) is rather short, in every HD patient the UHDRS should be performed. The Yale-Brown Obsessive Compulsive symptom scale (Y-BOCS) can be used to assess obsessive–compulsive disorder symptoms. In order to assess apathy, different rating scales are used: the Apathy Evaluation Scale (AES), the Apathy Inventory, the Lille Apathy Rating Scale (LARS), and the apathy sections of the Neuropsychiatric Inventory (NPI). It is strongly recommended to assess depression on a regular basis such as at each consultation using a structured questionnaire or other diagnostic instrument.

Therapy and Management

As depression is one of the most devastating symptoms to family life, the majority of drugs are prescribed for this condition. On the other hand, treatment of depression in HD has not been thoroughly studied and only open studies and expert recommendations are available. In general, depression in HD is treated like primary depression and depression in other affective disorders (for guidelines, refer to [40] for NICE guidelines or [41] for an overview). However, one should be aware that HD patients are likely to respond more sensitive to adverse central nervous system side effects than otherwise healthy individuals, and therefore, a slow titration and careful dosing is necessary. Furthermore, side effects of antidepressive therapies on motor functions or other psychiatric symptoms such as aggression or sleep disorders need to be considered and—vice versa—medications for motor symptoms, particularly chorea, might worsen depressive symptoms.

Open studies report beneficial effects on treating depression in HD for selective serotonin reuptake inhibitors (SSRIs), selective noradrenergic reuptake inhibitors (SNRIs), atypical antipsychotics, tetracyclic and tricyclic antidepressants, and monoamine oxidase inhibitors (MAO-I) [17]. There are no controlled data for the administration of MAO-I in HD depression and—notably—they are contraindicated in combined use with tetrabenazine. MAO-I should be thus used with caution in HD depression.

SSRIs are commonly used, which was also showed by a large study with 787 enrolled prodromal HD patients of whom 20 % received SSRIs. However, despite its frequent use, the effectiveness of SSRI treatment in HD-related depression has not been studied in controlled clinical trials [42]. Fluoxetine is an antidepressant of the SSRI class and was administered in combination with selegiline showing significant affective, behavioral, and motoric improvements in one patient without relevant adverse effects [43]. It is noted that fluoxetine has a long half-life and frequent drug interactions and is thus not recommended as a first-choice treatment in HD. Treatment with venlafaxine, an SSNRI, showed significant improvement during a 4-week observation period in patients with major depression, although side effects like nausea and irritability were reported [44]. Positive results were also noted for tricyclic antidepressants like imipramine [45] and tetracyclic antidepressants like mirtazapine [46].

There are some positive experiences with atypical antipsychotics in HD, not only for treating motor symptoms but also for depression therapy. Olanzapine, an atypical antipsychotic, which has been studied in an open-labelled study of 11 patients, with a daily-administered dosage of 5 mg/day, showed significant improvement in depression, anxiety, irritability, and obsessive behavior. Besides, olanzapine is used for treating motor symptoms, merely in a higher dosage of up to 30 mg/day [47].

For severe depressive symptoms, electroconvulsive therapy (ECT) can be a valuable treatment. In an HD case series, in all cases ECT was well tolerated and produced improvement in psychiatric and behavioral symptoms implying a positive risk–benefit ratio for ECT in patients with HD and severe depression [48]. Other nonmedical treatment for HD depression involves physical, occupational, and speech therapy. Such an intensive multidisciplinary approach focusing on structured physical training showed significant improvement in gait and balance but also a significant reduction in depression in a recently published clinical trial [49].

Since depression is a frequent but potentially treatable condition in HD patients that impairs quality of life and may exacerbate cognitive decline, early and sufficient treatment of depression is strongly recommended.

References

1. Huntington G. On chorea. Med Surg Rep Phila. 1872;26:317–21.
2. Group HsDCR. A novel gene containing a trinucleotide repeat that is expanded and unstable on Huntington's disease chromosomes. The Huntington's Disease Collaborative Research Group. Cell. 1993;72(6):971–83. Epub 1993/03/26.
3. Ridley RM, Frith CD, Crow TJ, Conneally PM. Anticipation in Huntington's disease is inherited through the male line but may originate in the female. J Med Genet. 1988;25(9):589–95. Epub 1988/09/01.
4. Duyao M, Ambrose C, Myers R, Novelletto A, Persichetti F, Frontali M, et al. Trinucleotide repeat length instability and age of onset in Huntington's disease. Nat Genet. 1993;4(4):387–92. Epub 1993/08/01.
5. Lee JM, Ramos EM, Lee JH, Gillis T, Mysore JS, Hayden MR, et al. CAG repeat expansion in Huntington disease determines age at onset in a fully dominant fashion. Neurology. 2012;78(10):690–5. Epub 2012/02/11.
6. Iizuka R, Hirayama K, Maehara KA. Dentato-rubro-pallido-luysian atrophy: a clinico-pathological study. J Neurol Neurosurg Psychiatry. 1984;47(12):1288–98. Epub 1984/12/01.
7. Cardoso F. Differential diagnosis of Huntington's disease: what the clinician should know. Neurodegener Dis Manag. 2014;4(1):67–72. Epub 2014/03/20.
8. Walker RH. Update on the Non-Huntington's disease choreas with comments on the current nomenclature. Tremor Other Hyperkinet Mov (N Y). 2012;2. Epub 2013/02/27.
9. Jung HH, Danek A, Walker RH. Neuroacanthocytosis syndromes. Orphanet J Rare Dis. 2011;6:68. Epub 2011/10/27.
10. Harper PS. The epidemiology of Huntington's disease. Hum Genet. 1992;89(4):365–76. Epub 1992/06/01.
11. Lovestone S, Hodgson S, Sham P, Differ AM, Levy R. Familial psychiatric presentation of Huntington's disease. J Med Genet. 1996;33(2):128–31. Epub 1996/02/01.

12. Beglinger LJ, Paulsen JS, Watson DB, Wang C, Duff K, Langbehn DR, et al. Obsessive and compulsive symptoms in prediagnosed Huntington's disease. J Clin Psychiatry. 2008;69(11):1758–65. Epub 2008/11/18.
13. van Duijn E, Kingma EM, van der Mast RC. Psychopathology in verified Huntington's disease gene carriers. J Neuropsychiatry Clin Neurosci. 2007;19(4):441–8. Epub 2007/12/12.
14. Roos RA. Huntington's disease: a clinical review. Orphanet J Rare Dis. 2010;5(1):40. Epub 2010/12/22.
15. Shiwach R. Psychopathology in Huntington's disease patients. Acta Psychiatr Scand. 1994;90(4):241–6. Epub 1994/10/01.
16. Naarding P, Kremer HP, Zitman FG. Huntington's disease: a review of the literature on prevalence and treatment of neuropsychiatric phenomena. Eur Psychiatry. 2001;16(8):439–45. Epub 2002/01/05.
17. Du X, Pang TY, Hannan AJ. A tale of two maladies? Pathogenesis of depression with and without the Huntington's disease gene mutation. Front Neurol. 2013;4:81. Epub 2013/07/13.
18. Larsson MU, Luszcz MA, Bui TH, Wahlin TB. Depression and suicidal ideation after predictive testing for Huntington's disease: a two-year follow-up study. J Genet Couns. 2006;15(5):361–74. Epub 2006/09/13.
19. Julien CL, Thompson JC, Wild S, Yardumian P, Snowden JS, Turner G, et al. Psychiatric disorders in preclinical Huntington's disease. J Neurol Neurosurg Psychiatry. 2007;78(9):939–43. Epub 2006/12/21.
20. Koponen S, Taiminen T, Portin R, Himanen L, Isoniemi H, Heinonen H, et al. Axis I and II psychiatric disorders after traumatic brain injury: a 30-year follow-up study. Am J Psychiatry. 2002;159(8):1315–21. Epub 2002/08/03.
21. Rabins PV, Pearlson GD, Aylward E, Kumar AJ, Dowell K. Cortical magnetic resonance imaging changes in elderly inpatients with major depression. Am J Psychiatry. 1991;148(5):617–20. Epub 1991/05/01.
22. Kulisevsky J, Litvan I, Berthier ML, Pascual-Sedano B, Paulsen JS, Cummings JL. Neuropsychiatric assessment of Gilles de la Tourette patients: comparative study with other hyperkinetic and hypokinetic movement disorders. Mov Disord. 2001;16(6):1098–104. Epub 2001/12/19.
23. Leroi I, O'Hearn E, Marsh L, Lyketsos CG, Rosenblatt A, Ross CA, et al. Psychopathology in patients with degenerative cerebellar diseases: a comparison to Huntington's disease. Am J Psychiatry. 2002;159(8):1306–14. Epub 2002/08/03.
24. Kessler RC, Berglund P, Demler O, Jin R, Merikangas KR, Walters EE. Lifetime prevalence and age-of-onset distributions of DSM-IV disorders in the National Comorbidity Survey Replication. Arch Gen Psychiatry. 2005;62(6):593–602. Epub 2005/06/09.
25. Paulsen JS, Nehl C, Hoth KF, Kanz JE, Benjamin M, Conybeare R, et al. Depression and stages of Huntington's disease. J Neuropsychiatry Clin Neurosci. 2005;17(4):496–502. Epub 2006/01/03.
26. Paulsen JS, Langbehn DR, Stout JC, Aylward E, Ross CA, Nance M, et al. Detection of Huntington's disease decades before diagnosis: the Predict-HD study. J Neurol Neurosurg Psychiatry. 2008;79(8):874–80. Epub 2007/12/22.
27. Ho AK, Gilbert AS, Mason SL, Goodman AO, Barker RA. Health-related quality of life in Huntington's disease: which factors matter most? Mov Disord. 2009;24(4):574–8. Epub 2008/12/20.
28. Murgod UA, Saleem Q, Anand A, Brahmachari SK, Jain S, Muthane UB. A clinical study of patients with genetically confirmed Huntington's disease from India. J Neurol Sci. 2001;190(1–2):73–8. Epub 2001/09/28.
29. Farrer LA. Suicide and attempted suicide in Huntington disease: implications for preclinical testing of persons at risk. Am J Med Genet. 1986;24(2):305–11. Epub 1986/06/01.
30. Paulsen JS, Hoth KF, Nehl C, Stierman L. Critical periods of suicide risk in Huntington's disease. Am J Psychiatry. 2005;162(4):725–31. Epub 2005/04/01.

31. Levy ML, Cummings JL, Fairbanks LA, Masterman D, Miller BL, Craig AH, et al. Apathy is not depression. J Neuropsychiatry Clin Neurosci. 1998;10(3):314–9. Epub 1998/08/26.
32. Naarding P, Janzing JG, Eling P, van der Werf S, Kremer B. Apathy is not depression in Huntington's disease. J Neuropsychiatry Clin Neurosci. 2009;21(3):266–70. Epub 2009/09/25.
33. Zappacosta B, Monza D, Meoni C, Austoni L, Soliveri P, Gellera C, et al. Psychiatric symptoms do not correlate with cognitive decline, motor symptoms, or CAG repeat length in Huntington's disease. Arch Neurol. 1996;53(6):493–7. Epub 1996/06/01.
34. Nehl C, Ready RE, Hamilton J, Paulsen JS. Effects of depression on working memory in presymptomatic Huntington's disease. J Neuropsychiatry Clin Neurosci. 2001;13(3):342–6. Epub 2001/08/22.
35. Mayberg HS, Starkstein SE, Peyser CE, Brandt J, Dannals RF, Folstein SE. Paralimbic frontal lobe hypometabolism in depression associated with Huntington's disease. Neurology. 1992;42(9):1791–7. Epub 1992/09/01.
36. Mega MS, Cummings JL. Frontal-subcortical circuits and neuropsychiatric disorders. J Neuropsychiatry Clin Neurosci. 1994;6(4):358–70. Epub 1994/01/01.
37. Kurlan R, Caine E, Rubin A, Nemeroff CB, Bissette G, Zaczek R, et al. Cerebrospinal fluid correlates of depression in Huntington's disease. Arch Neurol. 1988;45(8):881–3. Epub 1988/08/01.
38. Killoran A, Biglan KM. Therapeutics in Huntington's disease. Curr Treat Options Neurol. 2012;14:137–49.
39. Marsh L, McDonald WM, Cummings J, Ravina B. Provisional diagnostic criteria for depression in Parkinson's disease: report of an NINDS/NIMH Work Group. Mov Disord. 2006;21(2):148–58. Epub 2005/10/08.
40. McAllister-Williams RH. NICE guidelines for the management of depression. Br J Hosp Med (Lond). 2006;67(2):60–1. Epub 2006/02/28.
41. Gelenberg AJ. A review of the current guidelines for depression treatment. J Clin Psychiatry. 2010;71(7):e15. Epub 2010/07/30.
42. Rowe KC, Paulsen JS, Langbehn DR, Wang C, Mills J, Beglinger LJ, et al. Patterns of serotonergic antidepressant usage in prodromal Huntington disease. Psychiatry Res. 2012;196(2–3):309–14. Epub 2012/03/09.
43. Patel SV, Tariot PN, Asnis J. L-Deprenyl augmentation of fluoxetine in a patient with Huntington's disease. Ann Clin Psychiatry. 1996;8(1):23–6. Epub 1996/03/01.
44. Holl AK, Wilkinson L, Painold A, Holl EM, Bonelli RM. Combating depression in Huntington's disease: effective antidepressive treatment with venlafaxine XR. Int Clin Psychopharmacol. 2010;25(1):46–50. Epub 2009/12/10.
45. Whittier J, Haydu G, Crawford J. Effect of imipramine (Tofranil) on depression and hyperkinesia in Huntington's disease. Am J Psychiatry. 1961;118:79. Epub 1961/07/01.
46. Bonelli RM. Mirtazapine in suicidal Huntington's disease. Ann Pharmacother. 2003;37(3):452. Epub 2003/03/18.
47. Squitieri F, Cannella M, Piorcellini A, Brusa L, Simonelli M, Ruggieri S. Short-term effects of olanzapine in Huntington disease. Neuropsychiatr Neuropsychol Behav Neurol. 2001;14(1):69–72. Epub 2001/03/10.
48. Cucsin C, Franco FB, Fernandez-Robles C, DuBois CM, Welch CA. Rapid improvement of depression and psychotic symptoms in Huntington's disease: a retrospective chart review of seven patients treated with electroconvulsive therapy. Gen Hosp Psychiatry. 2013;35(6):678. e3-5. Epub 2013/04/02.
49. Piira A, van Walsem MR, Mikalsen G, Nilsen KH, Knutsen S, Frich JC. Effects of a one year intensive multidisciplinary rehabilitation program for patients with Huntington's Disease: a prospective intervention study. PLoS Curr. 2013;5. Epub 2014/01/25.

Chapter 10
Cognitive Impairment and Dementia (Mild or Major Neurocognitive Disorder) in Huntington's Disease

Cristina Sampaio and Beth Borowsky

Phenomenology of Cognitive Dysfunction in HD

Huntington's disease (HD) is an autosomal dominant neurodegenerative disease that affects approximately five to seven in 100,000 people, in Western Caucasian populations. Recent studies suggest that these estimates might be too low and the correct prevalence might be as high as 14 in 100,000. The disease is caused by an expanded trinucleotide (CAG) repeat in the Huntington gene on the short arm of chromosome 4. HD is commonly considered to be primarily a disorder of movement, which is a mistake. In fact, it is characterized by a triad of symptoms, including impairments in motor, cognitive, and psychiatric function. While the clinical diagnosis of HD requires the unequivocal presence of motor signs, the presence of other clinical signs, such as cognitive and psychiatric changes, as well as brain atrophy, has been clearly documented many years in advance of diagnosis [1–3]. Further, evidence suggests that the nonmotor symptoms of HD are the most debilitating to the patients [4, 5]. This is similar to what is reported in Parkinson's disease (PD) which speaks to the overall importance of these types of symptoms in determination of disability [6].

HD is a fully penetrant, autosomal dominant, inherited disorder. Therefore, the carrier of an expansion greater than 39 CAG repeats is genetically diagnosed as a bearer of the disease. The current standard for clinical diagnosis of HD, which is distinct from genetic diagnosis, is based on the unequivocal presence of motor signs. These signs appear chronologically late compared with other manifestations,

C. Sampaio, MD, PhD (✉) • B. Borowsky, PhD
Department of Clinical Research and Development, CHDI Management/CHDI Foundation, 155 Village Boulevard, Suite 200, Princeton, NJ 08822, USA
e-mail: cristina.sampaio@chdifoundation.org; beth.borowsky@chdifoundation.org

H. Reichmann (ed.), *Neuropsychiatric Symptoms of Movement Disorders*, Neuropsychiatric Symptoms of Neurological Disease,
DOI 10.1007/978-3-319-09537-0_10

creating different phases in the timeline of the disease. For practical reasons, it is common to refer to the period before the appearance of unequivocal motor signs as the premanifest stage and the period after such signs appear as the manifest stage. The premanifest period lasts for several decades. The years close to the appearance of the motor signs are of great interest for the understanding of the disease – this is called the late premanifest period and typically lasts about 5–7 years.

Cognitive decline is one of the most commonly reported complaints by HD patients. Despite the clear need, there are currently no treatments for improving cognition or slowing cognitive decline in HD or other neurological diseases. The progressive decline in cognitive functioning in HD has been very well characterized by a few prospective, longitudinal, observational studies [7–9]. These studies demonstrate a progressive decline in cognitive function that begins prior to clinical diagnosis of motor symptoms, in the premotor manifest or premanifest period, and progresses throughout the course of the disease [7–9]. While cognitive dysfunction occurs in many neurological and psychiatric diseases, it is important to note that both the course of decline and the specific domains of cognition that are impaired vary across different diseases.

There is a considerable amount of data on how premanifest and early manifest patients perform on a variety of cognitive tests, both cross-sectionally and longitudinally [7, 9–11]. These data provide evidence that HD differentially impacts specific domains of cognition throughout the course of the disease. The domains of cognition impaired in HD include executive function, psychomotor performance, emotion recognition, attention, and working memory. Tests that have shown the largest cross-sectional effect sizes between early manifest HD and controls include tests of processing speed, executive function, attention, memory, visuospatial processing, timing, and emotion processing [7, 9, 12–15]. Examples of such tests include Symbol Digit Modalities Test (SDMT), Stroop, Trail Making Test A and B (TRAILS), paced and speeded tapping tasks, Emotion Recognition (EMO), One Touch Stocking (OTS), University of Pennsylvania Smell Identification Test (UPSIT), Hopkins Verbal Learning Test (HVLT), Map Search, and the Montreal Cognitive Assessment (MoCA). Of these, paced and speeded tapping, Stroop, SDMT, EMO, HVLT, Map Search, UPSIT, OTS, and TRAILS also show some sensitivity in the premanifest population. In terms of longitudinal decline, tests such as SDMT, Stroop, Emotion Recognition, and Circle Tracing show the biggest decline over time in the early manifest group, while it has been more difficult to measure a significant change over time in the premanifest population. It should be noted that while cognitive deficits are detectable in the premanifest population, these deficits are subtle and more easily detected in those closer to disease onset compared to those farther from onset. There is no evidence of measurable cognitive deficits as a trait marker in HD, but rather the deficit develops slowly during the late premanifest period. A factor analysis approach suggests that motor planning/speed and sensory-perceptual processing are cognitive domains that may be important for predicting progression in the premanifest population [11].

The clear need for treatments to improve cognitive functioning in HD has led to increased research and development leading toward such therapies. This work includes the development of clinical tools to evaluate the effectiveness of new treatments on cognitive functioning in HD. Stout and colleagues [16] have recently developed a cognitive assessment battery, the HD-CAB, for use in clinical trials in late premanifest and early-stage HD patients. The battery was designed to measure both improvements in cognitive performance over shorter time periods and a reduction in the decline of cognitive functioning over longer periods of time. This battery will be an important tool to evaluate novel therapies designed to improve cognitive function in HD.

Since people with Huntington's disease have not only cognitive symptoms but also motor and mood disturbances, it is important to keep in mind that there is a reciprocal relationship between cognitive performance and both mood and motor functioning. In other words, cognitive performance can both affect and be affected by mood and motor functioning. This relationship can complicate assessment of symptoms in patients, as many cognitive tests require a level of motor performance and many motor tests require a level of cognitive competence. Further, performance on cognitive tests has been shown to be influenced by mood [17]. Thus, changes in performance in a given test can be influenced by changes in unrelated domains. Good clinical practice in HD should include evaluations of all domains: cognition, motor, and mood.

Functional Impact of the Neurocognitive Disorder in HD

Dementia refers to a progressive decline in cognitive abilities resulting in deficits in social and occupational functioning. The *Diagnostic and Statistical Manual of Mental Disorders,* 4th edition, defines a diagnosis of dementia as requiring a decline from a previous level of social or occupational functioning [18]. The most recent version of this manual, *DSM-5*, includes revisions to this terminology with the introduction of the category "Neurocognitive Disorder mild and major" to refer to mild cognitive impairment and dementia, respectively [19]. Furthermore in *DSM-5*, major or mild neurocognitive disorder due to Huntington's disease is now an independent entry that did not exist in previous editions, where HD was considered an etiological diagnosis after the exclusion of others.

The recognition of the specificity of neurocognitive disorder of HD is important. Cognitive impairment or dementia is common to many neurodegenerative and psychiatric diseases. However, the specific domains of cognition that are impaired and the presentation of the impairment over the course of the illness differ for each disease. Criteria for HD dementia have been based largely on features of the dementia associated with Alzheimer's disease (AD) [20]. However, the pattern of spared and impaired cognitive abilities observed in HD is distinct from that in AD [21, 22]. As described above, HD patients typically show a profile characterized as "subcortical," with attention deficits, cognitive slowing, impaired planning and problem solving, and visuoperceptual and emotion recognition deficits, while the dementia associated with AD is more "cortical" in nature, characterized predominantly by memory loss.

In order to determine the best criteria for diagnosing dementia in HD, Pevey and colleagues [20] assessed which cognitive measures accounted for the largest proportion of variance in functional ability. Their analysis provides evidence that cognitive measures of speed of processing and attention/initiation account for a significant amount of the variability in functional independence in HD. They propose the following definition for dementia in HD: cognitive impairment in at least two areas of cognition but does not require a memory deficit, in the context of impaired functional abilities and a deteriorating course.

The wealth of data collected on cognitive performance in HD clearly demonstrates that tools exist to measure a decline in cognitive functioning throughout the course of HD. Thus, it is very important to evaluate the functional impact that a decline in cognitive functioning places on patients and caregivers. A few important points to keep in mind are that physicians tend to focus on motor disturbances, rather than mood and cognitive disturbances when considering treatment, probably because they are the most visible symptoms, even though most HD patients are unaware of their involuntary movements [23, 24]. Thus, it is important to assess disability from the patient's and caregiver's perspective in addition to the physician's. Further, lack of insight into one's cognitive deterioration may limit the effectiveness of self-reporting of cognitive symptoms.

Several important studies have probed the differential impact of cognitive, motor, and mood symptoms on patients and caretakers. Banaskiewicz and colleagues sought to identify determinants of functional disability, patient's quality of life, and caregivers' burden [25]. They found that motor disturbances, cognitive impairment, apathy, and duration of illness were independent predictors of disability. Further, they found that depression and cognitive disturbances determined patient's quality of life, while motor disturbances and depression were the predictors of caregiver burden. These findings are consistent with previous reports indicating cognitive impairment, motor disturbances, and apathy as important factors affecting activities of daily living in HD patients [26]. The lower impact of cognitive disturbance on caregivers in the Banaskeiwicz [25] study is in contrast to studies in Parkinson's [27] and Alzheimer's disease [28], where cognitive impairment was the key predictor of caregiver burden.

In another study, Ho and colleagues did a semi-structured interview with a small HD cohort to examine the frequency in which various categories of health-related quality of life concerns were mentioned [29]. Cognitive-related concerns were mentioned rarely by those in the premanifest stage and those in advanced disease (Stage 5) but were mentioned frequently by those in Stages 1–4. As part of the development of Functional Rating Scale for premanifest and early-stage Huntington's disease (FuRST-pHD), Vaccarino and colleagues conducted focus groups with patients and companions [30]. They assessed which cognitive-related symptoms were reported as frequently occurring and which were reported to interfere with day-to-day function. Cognitive symptoms were reported frequently and were ranked among the highest for interfering with daily function. The most frequently reported cognitive symptoms were concentration, memory and executive function, with cognitive and finding the right words somewhat less frequent. Memory and executive function were reported to interfere the most with daily function, with concentration and cognitive interfering to lesser degrees.

Clinical Course of Cognitive Dysfunction in HD

There are a number of challenges in attempting to define the course of cognitive deficits along the protracted evolution of HD. In the concrete case of HD prior to the existence of a reliable diagnostic test, which was developed in 1993, it was not possible to make clear distinction of who was at risk and who was a control before the clinical diagnosis. Therefore data on studies done prior to the use of genetic testing in premanifest individuals is not informative. However, in the time since the definitive diagnostic test became available, the HD field has been in the unique position to be able to study the progression of the disease prior to clinical diagnosis. The HD field still faces the same challenges as other disorders in studies aiming to characterize the patterns of cognitive impairments. In particular, methodological issues associated with the standardization of the testing conditions and practice effects can confound some testing paradigms. While the ability to include premanifest subjects offers a unique glimpse into the onset of cognitive impairment, it can be very challenging to detect cognitive deficits in those far from the clinical diagnosis, when cognitive impairments are subtle. To detect deficits in individuals far from expected onset of motor symptoms, very sensitive tests must be used. When group effects are looked for in analysis that compares affected versus controls, large sample sizes are required since the effect size is small. Many of the studies published that could not find differences between Huntington's disease gene expansion carriers (HDGECs) and controls were underpowered (for review, see Dumas et al. [15]). It is also important to acknowledge the confounding effects when concurrent depression or other behavior or mood disturbances are present, which may happen frequently.

To inform on the evolution of the cognitive deficits over time, the best sources of data are the natural history, observational studies of PREDICT-HD [31] and TRACK-HD [8, 9], and systematic reviews of all studies conducted along the years as the one published by Dumas et al. [15].

The PREDICT study [31] is the largest and longest prospective, observational study that to date has collected data on more than 1,000 premanifest individuals and controls for more than 10 years. It was the first to show indisputably the presence of consistent impairments in the premanifest population and to follow-up longitudinally those individuals to define clearly the pattern of those impairments. TRACK-HD, although smaller in size, complements nicely the PREDICT data given that it includes a relevant group of early HD patients that were evaluated alongside with the premanifest cohort and was executed with the guiding principles of a clinical trial.

Dumas et al. [15] conducted a systematic review of clinical studies that evaluated cognition in HD in comparison with a control group and were published after the availability of the genetic of diagnostic test and before 2011.

Considerable effort has been made to characterize the different types of cognitive impairments, the manifestation of these deficits in the course of the disease, how large the effect size is when measured in standardized testing, and how much they progress along time. These aspects are important features to define the suitability of a deficit and its associated measurement to be used in an interventional trial. These efforts largely envisaged trials designed to delay or slow the disease progression, but the data generated can also be used to design trials focused on symptomatically enhancing cognition, as has been done in other diseases such as schizophrenia.

Assessing the wealth of data on cognitive impairment in HD, we can start to identify what impairments are sufficiently frequent to perturb and change the life of the subjects that bare them. Cognition is an array of extremely complex and interconnected processes. To individualize specific cognitive domains or to establish particular deficits in one of them and not in other is a difficult process. High-level domains of neurocognitive function are recognized. DSM-5 enumerates six as follows: complex attention, executive function, learning and memory, language, perceptual-motor, and social cognition. Neuropsychological tests or batteries of tests might preferentially target one of the domains, but rarely do they engage only one domain. Since experimental studies use large batteries of neuropsychological tests, it is useful to make an effort to understand which domains they represent.

The clinical studies mentioned above together reveal a pattern for the cognitive decline in HD that is summarized in Fig. 10.1. We attempted to aggregate the information in the figure by cognitive domains or subdomains affected rather than by test.

It is now well accepted that premanifest HD subjects, particularly those closer to predicted onset, show poorer performance in measures of attention, processing speed, psychomotor functions, episodic learning and memory, emotion processing,

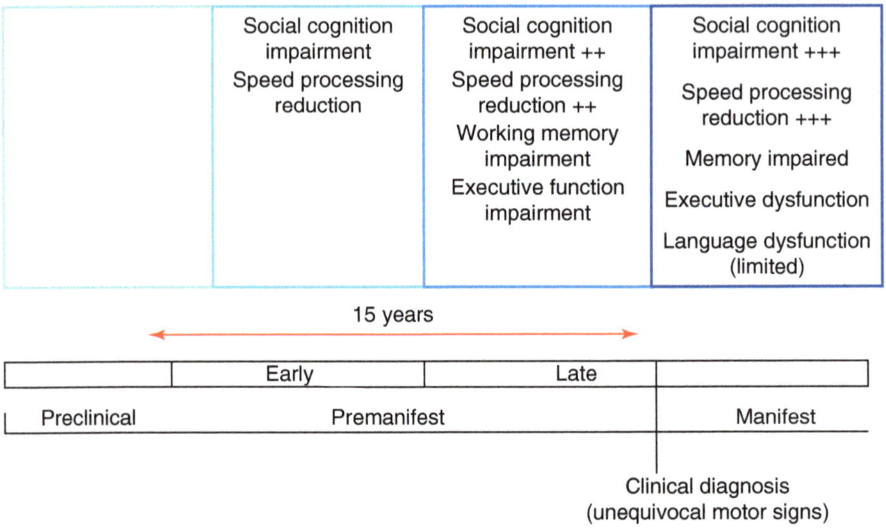

Fig. 10.1 Sequence of occurrence of cognitive deficits during the course of Huntington's disease

sensory-perceptual functions, and executive function in comparison to controls. The systematic review of studies on cognitive function allows the conclusion that cognitive decline shows a differential progression. During late disease stages all cognitive domains show moderate or severe disturbances. The global profile of cognitive functioning in premanifest HD is characterized by subtle deficits of psychomotor speed, negative emotion recognition, and executive functions. In manifest HD these deficits progressively worsen and are eventually accompanied by memory dysfunction. Global cognitive abilities and language capacities are the last to show deterioration. Eventually, these cognitive deficits in HD result in generalized dementia.

Cognitive and behavioral symptoms/signs of HD have been shown to be evident at least 15 years prior to the time at which motor diagnosis is typically given. The earliest deficit detected is emotion recognition, particularly with negative emotions. This equates well with the deterioration in social and familiar relationships frequently reported in HD environments. Although not formally demonstrated yet, it is reasonable to suggest the impaired ability to read nonverbal cues expressed by emotional expressions will contribute to relational tensions.

Another early and sensitive indicator of the early signs of HD includes changes to the speed of thinking and motor skills. A premanifest HD subject will begin to notice that completion of ordinary mental tasks is more tiring and takes more time to achieve the same outcome.

Memory impairments occur later than the changes in speeded processing and emotion recognition. Typically differences in attention/working memory are more reliably detected in those within 5 years of clinical onset of motor symptoms. The rate of decline of memory functioning is not pronounced. Throughout the course of HD, there are two primary memory difficulties: learning new information and recalling stored information. Overall memory decline does occur in manifest HD, and while for specific sub-domains there is a relative consensus in terms of decline in visual memory, there is less certainty about verbal memory.

One aspect that is particular to HD is the impairment of procedural memories, which is usually called implicit memory. These impact motor routines such as driving a car or a bicycle or tying shoes. The impairment of these motor memories means that a person has to rely on "conscious memory" to perform these tasks, which requires more concentration.

Executive Function

Executive function is a complex and critical component of a successful human life. Executive functions include prioritization, problem solving, judgment, abstract thinking, controlling emotions, and awareness of self and others.

Executive processes are universally and significantly impacted in HD. The aggregate of alterations in cognition stemming from impairments in the executive functions results in a constellation of behavioral and personality changes which is sometimes referred to as the "dysexecutive syndrome."

HD patients show impairments in set shifting ability, which is the cognitive ability to dynamically change focus between points of fixation based on changing goals and environmental stimuli. This contributes to the common occurrence of impulsive, hyperactive, disorganized, and aggressive behavior.

Language

Huntington's disease does not cause primary language dysfunction such as the word-finding difficulties, paraphasic errors, or receptive disorders that are typically associated with Alzheimer's disease and other cortical dementias. Care should be taken to distinguish language function, which is relatively preserved, from impairment in the motor production of speech. In the latter stages of the illness, most patients become unintelligible, although this does not signify a lack of comprehension, and therefore clinicians should maintain communication with patients, even in the absence of a response.

An impressive body of data is accumulating relating the cognitive deficits that are demonstrable by testing to the changes in brain structure as visualized by MRI or to changes in connectivity as studied by fMRI and DTI. The review of this data is outside the scope of this chapter. Suffice it to say that a congruent and consistent body of evidence is emerging relating temporal and functional changes in structure with correlate functional outputs [32, 33].

How does a HDGEC subject typically present? Most health professionals who do not work in specialized clinics dedicated to HD rarely see subjects at risk in a professional context. They might interact socially with a HDGEC without even being aware of HD carrier status. However a clue to it may be given if he or she complains that recently work has started to take longer and longer to complete, a sign of reduced speed processing.

In clinical terms, a subject that has been diagnosed with HD, and therefore has unequivocal motor signs, has his or her presence dominated by the almost omnipresence of those motor signs, which are eye-catching. It takes some training and effort to evaluate appropriately the patient that most of the time has difficulties in communicating and is perturbed by the ongoing decline of his or hers cognitive abilities. It is also common in this stage that the patient does not make any particular effort to complain since he or she is in denial or apathy or both. Thus, it is important to recognize that the affection of cognitive abilities in these patients is important and disabling, but it does not make them unaware of the surrounding world, as happens when Alzheimer's disease progresses.

Before developing motor signs, HDGECs experience several difficulties in going about their everyday lives and keeping their jobs in relation with the subtle impairments we describe. There is the schoolteacher that at 40 years of age becomes progressively more irritated and unable to cope with the indiscipline of her teenager students. It takes a good deal of insight to pursue this type of complaint given the current level overall discipline in high schools. Or there is the accountant, known to be meticulous and trustworthy, that starts to miss deadlines and to show lapses in the spreadsheets. These people will not complain specifically of the exact work issues but rather of the consequences that these have in their lives. If and when they do come to medical attention, there has been already a spiral of downstream events, like loss of a long-term job with an important impact in the self-esteem, or consequences in the marital relationship.

Therapeutic Possibilities and Perspectives

Managing Huntington's disease is challenging given the complexity of interconnected deficits resulting from the neurodegenerative process and the paucity of interventional tools currently available. Notwithstanding, there are a number of potential venues to be explored on the horizon.

Clinical trials with DNA-/RNA-based technologies [34] aiming to lower the production of mutant huntingtin protein are expected to be started in 2015. If successful, these interventions are likely to be beneficial to all domains affected by the disease, including cognition.

In the domain of small chemical molecules, the class of phosphodiesterase 10A inhibitors is in early phase II clinical trials [35]. This approach has the potential to have a beneficial effect on cognition mediated through a reinvigoration of the corticostriatal circuitry.

As described in this chapter, the nature of the cognitive impairment in HD is phenomenologically very different from the one seen in Alzheimer's disease, as would be expected from the distinct physiopathology of the neurodegenerative process in these two diseases. AD and HD are both misfolded proteinopathies, and as such, they share a number of common molecular dysfunctions. However, at a receptor level there are important differences and these limit the potential to bridge interventions across dementia disorders just based on analogy. The proposals for testing cognitive enhancers in HD must have a well-grounded rationale in HD pathophysiopathology. HD is a very protracted disease that evolves during decades with minor subtle deficits that are nevertheless impactful in individual lives. Potentially these can be ameliorated. There are a large number of CNS targets being investigated as potential cognitive enhancers to improve cognition [36]. Among these, at least the 5-HT6 antagonists and the H3 antagonists are being considered for HD.

To date five drugs have been tested in clinical trials to evaluate their potential to ameliorate cognitive deterioration in early HD. Donepezil, an inhibitor of acetylcholinesterase formally approved for the treatment of Alzheimer's disease, failed to show an improvement in cognition in HD [37]. This was a very small size trial ($n=30$) designed to evaluated the effect of donepezil in chorea; thus, the absence of an effect in the cognitive measurements is at best inconclusive.

Atomoxetine, a norepinephrine reuptake inhibitor commonly used for attention-deficit hyperactivity disorder, failed to show a benefit in attention as well as in executive/neuropsychological measures in a small ($n=20$) crossover study [38]. Modafinil has also been studied for cognition, and, while it was associated with increased alertness at a dose of 200 mg day, it failed to demonstrate any significant improvement in executive function and showed detrimental effects on visual recognition and working memory [39]. Latrepirdine was studied in a full clinical development plan. First, in a pilot phase II study [40], latrepirdine showed a beneficial effect in the nonspecific Mini-Mental State Examination, but had no effect in other cognitive rating scales such as the UHDRS cognitive tests or the ADAS-cog. The results of the phase III study (HORIZON) of latrepirdine did not confirm the potential beneficial effect. In co-primary outcomes, the Mini-Mental State Examination and the Clinician's Interview-Based Impression of Change, Plus Caregiver Input (CIBIC-Plus), the results did not reach statistical significance [41].

Citalopram was also tested to explore a potential procognitive effect in a randomized controlled trial in non-depressed HD patients ($n=33$). The trial did not find an effect in the primary outcome measure, executive function, but there was an improvement in depression scores despite the condition of patients not being depressed at baseline [42].

It is obvious the development of interventions for cognition in HD has not been systematic. In fact most of the studies in HD so far target motor endpoints. However, the field is now opening with new types of interventions marshaling in, namely, exercise [43], neural retraining [44], and magnetic stimulation [45] among others, that need proper evaluation and the drug-based treatments already mentioned.

There is a need for greater investment in proper trial methodology in terms of sample size, outcomes measures, and selection of populations if this new generation of efforts is to be successful. The recent investment into the development of a standard battery, the HD-CAB, for assessing cognition in HD clinical trials is a good step in that direction [16]. This will hopefully let us avoid the perils that have plagued other fields, where, in the absence of appropriate tools, clinical efficacy has been evaluated using assessments designed for other purposes. Because of the differences in the presentations and patterns of cognitive dysfunction across neurological and psychiatric diseases, tools developed for Alzheimer's disease or schizophrenia may not be suitable for HD. A recent systematic review of clinical trials in HD revealed that, in the absence of an accepted standard battery, a wide variety of cognitive tests have been used in HD clinical trials including the Mini-Mental State Examination (MMSE), the Unified Huntington's Disease Rating Scale (UHDRS) cognitive assessment battery (phonetic verbal fluency test, Symbol Digit Modalities Test and Stroop Test), Buschke Selective Reading Test, Benton Visual Retention Test, Grooved Pegboard, Wechsler Adult Intelligence Scale (WAIS), and Trail Making Test [46]. Implementation of the HD-CAB in future clinical trials will help to compare across studies and maximize the potential to see treatment effect.

References

1. Marder K, Zhao H, Myers RH, et al. Rate of functional decline in Huntington's disease. Huntington Study Group. Neurology. 2000;54(2):452–8.
2. Novak MJ, Tabrizi SJ. Huntington's disease: clinical presentation and treatment. Int Rev Neurobiol. 2011;98:297–323.
3. Roos RA. Huntington's disease: a clinical review. Orphanet J Rare Dis. 2010;5(1):40.

4. Mayeux R, Stern Y, Herman A, Greenbaum L, Fahn S. Correlates of early disability in Huntington's disease. Ann Neurol. 1986;20:727–31.
5. Bamford KA, Caine ED, Kido DK, et al. Clinical-pathologic correlation in Huntington's disease: a neuropsychological and computed tomography study. Neurology. 1989;39:796–801.
6. Antonini A, Barone P, Marconi R, et al. The progression of non-motor symptoms in Parkinson's disease and their contribution to motor disability and quality of life. J Neurol. 2012;259(12):2621–31.
7. Stout JC, Jones R, Labuschagne I, et al. Evaluation of longitudinal 12 and 24 month cognitive outcomes in premanifest and early Huntington's disease. J Neurol Neurosurg Ps. 2012; 83(7):687–94.
8. Tabrizi SJ, Scahill RI, Durr A, et al. Biological and clinical changes in premanifest and early stage Huntington's disease in the TRACK-HD study: the 12-month longitudinal analysis. Lancet Neurol. 2011;10(1):31–42.
9. Tabrizi SJ, Scahill RI, Owen G, et al. Predictors of phenotypic progression and disease onset in premanifest and early-stage Huntington's disease in the TRACK-HD study: analysis of 36-month observational data. Lancet Neurol. 2013;12(7):637–49.
10. Tabrizi SJ, Langbehn DR, Leavitt BR, et al. Biological and clinical manifestations of Huntington's disease in the longitudinal TRACK-HD study: cross-sectional analysis of baseline data. Lancet Neurol. 2009;8:791–801.
11. Harrington DL, Smith MM, Zhang Y, et al. Cognitive domains that predict time to diagnosis in prodromal Huntington disease. J Neurol Neurosurg Psychiatry. 2012;83(6):612–9.
12. Stout JC, Paulsen JS, Queller S, et al. Neurocognitive signs in prodromal Huntington disease. Neuropsychology. 2011;25(1):1–14.
13. Stout JC, Carlozzi NE, Queller S, et al. Candidates for neurocognitive markers in pre-HD: longitudinal assessment from the predict-HD cohort. Neurotherapeutics. 2008;5(2):372.
14. Paulsen JS. Cognitive impairment in Huntington disease: diagnosis and treatment. Curr Neurol Neurosci Rep. 2011;11(5):474–83.
15. Dumas EM, van den Bogaard SJ, Middelkoop HA, Roos RA. A review of cognition in Huntington's disease. Front Biosci. 2013;5:1–18 (Scholar edition).
16. Stout JC, Queller S, Baker KN, et al. HD-CAB: a cognitive assessment battery for clinical trials in Huntington's disease. Mov Disord. 2014; in press.
17. Iosifescu DV. The relation between mood, cognition and psychosocial functioning in psychiatric disorders. Eur Neuropsychopharmacol. 2012;22 Suppl 3:S499–504.
18. American Psychiatric Association. Diagnostic and statistical manual of mental disorders. 4th ed. Arlington: American Psychiatric Publishing; 2000.
19. American Psychiatric Association. Diagnostic and statistical manual of mental disorders. 5th ed. Arlington: American Psychiatric Publishing; 2013.
20. Peavy GM, Jacobson MW, Goldstein JL, et al. Cognitive and functional decline in Huntington's disease: dementia criteria revisited. Mov Disord. 2010;25(9):1163–9.
21. Butters N, Delis DC, Lucas JA. Clinical assessment of memory disorders in amnesia and dementia. Annu Rev Psychol. 1995;46:493–523.
22. Salmon DP, Kwo-on-Yuen PF, Heindel WC, et al. Differentiation of Alzheimer's disease and Huntington's disease with the dementia rating scale. Arch Neurol. 1989;46(11):1204–8.
23. Snowden JS, Craufurd D, Griffiths HL, Neary D. Awareness of involuntary movements in Huntington disease. Arch Neurol. 1998;55(6):801–5.
24. Sitek EJ, Sołtan W, Wieczorek D, et al. Self-awareness of motor dysfunction in patients with Huntington's disease in comparison to Parkinson's disease and cervical dystonia. J Int Neuropsychol Soc. 2011;17(5):788–95.
25. Banaszkiewicz K, Sitek EJ, Rudzińska M, Sołtan W, et al. Huntington's disease from the patient, caregiver and physician's perspectives: three sides of the same coin? J Neural Transm. 2012;119(11):1361–5.
26. Hamilton JM, Salmon DP, Corey-Bloom J, et al. Behavioural abnormalities contribute to functional decline in Huntington's disease. J Neurol Neurosurg Psychiatry. 2003;74(1):120–2.
27. D'Amelio M, Terruso V, Palmeri B, et al. Predictors of caregiver burden in partners of patients with Parkinson's disease. Neurol Sci. 2009;30(2):171–4.

28. Razani J, Kakos B, Orieta-Barbalace C, et al. Predicting caregiver burden from daily functional abilities of patients with mild dementia. J Am Geriatr Soc. 2007;55(9):1415–20.
29. Ho AK, Hocaoglu MB, European Huntington's Disease Network Quality of Life Working Group. Impact of Huntington disease across the entire disease spectrum: the phases and stages of disease from the patient perspective. Clin Genet. 2011;80:235–9.
30. Vaccarino AL, Sills T, Anderson KE, et al. Assessment of cognitive symptoms in prodromal and early Huntington disease. PLoS Curr. 2011;3:RRN1250.
31. Paulsen JS, Long JD, Johnson HD, et al. Clinical and biomarker changes in premanifest Huntington disease show Trial feasibility: a decade of the predict-HD study. Front Aging Neurosci. 2014;6:78.
32. Ross CA, Aylward EH, Wild EJ. Huntington disease: natural history, biomarkers and prospects for therapeutics. Nat Rev Neurol. 2014;10:204–16.
33. Poudel GR, Stout JC, Dominguez DJF, et al. White matter connectivity reflects clinical and cognitive status in Huntington's disease. Neurobiol Dis. 2014;65:180–7.
34. Yu S, Liang Y, Palacino J, Difiglia M, Lu B. Drugging unconventional targets: insights from Huntington's disease. Trends Pharmacol Sci. 2014;35:53–62.
35. Chappie TA, Helal CJ, Hou X. Current landscape of phosphodiesterase 10A (PDE10A) inhibition. J Med Chem. 2012;55:7299–331.
36. Wallace TL, Ballard TM, Pouzet B, et al. Drug targets for cognitive enhancement in neuropsychiatric disorders. Pharmacol Biochem Behav. 2011;99:130–45.
37. Cubo E, Shannon KM, Tracy D, Jaglin JA, Bernard BA, Wuu J, Leurgans SE. Effect of donepezil on motor and cognitive function in Huntington disease. Neurology. 2006;67:1268–71.
38. Beglinger LJ, Adams WH, Paulson H, Fiedorowicz JG, Langbehn DR, Duff K, et al. Randomized controlled trial of atomoxetine for cognitive dysfunction in early Huntington disease. J Clin Psychopharmacol. 2009;29:484–7.
39. Blackwell AD, Paterson NS, Barker RA, Robbins TW, Sahakian BJ. The effects of modafinil on mood and cognition in Huntington's disease. Psychopharmacology (Berl). 2008;199:29–36.
40. Kieburtz K, McDermott MP, Voss TS, et al. A randomized, placebo-controlled trial of latrepirdine in Huntington disease. Arch Neurol. 2010;67:154–60.
41. HORIZON Investigators of the Huntington Study Group and European Huntington's Disease Network. A randomized, double-blind, placebo-controlled study of latrepirdine in patients with mild to moderate Huntington disease. JAMA Neurol. 2013;70:25–33.
42. Beglinger LJ, Adams WH, Langbehn D, Fiedorowicz JG, Jorge R, Biglan K, Caviness J, Olson B, Robinson RG, Kieburtz K, Paulsen JS. Results of the citalopram to enhance cognition in Huntington disease trial. Mov Disord. 2014;29:401–5.
43. Khalil H, Quinn L, van Deursen R, et al. What effect does a structured home-based exercise programme have on people with Huntington's disease? A randomized, controlled pilot study. Clin Rehabil. 2013;27(7):646–58.
44. Enriquez-Geppert S, Huster RJ, Herrmann CS. Boosting brain functions: improving executive functions with behavioral training, neurostimulation, and neurofeedback. Int J Psychophysiol. 2013;88:1–16.
45. Nouchi R, Taki Y, Takeuchi H, et al. Brain training game boosts executive functions, working memory and processing speed in the young adults: a randomized controlled trial. PLoS ONE. 2013. doi:10.1371/journal.pone.0055518.
46. Mestre T, Ferreira J, Coelho MM, Rosa M, Sampaio C. Therapeutic interventions for symptomatic treatment in Huntington's disease. The Cochrane database of systematic reviews. 2009;(3):CD006456. doi:10.1002/14651858.CD006456.pub2.

Chapter 11
Tics

Valerie C. Brandt and Alexander Münchau

Abbreviations

ADHD	Attention deficit hyperactivity disorder
BG	Basal ganglia
CSTC	Cortico-striatal-thalamo-cortical
DA	Dopamine
DSM	Diagnostic and Statistical Manual
DTI	Diffusion-tensor imaging
GABA	γ-Aminobutyric acid
GPe	Globus pallidus externus
GPi	Globus pallidus internus
HRT	Habit reversal therapy
ICD	International classification of diseases
MPH	Methylphenidate
MSN	Medium spiny neurons
OCD	Obsessive-compulsive disorder
OFC	Orbitofrontal cortex
PANDAS	Pediatric autoimmune neuropsychiatric disorder associated with streptococcal infections
PFC	Prefrontal cortex
RCT	Randomized controlled trial
REM	Rapid eye movements
SMA	Supplementary motor area

V.C. Brandt, Dipl.-Psych, MPhil (CANTAB) (✉) • A. Münchau
Paediatric and Adult Movement Disorders and Neuropsychiatry, Institute of Neurogenetics, University of Lübeck, Maria-Goeppert-Str. 1, Lübeck 23562, Germany
e-mail: valerie.brandt@neuro.uni-luebeck.de; alexander.muenchau@neuro.uni-luebeck.de

H. Reichmann (ed.), *Neuropsychiatric Symptoms of Movement Disorders*,
Neuropsychiatric Symptoms of Neurological Disease,
DOI 10.1007/978-3-319-09537-0_11

THC Tetrahydrocannabinol
TMS Transcranial magnetic stimulation
TS Tourette syndrome

Tics: Diagnosis and Classification

Tics are sudden, patterned, repetitive movements (or sounds) resembling voluntary movements but are misplaced in context and time [1]. Single tics cannot easily be distinguished from voluntary movements phenomenologically or electrophysiologically [1]. They mainly affect the face, head, shoulders, and neck [2]. Tics can be simple involving single muscle groups (eye blinking, eye rolling, throat clearing) and complex, e.g., actions appearing intentional or compulsion-like (gestures, single words or sentences, squatting, jumping, repetitive touching) but are not goal directed [2]. Two characteristics that distinguish tics from other hyperkinetic movement disorders (except for psychogenic movement disorders and akathisia) are partial suppressibility and the fact that most TS patients, particularly affected adolescents and adults, experience tics as voluntary, intentional movements that are executed to transiently relieve an uncontrollable urge to tic [3, 4]. Tics can be subdivided into motor, phonic (vocal), cognitive, and sensory tics [5].

Phonic or vocal tics are sounds that are produced by air movement through the vocal cords, nose, or mouth such as throat clearing, barking, grunting, high-pitched sounds, or sniffing [6].

Cognitive tics or "impulsions" are repetitive thoughts, but contrary to obsessions typically observed in OCD; they are not anxiety-driven but occur as a reaction to auditory, visual, tactile, or inner stimuli that trigger the urge to tic [7, 8]. Strictly speaking, sensory tics are not tics as such but are sensations preceding a tic and are explained in more detail below (see section "Premonitory urges").

Tics are usually easy to identify and discern from other extra movements. To avoid misclassification or misdiagnosis, a general physical and neurological examination by an experienced physician is recommended by a European panel of experts [6].

Tics can resemble stereotypies. However, the latter are typically more complex and are repeated consecutively. On the other hand, stereotypies are not preceded by an inner urge to move. Some brief tics can be difficult to distinguish from myoclonus, but again myoclonus is not preceded by an urge. Also, during writing or fine finger movements, tics usually subside, whereas myoclonus is either unchanged or becomes more prominent.

Sometimes it can be challenging to distinguish between rapid tics and chorea, particularly, with outstretched arms or raised legs. Chorea, though, is unpredictable, floating, and chaotic.

In some patients with longer-lasting tonic tics, particularly affecting the neck, tics can resemble dystonia. Electromyography may help. Cocontraction of agonist and antagonist is typical for dystonia but not for tics.

Diagnostic criteria for tic disorders were defined in a very similar manner both in the tenth edition of the European *International Classification of Diseases* (ICD)-10 and in the American *Diagnostic and Statistical Manual*, fifth edition (DSM-5).

Both classification systems specify that tic disorders first occur in infancy, childhood, or adolescence and provide the following four categories: (1) TS; (2) persistent/chronic motor or vocal tic disorder, the same criteria apply as in TS, but tics are limited to either motor or vocal tics; (3) provisional tic disorder, the same criteria apply as in chronic tic disorder, but the symptoms have been present for less than 12 months; and (4) tic disorder not otherwise specified.

Tics have very rarely been associated with structural brain lesions. The number of reported patients is very small, and their clinical details are scant. In particular, in many reports it is not clear whether "symptomatic tics" were associated with preceding urges.

Tics can be induced or exacerbated by drugs (e.g., cocaine, amphetamine, antidepressants, anticonvulsants, antihistamines). Cocaine abuse is probably the most common cause of adult-onset tics. Tics are also common in autism spectrum disorders. They are sometimes part of the clinical presentation of Huntington's disease and are very typical in neuroacanthocytosis. Complex tics have been described in pantothenate kinase-associated neurodegeneration and a number of X-chromosomal disorders [9].

If a patient exhibits uncommon symptoms such as severe deterioration or adult onset, additional investigations including neuroimaging or neurophysiological techniques are recommended. Also, if the physical examination reveals dysmorphic features, or if the patient presents with learning difficulties or symptoms and signs suggestive of an autism spectrum disorder, further advise by a clinical geneticist should be sought [6].

However, as a rule, the vast majority of tic disorders belong to the TS spectrum. TS will therefore be the main focus of this chapter.

Gilles de la Tourette Syndrome

Definition

TS was first described in 1825 by the French physician Jean-Marc Itard. However, the disorder was only later named after Georges Edouard Albert Brutus Gilles de la Tourette who described nine patients suffering from what he called "maladie des tics" at the time [10]. Today, TS is defined as a neuropsychiatric disorder, acknowledging the fact that it can be successfully treated with neuroleptics and deep brain stimulation, yet has a social component to it that expresses itself in various forms such as TS patient's ability to suppress tics if socially required, or coprolalia, i.e., socially inappropriate automatic swearing.

TS is defined by the presence of multiple motor and vocal tics (not necessarily at the same time) for more than 1 year, with an onset before the age of 18. According to the DSM-IV-TR and more recently the DSM-V, it is possible to diagnose TS in patients who experience all symptoms without reporting distress or impairment [11]. The DSM-V classifies TS as a motor disorder and groups it in the neurodevelopmental disorders category.

Defining Clinical Characteristic

Tics and Premonitory Urges

Tics in TS occur in bouts and wax and wane in frequency and intensity over hours, days, and years. The tic-repertoire typically varies across the life span in a given patient. Tics are suggestible [2] and "contagious" [12]. Patients frequently report that tics increase under stress and decrease when focused on a task, for instance, playing a musical instrument or exercising. Silva et al. (1995) identified 17 events that can cause tic exacerbation. Their main characteristic was strong emotional excitement, such as emotional trauma and social gatherings but also impending birthdays or a vacation trip [13]. Moreover, it has been shown that overall stress levels are higher in TS patients than in healthy controls [14]. However, a controlled study inducing stress experimentally in ten adolescents with TS found no increase in tic frequency under stress as compared to baseline. Tic suppression though was less effective under stress [15]. These results need to be interpreted with care due to the small sample size and the fact that only the effects of one task were measured.

Tics can be suppressed to a certain degree for a few minutes up to a few hours [2], and patients often report suppressing their tics in public or "diverting" their most obvious tic, such as facial grimacing, to less obvious movements, for instance, leg or foot movements.

For a long time it was assumed that tics are entirely automatic and uncontrollable motor phenomena. However, tics are often preceded by a premonitory sensation, an inner urge to move, which cannot be suppressed or controlled and may increase until transiently relieved by a tic [4, 16, 17]. Suppressing tics together with an increasing urge to tic can cause distress.

Premonitory sensations either can be experienced at the site where tics occur, can represent a more generalized inner tension or anxiety, or both. They are sometimes described as a pressure-like, tickling, cold, or warm sensation [18]. Overall, approximately 80 % of patients report to experience premonitory urges, depending on age and measure [19].

It is yet unclear whether urges precede, occur at the same time, or follow the onset of tics during development. Self-reports of adult TS patients suggest that first awareness of urges occurs around the age of 10, approximately 3 years after the onset of tics. However, Robertson, Leckman, and colleagues pointed out that this estimate may be due to difficulties of children at the age of 5–7 years to understand and describe the concept of urges [19, 20]. Moreover, awareness of premonitory sensations increases with age, not with tic duration, and may thus depend on cognitive development rather than time since tic onset [18].

It has been suggested that the awareness of premonitory urges improves the ability to suppress tics in some patients [20]. Banaschewski et al. (2003) investigated 254 children and adolescents aged 8–19 years. There was a significant increase in the number of children who reported premonitory sensations as well as an increasing ability to suppress tics with age. However, whereas 37 % reported premonitory sensations, 64 % were able to suppress tics. Also, only 60 % of children who gave unequivocal answers to both questions showed an overlap of premonitory sensations and the ability to suppress tics. Thus, the authors concluded that premonitory sensations are not a necessary prerequisite for tic suppression [18]. Moreover, it was shown in a sample of adults with uncomplicated TS that there was no correlation between the ability to suppress tics and the extent of premonitory urges further corroborating existing evidence that premonitory urges and the ability to suppress tics are not directly related [21].

A study investigating 100 TS patients established that premonitory urges are related to symptom severity. In patients with comorbid disorders, urges are most strongly related to OC symptoms and anxiety. Both in patients with complicated and uncomplicated TS, urges were negatively related to perceived quality of life [22].

Echo, Pali-, and Coprophenomena

In addition to tics, TS patients can have echo-, pali-, and coprophenomena. These are currently classified as complex tics, although there is some disagreement as to whether this definition is justified [23]. Paliphenomena include palipraxia, palilalia, and palilogia, i.e., the repetition of own gestures, syllables, or words [24]. Echophenomena encompass echopraxia and echolalia, i.e., the repetition of other people's gestures or sounds/words, and are relatively common in TS [12]. Imitation is considered normal in children (learning by imitation) and to a certain degree in healthy adults (e.g., contagious yawning). However, like tics, echophenomena are "exaggerated normality," misplaced in context and time [23]. Coprophenomena constitute obscene or offensive behavior such as coprolalia (involuntary swearing) and copropraxia (offensive gestures). They are extremely salient but occur only in 10–15 % of TS patients [19].

Sleep

Sleep patterns in TS patients differ from healthy controls. Adults and children with TS have lower sleep efficiency, which correlates negatively with symptom severity during the day [25, 26]. Adults have lower slow wave sleep percentage and percentage of stage 1, less number of awakenings and sleep stage changes, and increased sleep latency. Tics can occur during sleep, albeit less frequently than during the day. Also, overall movements are increased during sleep suggesting hyperarousal. This is in line with the assumption of reduced intracortical inhibition of motor pathways [25]. Rapid eye movement (REM) sleep irregularities in patients with comorbid ADHD are probably due to ADHD rather than tics [25, 26].

Comorbidities

Approximately 90 % of all TS patients suffer from comorbidities, the most common of which are ADHD (60 %) [19] and OCD (41 %) [27]. In patients with TS, OC symptoms typically occur after tic onset, around the age of 10, and remit in approximately 40 % of the patients [28]. In roughly two thirds of TS patients with comorbid ADHD, the ADHD symptoms occurred before tic onset and tend to decrease later than tics [29], while their persistence into adulthood is associated with poorer psychosocial functioning. Tic severity in childhood predicts tic severity in adulthood [27], while childhood intelligence quotient predicts the persistence of OC symptoms [27]. A smaller caudate volume in children predicts tic severity as well as OC symptoms in early adulthood [30]. The association between tics, OC symptoms, and ADHD has been assessed in a longitudinal study in a large sample ($n = 776$) that was randomly selected in the USA in 1975 [31]. The data show that tics in childhood predict an increase in OC symptoms in early adulthood. Furthermore, OC symptoms in childhood predict ADHD symptoms in adulthood, while ADHD symptoms in childhood predict OC symptoms in adulthood [31].

Less common are anger control problems, learning disability, mood and anxiety disorders, oppositional defiant and conduct disorders, self-injurious behavior, and autism. Males are more often affected by ADHD, conduct and oppositional defiant disorders, anger control problems, and learning disability than females, whereas females are more often affected by OCD and self-injurious behavior [32].

Fig. 11.1 Assessment of Tourette syndrome [33]. Thorough history taking including enquiring about symptoms indicative of comorbid attention deficit hyperactivity disorder (*ADHD*) and obsessive-compulsive disorder (*OCD*) is the most relevant part of the clinical assessment. It is followed by a neurological and neuropsychological examination with a particular view to signs of neurodegenerative disorders where tics might be part of the clinical presentation, e.g., Huntington's disease. Home videos can be very useful in cases where few or no tics occur in clinics. For standardized video assessment the *Rush Video protocol* has proven useful [34]. Other standardized tools include the *Diagnostic Confidence Index* (*DCI*) [35] estimating the likelihood of having Tourette syndrome, the *Yale Global Tic Severity Scale* (*YGTSS*) [36] assessing overall tic severity, the *Yale-Brown Obsessive Compulsive Scale* (*Y-BOCS*) [37] for the assessment of OCD, the *Premonitory Urge for Tics Scale* (*PUTS*) [38] addressing premonitory urges, and the TS quality of life (*GTS-QOL*) questionnaire [39]. If there are clinical indications of a comorbid disorder, further psychiatric evaluation or neuropsychological tests should be carried out. If on the grounds of the clinical examination [1, 2] or additional psychiatric/neuropsychological assessment [3], a secondary tic disorder or complex neuropsychiatric syndrome is suspected; further investigation including brain imaging, neurophysiology, and genetic testing is recommended. Following clinical assessment patients should be informed on the diagnoses and should be offered counseling. Then an individualized treatment plan is formulated. *HRT* habit reversal treatment; *DBS* deep brain stimulation (Adapted with permission from Depboylu et al. [33])

Clinical Assessment

General Approach

A diagnostic algorithm is suggested in Fig. 11.1. In children with TS, history taking should be carried out together with parents; in adult patients the partner should be present, provided patients do not wish otherwise. During clinical assessment it is of particular interest to determine which symptoms are most debilitating, when symptoms first occurred, how they developed over time, and whether there are potential

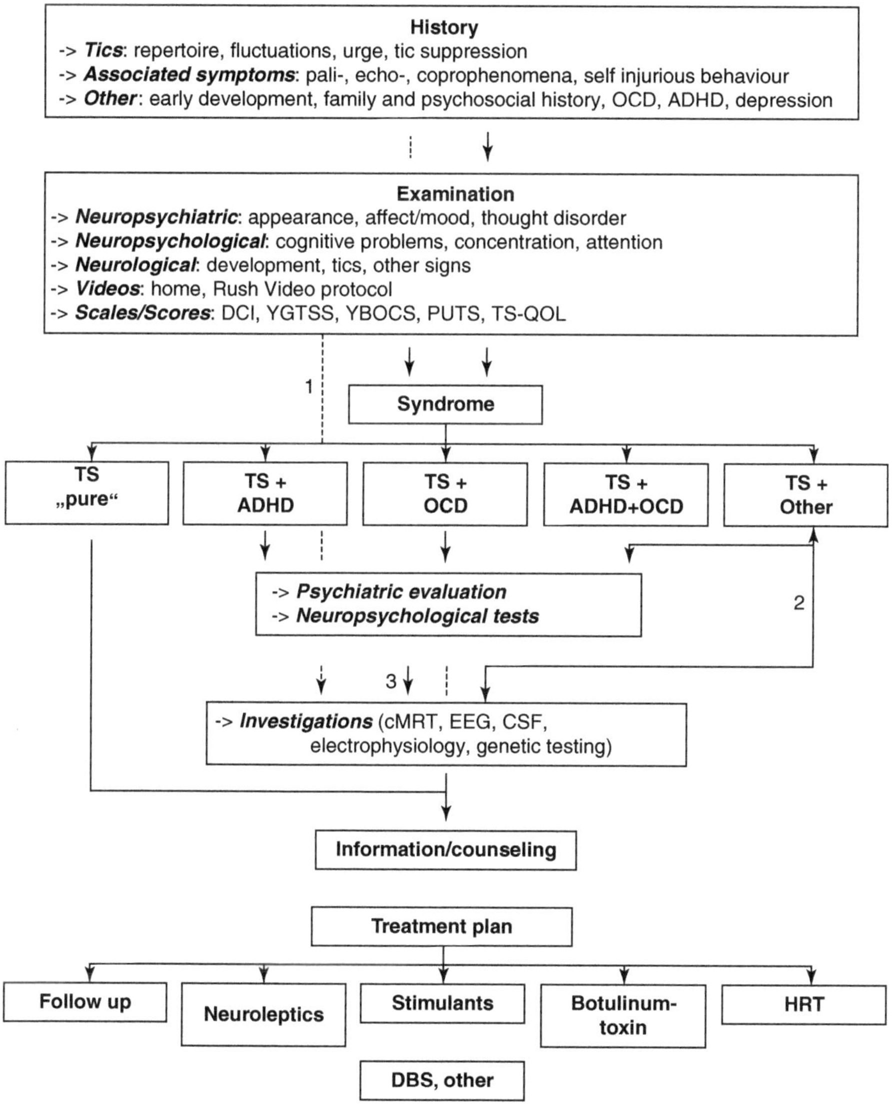

triggers and stressors. Psychosocial history should also be taken into account: how do parents or partners cope with the disorder, are there conflicts, how is the financial and housing situation, and is there a reliable social network? Complications during delivery, early development including motor milestones, and past medication and family history, particularly as regards neuropsychiatric diseases, should be documented.

Questionnaires

TS Questionnaires

For a summary of questionnaires, see Table 11.1. The number of motor and vocal tics, their severity, frequency, intensity, and complexity as well as overall impairment by these symptoms in TS and other tic disorders can be assessed with the Yale Global Tics Severity Scale (YGTSS), a clinician-rated instrument [36]. Of the existing scales, the YGTSS appears to have the best psychometric properties. It covers a broad range of symptoms. It exhibits high internal consistency, stability, and convergent as well as discriminant validity [40]. Administering the scale can take up to 20 min and requires some training on the part of the clinician. The Diagnostic Confidence Index (DCI) [35] is a questionnaire that assesses whether typical symptoms of TS are present or were present in the past. This index can be used to establish the lifetime likelihood of having TS. However, psychometric properties have yet to be investigated. The Shapiro Tourette Syndrome Severity Scale contains only five items and has high internal consistency and reliability [7]. However, it does not capture the broad phenomenology that characterizes TS. The Hopkins Motor/Vocal Tic Severity Scale is completed by clinicians and parents, assessing motor and vocal tics and associated impairment, but psychometric properties are unclear. Interrater reliability was similar for the YGTSS, Shapiro Tourette Syndrome Severity Scale, the Tourette's Syndrome-Clinical Global Impression Scale, and the Hopkins Motor/Vocal Tic Severity Scale in a sample of 20 TS patients [41].

Premonitory urges can be measured with the Premonitory Urges in Tic Disorders Scale (PUTS) [38]. The scale was originally developed for children but has recently also been evaluated in adults [42]. Psychometric properties are good, but only in individuals above the age of 10 years [17, 38]. Although the YGTSS, the DCI, and the PUTS can be recommended for clinical use, a lot more research with different age groups and larger samples is necessary to establish firm knowledge about their psychometric properties.

The YGTSS also contains one item for a quick assessment of impairment [36]. Alternatively, there is a quality of life scale specifically developed for TS patients (Gilles de la Tourette Syndrome Quality of Life Scale; GTS-QOL), encompassing four subscales for psychological problems, cognitive problems, physical/activity of daily living problems, and OC problems [39]. The scale exhibits high internal consistency and test-retest reliability as well as good content validity (judged by experts) and convergent validity (correlations with related scales) [39, 43].

Table 11.1 Summary of questionnaires

Questionnaires		
Instrument	Content	Short description
Tourette syndrome (TS)		
Diagnostic Confidence Index (DCI)	TS – lifetime likelihood	Diagnostic criteria for TS
		Psychometric properties: unknown
Yale Global Tics Severity Scale (YGTSS)	TS – number, severity, frequency, intensity, and complexity of motor and vocal tics	Clinician-rated, approx. 20 min
		Psychometric properties: good
The Shapiro Tourette Syndrome Severity Scale	TS – noticeability to others and interference of daily life	5 items
		Psychometric properties: good
		Not sufficient for covering the range of TS symptoms
The Hopkins Motor/ Vocal Tic Severity Scale	TS – motor and vocal tics and associated impairment	Clinician-rated and parent-rated
		Psychometric properties: unclear
Premonitory Urges in Tic Disorders Scale (PUTS)	Tics – preceding bodily sensations/ urges	Self-rated, 10 items
		Psychometric properties: good
Gilles de la Tourette Syndrome Quality of Life Scale (GTS-QOL)	TS – problems: psychological, physical, cognitive, and obsessional	Self-rated, 27 items
		Psychometric properties: good
Attention deficit hyperactivity disorder (ADHD)		
Conners 3	ADHD children – general psychopathology, inattention, hyperactivity/impulsivity, learning problems, executive functioning, aggression, peer relations, family relations, ADHD inattentive, ADHD hyperactive-impulsive, ADHD combined, oppositional defiant disorder, conduct disorder	Self-report, parent-report, and teacher-report
		Long form: 99/110/115 items
		Short form: 39/43/39 items
		Screening: 10 items
		Psychometric properties: good
Conners Adults ADHD Rating Scale (CAARS)	ADHD adults – *factor-derived subscales*: inattention/memory problems, hyperactivity/restlessness, impulsivity/emotional lability, problems with self-concept	Self-report and other-report
	DSM-IV™ ADHD subscales: DSM-IV inattentive symptoms, DSM-IV hyperactive-impulsive symptoms, DSM-IV total ADHD symptoms, ADHD index, inconsistency index	Long form: 66 items
		Short form: 26 items
		Screening: 12/18 items
		Psychometric properties: good

(continued)

Table 11.1 (continued)

Questionnaires		
Instrument	Content	Short description
The Wender Utah Rating Scale (WURS)	ADHD adults – assesses symptoms of ADHD retrospectively	Self-rating
		Long form: 61 items
		Short form: 25 items
		Psychometric properties: good
Obsessive-compulsive disorder (OCD)		
Yale-Brown Obsessive Compulsive Scale for adults (Y-BOCS) and children (CY-BOCS)	OCD adults/children – lifetime obsessive and compulsive symptoms: checking, washing and contamination, symmetry/ordering behavior, and hoarding	Clinician-rated
		10 items
		+ symptom checklist: 58–80 items
		Psychometric properties: good
Obsessive Compulsive Inventory-revised version (OCI-R)	OCD adults – doubting/checking, washing, ordering, hoarding and neutralizing	Self-rated
		18 items
		Psychometric properties: good
Obsessive-Compulsive Inventory for children (OCI-CV)	OCD children – doubting/checking, washing, ordering, hoarding, and neutralizing	21 items
		Psychometric properties: acceptable
Leyton Obsessional Inventory (LOI)	OCD adults – assesses obsessional symptoms	Self-report
		69 items
Leyton Obsessional Inventory for children (LOI-CV)	OCD children – assesses obsessional symptoms	Self-report and parent-report
		Long: 20 items
		Short: 11 items
Revised Children's Obsessive-Compulsive Inventory (CHOCI-R)	OCD children – obsessive and compulsive symptoms, degree of impairment	Self-report and parent-report
		20 items
		Psychometric properties: good

ADHD Questionnaires

ADHD should be diagnosed using standard interviews, inquiring about present and past inattention, impulsivity, and hyperactivity (starting before age 7) and integrating information from different sources. Further information should be collected about the severity, frequency, chronicity, and pervasiveness of the symptoms as well as their childhood onset and associated impairment [44]. Although not sufficient for a diagnosis, rating scales can be a useful tool to screen for ADHD symptoms. For a comprehensive review of scales assessing ADHD in children and adolescents, see [45]. For adults, the scales with the best psychometric properties and the best content validity are Conners Adult ADHD Rating Scale (CAARS) and the short version of the Wender Utah Rating Scale (WURS) [46]. The WURS asks patients to complete questions retrospectively regarding ADHD symptoms in childhood. It is easy to use and has good psychometric properties [47].

The Conners Adult ADHD Rating Scale has several advantages over other ADHD rating scales [48]. First of all, it has a children's version, the Conners 3 (formerly Conners Rating Scale revised, CRS-R), and an adult's version, the CAARS. Secondly, it assesses impulsivity, inattention, and hyperactivity respectively in subscales and provides separate norms for different age groups and gender. Thirdly, it provides self-report scales (CAARS-S/Conners 3-SR) and observer-report scales (CAARS-O (observer)/Conners 3-P (parent)/Conners 3-T (teacher)) in a long version, a short version, and a screening for adults as well as for children. For children, Conners provides a 10-item screening instrument, the Conners 3 ADHD Index (Conners 3-AI), which can quickly identify children who should be assessed in more detail. Finally, internal consistency, interrater reliability, and validity are good.

OCD Questionnaires

The Yale-Brown Obsessive Compulsive Scale for adults (Y-BOCS) and children (CY-BOCS) encompasses ten clinician-rated items assessing obsessive and compulsive symptom severity with regard to time spent with OC symptoms, distress, interference, resistance, and degree of control over them [37]. Additionally, there is a symptom checklist of 58–80 items dealing with lifetime obsessive and compulsive symptoms concerning checking, washing and contamination, symmetry/ordering behavior, and hoarding. For adults, there is an interview version and a self-report version. Both have good psychometric properties and are equally sensitive and specific [49]. Parents are asked to complete the scale for their affected children. The Dimensional Y-BOCS (DY-BOCS) assesses symptom severity separately for each symptom cluster and adds avoidance ratings [50]. Although all three questionnaires can be recommended for clinical use, they are time consuming. Shorter alternatives are the 18-item Obsessive-Compulsive Inventory-revised version (OCI-R) [51] for adults and the 21-item OCI-CV [52] for children. The OCI-R/OCI-CV assesses six symptom domains including doubting/checking, washing, ordering, hoarding, and neutralizing. Psychometric properties are good for the OCI-R [51], but only acceptable for the OCI-CV [53].

In clinical samples, the Leyton Obsessional Inventory for both adults (LOI) and children is commonly used (LOI-CV) [54, 55]. The LOI-CV provides a self-report and a parent-report version. Sensitivity is higher in the parent-report form [56]. Self-report and parent-report versions of the revised Children's Obsessive-Compulsive Inventory (CHOCI-R) have good internal consistency, criterion validity, and convergent validity and are strongly related to each other [57]. With 14 symptom items and 6 severity items, the CHOCI is a relatively quick, but not exhaustive, measure. It is better at discriminating at the mild–moderate end of OCD in children, while the CY-BOCS discriminates better at the severe end of the disorder [57].

Neuropsychological Assessment

Motor behavior, cognitive functions, and inhibitory control are essentially normal in TS [32]. Tasks testing for manual dexterity (Purdue pegboard test) and visuomotor integration (Beery visual-motor integration test) have shown abnormalities in TS [58]. Children with uncomplicated TS exhibit enhanced cognitive control in tasks of response inhibition, such as oculomotor switching tasks, probably because tic suppression improves inhibitory control over time [59]. However, coexisting ADHD has a negative impact on cognitive performance [60]. The neuropsychological profile of coexisting TS and OCD has not been well established. However, executive function deficits have been documented in response inhibition [61] and set shifting paradigms [62]. Clinical neuropsychological assessment should be tailored to clinical needs.

Prevalence and Course

TS is 3:1 (USA) to 4.3:1 (UK) times more likely to occur in males than in females [63, 64]. It is a common disorder with a prevalence of approximately 0.3–1 % depending on the population investigated and the measures used [63–65]. Estimations of prevalence rates vary widely, due to changing definitions of TS, waxing and waning of tics, the ability to suppress tics, the decrease of tic severity over time in most affected individuals, and possibly the masking effects of comorbidities [66]. The 2007 US National Survey of Children's Health has estimated a lifetime prevalence of 0.3 % by parent report [64]. Estimates based on epidemiological studies in the UK suggest a prevalence of tic disorders in the range of 3.4–24.4 % and of TS between 0.4 and 3.8 % in children and adolescents aged 5–18 [63]. The overall international lifetime prevalence of TS is estimated to be approximately 1 % [19, 63]. TS seems to occur less frequently in Hispanics, African-Americans, and sub-Saharan black Africans [63]. Data concerning the administrative 12-month prevalence in a sample of 2.2 million individuals in Germany found a prevalence of 0.8 % for all tic disorders, indicating that TS might generally be underdiagnosed and undertreated [65]. Because most parents do not correctly classify tics as a neurological symptom, the average time until TS is diagnosed (if at all) is at least 5 years and is often followed by great relief on part of the patient [67].

The first tics typically occur around the age of 5–7 years, with vocal tics developing several months to years later [19]. Prevalence rates are highest around the age of 10 and then decrease markedly after the age of 12 [19, 65]. This probably reflects the finding that most patients experience their most severe symptoms at age 8–12 and then seek medical advice [68]. Clinical and epidemiological studies indicate that 59–85 % of patients with tic disorders are tic-free or only have mild tics upon entering adulthood [69, 70]. In the remaining 20 %, the symptoms continue or become even more pronounced after the age of 18 and often have a debilitating effect on work and social life [70]. Predictors of a worse long-term outcome include higher tic severity in childhood, smaller caudate volume, poorer fine motor skills, and untreated comorbidities [69].

Etiology

Genetic Factors

A number of findings point towards a prominent role of genetic factors, but the precise background is complex, probably polygenetic and largely unclear [71]. Family studies showed that TS and tics are 10–100 times more likely to develop in individuals who have a first-degree relative with TS [72]. TS patients are more likely than healthy controls to have first-degree family members with TS, chronic tics, and early-onset OCD, irrespective of whether patients have OC symptoms or not [72]. Interestingly, OCD is more likely to occur in female relatives, while TS is more likely to occur in male relatives. Moreover, OCD patients are more likely than healthy controls to have a family history of tics indicating that some forms of OCD and TS may share genetic influences. However, the genetic architecture (number, frequency, and distribution of genetic risk factors) of the two disorders has not been decoded, probably because there are many different genetic variations associated with an elevated risk for developing TS and OCD [73]. Recent data suggest a heritability point estimate of 0.58 for TS and 0.37 for OCD. Rare alleles (frequency <5 %) explained 21 % of the variance of TS heritability but 0 % in OCD heritability. The genetic correlation between TS and OCD was 41, confirming that there is some genetic overlap between the two disorders but that they might have distinct genetic architectures [74]. Although the DA neurotransmitter system appears to play a pivotal role in TS, no consistent association has been found between TS and DA candidate genes [75].

ADHD is also more common in family members of TS patients but is mostly accompanied by tics; hence, they may share some etiological basis but are not likely to be two phenotypical variants of the same genotype [73]. Large European and American genome studies are currently under way to identify genetic polymorphisms associated with TS (see TIC Genetics: https://tic-genetics.org).

Environmental Factors

By analogy to Sydenham's chorea, Swedo et al. suggested that tics and OCD may be sequelae of a preceding streptococcal infection [76, 77]. The acronym PANDAS (pediatric autoimmune neuropsychiatric disorder associated with streptococcal infection) was suggested for a TS-like syndrome with sudden onset following streptococcal infections and a monophasic rather than undulating course. However, a causal relationship between preceding streptococcal infections and clinical symptoms has not been proven yet. In addition, the fact that some children diagnosed with PANDAS also have chorea on clinical examination raises the question of whether at least some of these children suffer from Sydenham's chorea rather than PANDAS. The role of infections and inflammatory processes in general as etiological factors in TS is currently unclear. A collaborative research project, the "European

Multicentre Tics in Children Studies (EMTICS)," funded by the European Union (7th framework programme; HEALTH.2011.2.2.1–3), addressing these issues, is currently under way.

Severe nausea of the mother in the first trimester, severe maternal psychological stress during pregnancy, and maternal consumption of more than two cups of coffee per day or more than ten cigarettes per day during pregnancy have been suggested as possible epigenetic risk factors [78]. Birth-related risk factors encompass an identical twin with lower birth weight, low birth weight with ischemic parenchymal brain lesions or enlargement of the ventricles, transient perinatal hypoxia or ischemia, and low Apgar scores shortly after birth [78, 79].

The fact that the prevalence in men is higher than in women led to the assumption that androgenic hormones may play a role during certain stages of development. Moreover, in some TS patients symptoms may be caused or exacerbated by a heightened sensitivity of the hypothalamic-pituitary-adrenal axis and thereby the noradrenergic sympathetic systems [78]. However, with the exception of birth weight and maternal smoking, the association between the factors listed above and the development of TS is weak and inconsistent [79]. Motor tics, vocal tics, depression, and anxiety in children and adolescents with TS are correlated with the number of minor negative life events (e.g., relations with family/peers, school achievements), whereas the severity of compulsions, aggression, and ADHD symptoms is correlated with the subjective evaluation of major negative life events (e.g., divorce of parents) [80].

Pathophysiology

Abnormalities in the Basal Ganglia

TS has been repeatedly associated with structural and functional changes in the BG, the thalamus, and the frontal cortex, which are implicated in the formation of habits. Habits, like tics, are stimulus-driven actions that are not outcome dependent and do not require specific attention. They are also repetitive and change over time; hence, some authors have drawn parallels between these two motor phenomena and their neural substrates with a predominant focus on the BG [81, 82]. The BG consist of several nuclei that play an important role in action selection, implementation of learned motor and cognitive sequences, and performance monitoring in goal-directed behavior. The striatum (caudate and putamen) receives the majority of its input from the cortex and the intralaminar nuclei of the thalamus and projects back to the cortex in a feedback circle that has been termed the cortico-striatal-thalamo-cortical (CSTC) loop [83].

The CSTC loops are at least partially segregated into sensorimotor, associative, and limbic loops [84]. Dysfunction of the sensorimotor loop has been associated with the development of tics, while more complex behavioral disorders might be related to dysfunctions in the associative and limbic loops [85, 86]. Neurochemically, the striatum can be divided into two parts. The matrix consists of matrisomes and receives its input from sensorimotor areas. The striosomes receive their input from the orbitofrontal cortex (OFC), the cingulum, and the insula and are therefore part of the limbic-associative loop [87]. The neuronal population in both areas can be subdivided into 95 % medium spiny neurons (MSN), which mainly project to the globus pallidus internus (Gpi) both directly and indirectly via the globus pallidus externus (GPe) and the subthalamic nucleus, 3 % GABAergic (GABA, γ-aminobutyric acid) and 2 % cholinergic tonically firing inhibitory interneurons [87]. These inhibitory interneurons partly coordinate the activity of the MSNs throughout the striatum and thereby its output. The BG function as a break on the motor system. If inhibitory neurons, which project from the BG to the motor parts of the thalamus, increase their firing rates, motor activity will be more focused. If, on the other hand, these inhibitory neurons decrease their firing rate, more widespread motor output will be facilitated [88].

Neuropathological studies of TS have found a decreased number, as well as an abnormal distribution, of cholinergic and GABAergic inhibitory interneurons in the sensorimotor and associative areas of the striatum as compared to healthy controls [89, 90]. There seems to be an imbalance of parvalbumin-positive GABAergic interneurons with a decrease in number and density of neurons in the GPe and an increase in the GPi [89], which points to a disrupted inhibitory-excitatory balance between sensorimotor, associative, and limbic loops [90]. These alterations may foster the development of context-independent extra movements including tics. The imbalance in the BG may be caused by genetically determined aberrant neuronal migration of interneurons from the precursor of the GP to the precursor of the striatum, the cortex, and the hippocampus during embryogenesis [89].

These findings have been further corroborated by a multitude of studies employing a wide variety of research techniques. Single cell research shows that activity patterns of the MSNs and cholinergic interneurons in the putamen and GPi are correlated with tics and stimulation of the putamen can cause tic-like stereotypies in animals as well as humans (for review, please see [82]). Imaging techniques showed an abnormally high connectivity within the CSTC loops in TS patients. Changes in connectivity in the sensorimotor and associative loops were correlated with the occurrence of complex tics, while changes in the limbic and associative loops were correlated with OC symptoms [91]. Comparing tics to self-paced movements revealed increased activations in the somatosensory and premotor cortex, putamen, amygdala and hippocampus, correlating positively with tic severity and decreased activations in the caudate nucleus and anterior cingulate cortex correlating negatively with tic severity [92].

Structural and Functional Changes in Other Brain Areas

Differences in structure and function between healthy individuals and TS patients are subject to change during development [93, 94]. Resting state studies have revealed brain connectivity patterns in TS reminiscent of earlier stages of development, i.e., overall activity in adjacent areas was more strongly correlated, whereas activity between distant areas showed lower correlations resembling correlational patterns previously found in younger healthy children, as well as adolescents with autism and ADHD [95]. Volumetric MRI showed a reduction in caudate size in children and adults with TS, whereas volumes of the amygdala, hippocampus, and thalamus were increased in children [96]. In adults, amygdala and hippocampus volumes were decreased and inversely correlated with tic severity, OC symptoms, and ADHD symptoms [93]. Diffusivity weights in children and adults with TS were altered in the BG, thalamus, nucleus accumbens, and amygdala [97, 98]. However, a study with male adolescents without comorbidities, who had never been treated pharmacologically, showed no differences in brain volume as compared to healthy controls [99]. Thus, it is largely unclear whether and to what extent differences between TS patients and healthy controls are cause or consequence of TS, OCD, and ADHD; represent adaptive changes to these disorders; or are secondary to medication.

The areas most reliably found to be thinner in cortical thickness studies in TS than in healthy controls are motor and sensory cortices in children and adolescents. Moreover, in adolescents with TS thickness was inversely correlated with worst-ever tic severity [100]. Other areas showing cortical thinning include the right dorsolateral prefrontal cortex (PFC), entorhinal cortex, OFC, parietal cortex, and cingulate cortex. Thinning of these areas may reduce inhibitory control and cause aberrant sensorimotor gating, as well as an elevated vulnerability to coexisting OCD or depression [81, 82].

Diffusion-tensor imaging (DTI) corroborates existing evidence of abnormalities in the sensorimotor cortices, showing white matter changes in motor and somatosensory circuits and fronto-striatal areas [101, 102] White matter changes have also been found in interhemispheric and transcallosal connections and were associated with interhemispheric disinhibition [103], as well as tic severity [104]. Reduced inhibition at rest has also been demonstrated by transcranial magnetic stimulation (TMS) studies [105, 106] but inhibition was normalized during movement preparation possibly because activation in subcortical regions is biased by prefrontal structures during goal-directed behavior [107].

Although TS is commonly associated with disinhibition, several studies have shown that tic severity was associated with enhanced cognitive control as well as structural changes in the PFC [59, 108]. The PFC might serve to bias response competition in motor areas rather than exert inhibitory control over other brain areas and may be hyperactive in TS patients. This hyperactivity may be compensated for in adolescence by structural and functional changes in the long-range neural pathways that link the PFC to motor areas [109]. A recent DTI study in 19 unmedicated, uncomplicated male, adult TS patients confirmed this assumption, indicating that tics might be caused by changes in PFC, thalamus, and putamen. Changes in the cingulate gyrus, however, appear to be the result of compensatory changes [110]. Moreover, volumetric changes in the PFC do not appear to be related to the ability to suppress tics [111].

Structural and Functional Brain Changes Associated with Urges

One important feature distinguishing tics from habits is the experience of premonitory urges. These are difficult to investigate though because they are subjective experiences. Some researchers suggest that premonitory urges may develop on the basis of sensorimotor and primary motor cortical inputs converging on the MSNs in the striatum [78]. Studies investigating brain activity associated with premonitory urges have yielded mixed results. Tic suppression causes activation changes in a number of brain regions including cortical areas (PFC, primary sensorimotor, temporal, parietal, and cingulate) and subcortical areas (caudate nucleus, putamen, and thalamus) [112]. Activations in the somatosensory cortices, putamen, amygdala, and hippocampus were found in another study prior to tic onset, probably reflecting the intense sensory and emotional experience of premonitory urges [92]. Moreover, the extent of experienced premonitory urges correlates positively with thickness of the primary somatosensory cortex [113]. Overall, the most consistent area associated with sensory urges so far has been the supplementary motor area (SMA) [82]. Accordingly, repetitive TMS applied over the SMA but not the primary motor or premotor cortex led to tic reduction in a pilot study [114]. Maia and Frank (2011) suggested that motor tics might initially occur coincidentally together with certain (sensorimotor) states because the likelihood of an excitatory signal relative to an inhibitory signal in the BG is overall higher in TS. Every time a movement was coupled with a certain state, a set of motor plans would also be activated in the SMA and would, via Hebbian learning mechanisms, become linked to the state over time. After a few pairings of state, SMA motor plan and BG gated action, the state would automatically cause the activation of a motor plan in the SMA, thereby producing an urge to move [115].

In conclusion, TS brains differ from healthy brains in many cortical and subcortical regions, including areas associated with motor, behavioral, emotional, and executive control, as well as memory. Well-designed, large-sample longitudinal studies, controlling for comorbidities, will be necessary to disentangle which structural and functional changes are at the heart of the disorder and which are a consequence of having lived with TS for some time.

Dopamine

Among the neurotransmitter systems that are likely implicated in TS (dopamine (DA), serotonin, noradrenaline, glutamate, GABA, acetylcholine, and opioids), DA seems to be the key player. Interactions between the systems, especially DA and serotonin, may be crucial for the development of TS but have not yet received enough attention. Results from different lines of research suggest DA imbalance/ hyperactivity in TS. For instance, DA is highly active in PFC and striatum; both areas were most commonly found to be structurally and functionally altered in

TS. Direct evidence for the role of DA comes from successful pharmacological treatment of TS. While D2 DA receptor blockers (e.g., haloperidol) and DA reuptake inhibitors (e.g., tetrabenazine) improve tics, L-dopa and central nervous system stimulants such as cocaine can lead to tic exacerbation.

Precise delineation of abnormalities of dopaminergic neurotransmission in TS is difficult. First of all, DA levels in humans can only be measured indirectly. Secondly, any difference in the DA system in TS could be either the cause or the consequence of the disorder; cross-sectional data do not provide any information about causal effects. Thirdly, DA phasic and tonic levels as well as receptor density are regulated by complex feedback mechanisms. Therefore, most findings could be caused by a number of different factors. Phasic DA is released as the result of action potentials, i.e., spike dependent. Tonic DA levels represent relatively stable extracellular DA levels and depend on the diffusion rate and on DA transporters, pumping DA from the synaptic cleft back into the presynaptic neuron after an action potential occurred or releasing DA from neurons if required. Tonic DA levels stimulate autoreceptors of the presynaptic neuron, thereby regulating DA reuptake and amounts of phasic DA release. The density of D2 receptors is also regulated based on available extracellular DA concentration. Any of these factors could be altered and compensated for in TS [116]. A clear picture of whether TS symptoms are due to DA hyperinnervation, supersensitive DA receptors, presynaptic DA abnormalities, or DA tonic-phasic dysfunction, or a combination of these factors, is only starting to emerge [75, 81].

The DA hyperinnervation hypothesis postulates excessive innervation by DA terminals particularly in the striatum of TS patients. Increased DA transporter binding in the striatum in vivo and in postmortem tissue supports the notion of hyperinnervation by DA terminals. Contradictory null results in studies investigating vesicular monoamine binding, and mixed results from SPECT studies, however, suggest that the theory is not straightforward [75].

Regarding the supersensitivity of DA receptors, postmortem studies have found increased numbers of D2 receptors in the PFC of TS patients [117]. PET and SPECT studies found heightened D2 density in the caudate and left ventral striatum [118, 119], while a study investigating medication-naive TS patients found no difference [120]. Even decreased D2 binding has been reported for a number of extrastriatal regions [121].

Neuroimaging studies in humans have found increased DA transporter binding in the neostriatum and increased DA activity in the ventral striatum, increased numbers of striatal and cortical DA receptors, different binding properties in the BG, and a release of DA in TS patients after receiving a stimulant exceeding healthy controls by at least 90 % [118, 122, 123].

The most popular model is based on the tonic-phasic release of DA. Decreased tonic levels of DA in TS may lead to an increase in phasic DA release. It should also be pointed out that the brain is a homeostatic system and may adapt to dopaminergic medication over time [116]. Apart from possible side effects, this is another factor to consider and to communicate to patients when initiating treatment with antipsychotics.

To summarize, although DA appears to play an important role in the pathophysiology of TS, there is still a lot to be learned about which mechanisms are disrupted and how they interact with other neurotransmitter systems. Further insight may be gained by investigating more homogeneous samples in terms of age, TS with and without comorbidities, and medication intake.

Treatment

General Measures

Treatment should be tailored to the needs of an individual patient following thorough clinical assessment (see Fig. 11.1). Explaining the neurological background, possible comorbidities, the waxing and waning nature and the natural course of tics and TS, and its association with stress to patients and their families is the mainstay of management. Children with tics are often told to stop their tics and "behave." Therefore, communicating that tics are automatic and represent neurobiological and not psychological phenomena helps to decrease tension in families or at school. Similarly, counseling of teachers is important. A long-term relationship with a TS expert is helpful to support patients and families through the years.

TS cannot be cured. However, tic frequency and severity can be treated to a certain degree, and comorbid disorders such as OCD, ADHD, and depression can and should be treated to facilitate psychosocial functioning and support development in patients [6]. Until 2011, the only country providing explicit guidelines for the diagnosis and treatment of TS was Germany. On the basis of these, experts of the European Society for the Study of Tourette Syndrome (ESSTS) then developed the first European guidelines for the diagnosis and treatment of TS [6, 124–126]. TS can be treated with antidopaminergic medication, other drugs, THC [127], or deep brain stimulation [126]. Habit reversal therapy (HRT) has also been suggested as an option [128].

Two things should be taken into consideration before deciding on a treatment strategy. Firstly, subjective impairment does not correspond with tic severity and should be assessed independently. Secondly, for many children and adolescents, TS does not interfere with daily life. Therefore, not every tic needs to be treated.

Treatment is recommended predominantly in the following circumstances [6]. Tics are so severe that they cause pain or injuries. Pain can arise from repetitive brisk neck or limb tics leading to musculoskeletal pain. In severe cases, tics can damage joints or result in compressive myelopathy. Pain may also result directly from striking or being struck by body parts or self-injurious behavior. Some patients experience relief from tics by self-inflicted pain. Few patients report that they experience pain during tic suppression. Tics can also worsen pain such as headaches.

Tics can raise social problems such as bullying, cause stigmatization, withdrawal, depression, and anxiety, which may not be overcome by psychoeducation and counseling of patients, families, and peers alone. Salient motor and vocal tics, especially coprolalia, can cause social friction; hence, children with TS experience more social and educational problems than healthy controls. Comorbidities can additionally aggravate these problems [129].

Pharmacological Treatment of TS

The most commonly used drugs in TS are antipsychotics, also known as neuroleptics [130]. Neuroleptics unfold their effect by blocking D2 DA receptors. Surprisingly, there are few well-conducted, double-blind, randomized controlled trials (RTC) investigating the efficacy and safety of pharmacological treatment in TS. There are two Cochrane reviews on pharmacological treatment in TS, one on the effects of cannabinoids and one on the pharmacological treatment of children with ADHD and comorbid tics. Cochrane reviews are systematic reviews that only select studies with the highest standards (randomized, placebo-controlled, double-blind). It is difficult to make recommendations based solely on the Cochrane reviews. Therefore, the authors of the European clinical guidelines for TS and other tic disorders conducted a full review of all pharmacological studies from 1979 to 2010, regardless of their quality. Their results will be summarized in the following sections (for a full review and original publications, please see [124].

Typical Antipsychotics

Haloperidol and pimozide are D2 DA receptor antagonists.
Efficacy: Pimozide and haloperidol are the most thoroughly studied antipsychotics for tic treatment and show the most consistent effects of all drugs tested. Most studies have found that both haloperidol and pimozide significantly reduce tic severity. However, haloperidol seems to consistently lead to more side effects than pimozide.

According to the Cochrane reviews, haloperidol reduces tics significantly compared to placebo. Pimozide and risperidone were less effective than haloperidol but more effective than a placebo and had fewer side effects than haloperidol [131]. A more recent meta-analysis of five high-quality RCTs testing antipsychotics (risperidone, pimozide, haloperidol, and ziprazidone) and alpha-2 agonists (adrenergic stimulants) showed that antipsychotics reduced tic severity significantly as compared to a placebo group, irrespective of the type of antipsychotic [132]. Overall, pimozide causes fewer side effects than haloperidol, especially long term. Whereas pimozide is sometimes used and recommended by TS experts, haloperidol is only very rarely used in TS specialty clinics, predominantly because of its untoward side effects.

Side effects (of D2 blockers): drowsiness, sedation, headaches, acute dystonic reaction, akathisia, parkinsonism, anxiety, hyperprolactinemia, gynecomastia, galactorrhea, irregular menses, sexual dysfunction, and significant weight gain. A combination of pimozide with macrolides and sertraline can lead to fatal QTc prolongation.

Therefore, regular ECG is recommended. Additionally, a few case reports have drawn attention to the risk of inducing tardive dyskinesia. However, this is a contentious issue. A recent systematic review found no evidence for tardive phenomena in TS [133].

Recommended dose: Dosages used in studies range from 2 to 20 mg/day for haloperidol and from 2 to 20 mg/day for pimozide. For clinical use, however, recommended doses that are typically prescribed in TS start at 0.5 mg/day. Recommended average doses for adults taking haloperidol range between 1 and 10 mg/day, with a recommended maximum between 10 and 15 mg/day. For pimozide, the recommended average dose is up to 2–8 mg/day, with a recommended maximum of 8–12 mg/day [33, 134] (for details see Table 11.2).

Fluphenazine is a D2 DA receptor antagonist, mainly used in the USA.

Efficacy: It has been shown to be effective short term and long term. In addition, it appears to cause fewer side effects than haloperidol. However, study samples were too small to draw general conclusions from these findings [124].

Recommended dose: Initial doses should range from 0.5 to 1 mg/day; treatment doses should eventually range from 1.5 to 10 mg/day [33] (see Table 11.2).

Table 11.2 Recommended doses of medications [134]

Medication					
Drug	Initial dose (mg)	Average recommended dose for adults	Recommended maximum dose (mg)	Maximum approved dose (mg)	Intake
Typical antipsychotics					
Haloperidol	0.5	1–10	10–20	100	2–3×/day
Pimozide	0.5–1	2–8	8–12	16	1×/day in the evening
Fluphenazine	0.5–1	1.5–10			
Benzamides					
Tiapride	50–100	150–600	600–800	1200	2–3×/day
Sulpiride	50–100		800–1200	1600	2×/day
Atypical antipsychotics					
Risperidone	0.5–1	1–8	4–8	16	2×/day
Ziprazidone	5–10	10–80			
Aripiprazole	2.5		10–30	30	1×/day
Noradrenergic agents					
Clonidine	0.025–0.05	0.1–0.15			
Guanfacine	0.5	0.5–1	1–4		1×/day at bedtime
Tetrabenazine	12.5		75	200	3×/day
Tetrahydrocannabinol	2.5		20–30		2–3×/day

Adapted with permission from Ludolph et al. [134]

Benzamides

Tiapride is a D2 DA receptor antagonist with very low antipsychotic action. Tiapride is also assumed to bind to serotonergic 5HT3 and 5HT4 receptors.

Efficacy: The positive effects of tiapride on tic severity have been investigated in at least eight studies. All suggested that the drug reduces tics significantly. It has to be taken into account though that most of the studies were not placebo-controlled, only one was double-blind, and the sample sizes were small [124].

Side effects: limited; drowsiness, moderate transient hyperprolactinemia, and weight gain. Tiapride did not affect cognitive performance, neurosecretory, hypothalamic-hypophyseal regulation of the sex hormones, thyroid-stimulating hormone, growth hormone, or thyroid hormone [124].

Recommended dose: For adults, the recommended target dose of tiapride is 150–600 mg/day, starting from 50 to 100 mg/day with a recommended maximum of 600–800 mg/day. For children, doses up to 300 mg/day are typically used [33, 134] (see Table 11.2).

Tiapride is a useful and generally well-tolerated treatment for tics; however, more placebo-controlled, double-blind studies in larger samples preferably with longer follow-up are needed to judge its effects more reliably.

Sulpiride is a D2 DA antagonist. It is a weak antipsychotic and, in low dosages (50–200 mg/day), weak antidepressant, stimulating, and anxiolytic drug.

Efficacy: Sulpiride significantly reduced tics in children, adolescents, and adults [135, 136]. A double-blind, placebo-controlled crossover trial in 11 patients with TS and comorbid OCD showed that sulpiride reduces tics but not OC symptoms and that fluvoxamine alone or in combination with sulpiride alleviates OC symptoms but not tics. However, although the study was well designed, only 11 patients were included limiting its power [137].

Side effects: sedation/drowsiness; often increased appetite leading to weight gain, galactorrhea/amenorrhea, restlessness, sleep disturbances, and rarely depression. Adverse reactions such as hypotension, long-QT syndrome, dry mouth, sweating, nausea, allergic rash, or pruritus are less common, and tardive dyskinesia has only been reported in one case [124].

Recommended dose: Initial doses of sulpiride range from 50 to 100 mg/day; the maximum treatment dose should not exceed 800–1200 mg/day (see Table 11.2).

Overall, D2 DA antagonists appear to reduce tics in approximately 70 % of patients. However, the disadvantages of a treatment with D2 blockers, particularly at higher doses, are potentially severe side effects [124].

Atypical Antipsychotics

Risperidone is a predominant DA antagonist (D2) but also has antiserotonergic (5-HT2) effects.

Efficacy: Several studies and case reports in patients ranging from 6 to 62 years of age suggest that the efficacy of risperidone in TS is comparable to that of haloperidol and pimozide. However, severe side effects seem to be less common [124]. Risperidone appears to be as effective as clonidine and pimozide in reducing tics, but risperidone also reduces OC symptoms [130, 138]. Risperidone may also help to treat aggressive behavior in TS.

Side effects: depressive symptoms, fatigue, somnolence, and extrapyramidal symptoms (possibly fewer than in pimozide). Although side effects seem to occur less frequently with risperidone, depression can occur [124].

Recommended dose: Risperidone can be administered in doses starting from 0.5 to 1 mg/day, with recommended average treatment doses between 1 and 8 mg/day [134] (see Table 11.2).

Clozapine cannot be recommended for treatment of TS. It can lead to increased tic severity and has potentially severe side effects [124].

Ziprazidone mainly acts as an antagonist to a variety of serotonin and DA receptors.

Efficacy: It has only been tested in one double-blind RCT and in an open-label study and reduced tics significantly compared to a placebo group [124].

Side effects: The most common adverse reaction at low doses (5–20 mg/day) was somnolence. None of the patients experienced weight gain, extrapyramidal symptoms, akathisia, tardive dyskinesia, or QT prolongation. Laboratory parameters were normal, except for prolactin. These are promising results, especially with regard to side effects. However, studies on higher doses and long-term intake of ziprazidone will be needed to determine its effects in more detail [124].

Recommended dose: Initial doses range from 5 to 10 mg/day; recommended target doses vary between 10 and 80 mg/day [33] (see Table 11.2).

Aripiprazole acts as a partial D2 DA receptor agonist, a partial agonist at 5-HT1A receptors, and as an antagonist at 5-HT2A receptors.

Efficacy: Aripiprazole has been described as effective in reducing tics in more than 200 cases. Four studies found aripiprazole unequivocally efficacious in reducing tics. Case reports suggest that aripiprazole might be a promising drug, even in TS patients who have not responded to previous pharmacological treatment. However, none of the studies was blinded or included a placebo group [124].

Side effects: weight gain, akathisia, sedation, and nausea.

Recommended dose: Aripiprazole is typically administered from 2.5 mg/day initially to 10–30 mg/day as clinically useful doses in adults [134] (see Table 11.2).

Noradrenergic Agents

Noradrenergic drugs include clonidine, guanfacine, and atomoxetine. They are most commonly used in children and adolescents with ADHD and comorbid tics. They are not as effective as antipsychotics in reducing tics.

Clonidine is an alpha-2 adrenergic drug and is used more often in the USA than in Europe.

Efficacy: The number of studies that have found a significant effect of clonidine about equals the number of studies that have not. However, a large multicenter, randomized, double-blind placebo-controlled study investigating 136 children with ADHD and comorbid chronic tic disorder showed that clonidine reduced ADHD symptoms and tic severity and was well tolerated with the exception of 28 % of patients who experienced moderate to severe sedation [139]. A randomized, double-blind, placebo-controlled multicenter study investigating a very large sample showed a significant reduction of tic severity in children and adolescents [140].

Side effects: sedation, dry mouth, headache, irritability, hypotension, and disturbed sleep. Blood pressure, heart rate, and symptoms suggestive of cardiovascular problems should be monitored during dose adjustments. Some practice guidelines specifically recommend follow-up electrocardiograms. Abrupt discontinuation can cause rebound hypertension, tics, and anxiety. There is some disagreement in the field as to the overall severity of side effects, especially with higher dosages [124].

Recommended dose: Clonidine should be started at approximately 0.025 mg/day and gradually increased until a dose of 0.1–0.15 mg/day is reached [33] (see Table 11.2).

Guanfacine is an α-2 adrenergic agonist.

Efficacy: It reduces tics and ADHD symptoms in children, but effects are small. However, its efficacy and usefulness in clinical practice remains somewhat unclear, as evidence is contradictory.

Side effects: somnolence, headache, fatigue, sedation, dizziness, irritability, upper abdominal pain, and nausea, which typically occur within the first 2 weeks of intake and then remit. Guanfacine can cause mania in susceptible children with a personal or family history of bipolar disorder. Furthermore, guanfacine can induce syncopes possibly because it can cause hypotension or bradycardia [124].

Recommended dose: Guanfacine is typically administered from 0.5 to 4 mg/day (see Table 11.2).

Atomoxetine is a selective noradrenaline reuptake inhibitor.

Efficacy: Atomoxetine has been shown to successfully reduce ADHD symptoms and tics in comorbid TS in children [141]. However, a number of case studies have reported new onset or recurrence of tics or an increase in tic severity in children treated with atomoxetine. One problem with atomoxetine is delay of onset of action, requiring 2–4 weeks of therapy before optimal therapeutic responses are achieved. Also, combination treatment with selective serotonin reuptake inhibitors must be approached very cautiously. For now, atomoxetine's effect on tics is unclear. Further studies are needed.

Side effects: increase of mean heart rate, nausea, decreased appetite, and decreased body weight [124].

Other Drugs

Tetrabenazine is a vesicular monoamine transporter type 2 antagonist. It depletes presynaptic DA and serotonin stores and blocks postsynaptic DA receptors.

Efficacy: A retrospective chart review of 77 TS patients showed a moderate to high reduction in TS symptoms in more than 80 % of patients [142].

Side effects: drowsiness/fatigue, nausea, depression, insomnia, akathisia/parkinsonism, and weight gain, but less than typically found in patients that are treated with antipsychotics. Side effects improved with lower doses. No study has reported tardive dystonia or other serious adverse reactions yet [124].

Recommended dose: Tetrabenazine is usually started at a dose of 12.5 mg/day up to 75 mg/day as an average treatment dose (see Table 11.2).

Clonazepam, a benzodiazepine, is a GABA-A receptor agonist.

Efficacy: Several studies have shown clonazepam to be effective and possibly more effective than clonidine in children. However, study samples were relatively small and no well-designed RCTs have been conducted yet.

Side effects: sedation, short-term memory problems, ataxia, paradoxic disinhibition, and dependency [124].

Because of sedation and the risk of dependency, clonazepam is not recommended as a tic treatment.

Baclofen is a GABA-B receptor agonist.

Efficacy: Baclofen reduced tics significantly in a large sample of children with TS. However, the results of a small double-blind RCT remain inconclusive [143]; hence, more evidence is needed in order to determine whether baclofen is a useful treatment for TS or not.

Side effects: sedation and drowsiness [124].

Baclofen is currently not recommended for treatment of tics.

Levetiracetam is a GABAergic drug and currently mainly used as an anticonvulsant.

Efficacy: Levetiracetam is most likely not effective as a treatment for TS [144].

Naloxone is an opioid receptor antagonist.

Efficacy: It ameliorated tics significantly in a small double-blind RCT of ten adult patients and single cases. However, doses have to be handled with care since lower doses seem to cause a decrease but higher doses may cause an increase in tics [145].

Naloxone is currently not recommended for the treatment of tics.

Nicotine can be administered as a chewing gum or a transdermal patch, and both can potentiate the effects of antipsychotic drugs, even in poor responders.

Efficacy: Randomized, double-blind placebo-controlled trials show that given together with antipsychotic agents over a timespan of approximately 2 weeks, nicotine further reduced tic severity and improved attention in adults and children/adolescents [146, 147].

Side effects: adverse gastrointestinal reactions, nausea, vomiting, and less frequently headache and sedation [124].

Nicotine is currently not recommended for the treatment of tics.

THC: Based on anecdotal evidence suggesting that consuming marijuana can attenuate symptoms in TS patients, several studies systematically investigated the effects of THC in TS and found that it alleviates symptoms without affecting cognitive performance [127]. A Cochrane review on the effectiveness of delta 9-THC reported that the effects on tic frequency and severity were small but significant [148].

Side effects: Dizziness, tiredness, and dry mouth.

Recommended dose: Up to 20–30 mg/day.

Botulinum Toxin

Local injections can be used to treat well-localized, simple motor, and vocal tics in adults and children from the age of 8. In addition to reducing tics, the treatment sometimes also reduces premonitory urges. It should be noted that the average time to response is approximately 6 days with an average response duration of about 3 months. There is good evidence that standardized treatment is objectively effective [149], but there is only a weak relation between such objective tic reduction and subjective improvement. The latter can often be achieved through individually tailored injection protocols [150]. Patients sometimes report that the treated tic "moved" to a different body region.

Side effects: temporary soreness, mild muscle weakness, and hypophonia (common in vocal tic treatment) [124].

Overall Recommendations for Pharmacological Treatment of TS

Among TS specialists, tiapride and aripiprazole are currently considered the most useful drugs for the treatment of both children and adults with TS followed by sulpiride and risperidone. Pimozide is an option in severely affected patients but has more side effects than the aforementioned drugs. In particular, QT prolongation has to be monitored. Tetrabenazine is an alternative that can be very helpful in some patients. The main limitation of this drug though is depression occurring in a considerable proportion of patients. Noradrenergic drugs including clonidine, guanfacine, and atomoxetine can be useful, particularly in children with comorbid ADHD, but their anti-tic potency is relatively weak. Although currently the only drug licensed for the treatment of TS, haloperidol is only very rarely prescribed in clinical practice. It is effective but has many side effects and is often not well tolerated. THC is a choice when other drugs have failed; it is sometimes very useful. The effectiveness of *ziprazidone is questionable. Fluphenazine, clozapine, clonazepam, baclofen, levetiracetam,* and *naloxone are not recommended. Also, nicotine is currently considered an experimental drug only.*

Behavioral Therapy

The predominant behavioral therapy for tics is the Comprehensive Behavioral Intervention for Tics. This approach combines HRT with function-based interventions that target daily life events, which typically increase tic severity. TS patients are taught to pay early attention to premonitory urges (awareness training) and use them to suppress tics by performing a competing motor response, a response that is physically incompatible with the targeted tic. Additional therapeutic elements consist of self-monitoring, relaxation training, contingency management, motivational procedures, and generalization training [151]. Exposure and response prevention interventions expose patients to the urge to tic while keeping the patient from performing the tic, to achieve habituation to the urge.

A recent meta-analysis of eight studies comprising 438 patients suggested that behavioral therapies have a significant effect over comparison conditions, which was comparable to the effect sizes found in pharmacological treatment studies [151]. Larger treatment effects were found in older patients, patients who received more therapy sessions, and patients with fewer ADHD symptoms [151]. Furthermore, an overview over five studies investigating HRT indicated that it might be more effective than a control treatment. However, one study showed that 10 months after treatment, there was no difference between treatment and control group, and another study even showed that 6 months post-treatment, the placebo group had experienced greater improvement (57.7 %) than the HRT group (46.2 %), yet the high dropout rate in this study does not allow any firm conclusions [128]. Although it has been repeatedly proposed that HRT constitutes an effective therapeutic approach, high-quality longitudinal data on the long-term effects of HRT are still lacking. Most studies suffer from small sample sizes, high dropout rates, raters not blinded to the conditions, inclusion in follow-up studies only of patients who responded positively to the treatment, and comparison of the treatment group to itself at baseline. Given the natural course of tics, it is necessary to include a control group into longitudinal designs.

Deep Brain Stimulation

Deep brain stimulation (DBS) has been introduced as an alternative treatment option for patients suffering from severe treatment refractory TS about 10 years ago. Case reports and small, uncontrolled trials suggest some efficacy of DBS, particularly of the intralaminar nuclei of the thalamus and the GPi. However, optimal target location, stimulation parameters, and inclusion/exclusion criteria for surgery are still unclear. There are no RTCs including larger numbers of patients. Although persistent serious adverse effects are uncommon, surgery- and stimulation-related adverse events including sedation, anxiety, and apathy can occur. Among European TS and DBS experts, there is general agreement that, at the present time, DBS should only be used in adult, treatment-resistant, and severely affected TS patients, preferably in the context of controlled trials.

Treatment of Comorbidities

Comorbidities, most commonly ADHD and OCD, are present in the majority of TS patients and have to be taken into account when considering treatment goals, especially because comorbidities cause impairment more often than TS. Also, in many cases comorbid disorders are more responsive to treatment. It is often not necessary or recommendable to treat both tics and ADHD/OCD separately. An improvement in comorbidities can reduce stress and improve attention, thereby reducing tic severity. Coexisting TS does not necessarily change the treating algorithms for OCD and ADHD. Neither the treatment with stimulants, such as methylphenidate (MPH), nor its discontinuation appears to affect tic frequency or severity in children with TS. Only very high doses may lead to transient tic exacerbation [124].

A recent review on the most effective treatment of TS and coexisting ADHD concluded that, keeping the risk-benefit profile in mind, noradrenergic agents (clonidine) could be used as a first-line treatment. Reuptake inhibitors (atomoxetine) and stimulants (MPH) also appeared to be effective, but rigorous studies are still lacking [152]. A Cochrane review of 8 studies concluded that in comorbid TS and ADHD, MPH, clonidine, desipramine, dextroamphetamine, guanfacine, and atomoxetine reduced ADHD symptoms, while guanfacine, desipramine, MPH, clonidine, and the combination of MPH and clonidine improved tics significantly in children [153].

Patients with TS and comorbid OCD may not be as responsive to fluvoxamine as are uncomplicated OCD patients. In this case, coadministration of an antipsychotic should be considered.

Case Report

A 25-year-old patient presents to the TS specialty clinic. She reports that around the age of 8 years, her mother had first noticed increased coughing that persisted for several weeks to months without a throat infection. Since the age of 10 she had various extra movements including eye blinking, facial grimacing, raising eyebrows, eyes to the side, head and shoulder movements, and also noises including guinea pig whistling, throat clearing, and coughing. Symptoms fluctuated with good and bad periods that appeared to be season related. Movements were preceded by inner tension and an urge to move which was lessened after the movements. There was an increase of symptoms when she was tensed, stressed, or tired and a decrease during concentration. The patient also described forced touching of objects and bodies with a preference to do so three or five times because, as she said, she liked these numbers. Also, sometimes she would repeat words repeatedly (again three to five times). No echophenomena or coprophenomena were reported. As regards obsessive-compulsive symptoms, she had always had a habit to wash her hands three times in a row, but frequency of hand washing was not increased. She used to click on the glass with a teaspoon when drinking tea or coffee. No other obsessive thoughts or behaviors were reported. She never had any problems with concentration or attention. She reported good school performance. Occasionally, she is slightly irritated when asked to abstain from certain movements. There are no aggressive behaviors and no rage attacks. Past medical history is unremarkable.

The patient is currently studying economics. She is married and has a 4-year-old healthy daughter. Her father also had facial and neck tics when he was younger and still excessively blinks at times. Her mother is described as a very orderly person. She regularly spends several hours a week evening up household items in addition to keeping the house very tidy. There is no other family history of note. The patient has not tried medication yet.

On examination she is friendly, but slightly guarded and tensed with variable eye contact. She is euthymic and there is no thought disorder. She has multiple motor and phonic tics including facial grimacing, raising eyebrows, head to the side, head and shoulder movements, trunk movements, and also complex arm movements like raising the hand, putting it in front of the shoulder, throat clearing, and coughing. There are also echophenomena when facial tics were imitated by the examiner. The remainder of the neurological examination is normal.

In summary, this patient has a typical history of multiple motor and phonic tics with onset before the age of 18 and a duration of more than 1 year. Also, tics are preceded by premonitory sensations and fluctuate in a typical way so that a diagnosis of TS can be made. The patient also has palilalia, echolalia, and several "just right phenomena." There is no indication that she has comorbid OCD or ADHD, but family history is suggestive of OCD in the mother and TS in the father.

In clinics, the neurobiological basis of tics and associated phenomena is discussed and the diagnosis of TS explained. It is pointed out that currently the underlying cause of TS is unclear with genetic factors likely playing a prominent role. Given the patient's concern that her symptoms might solely be caused by stress, it is clarified that tics are no psychological phenomena. The patient wishes medical treatment. As first-line drug tiapride is recommended with an initial dose of 50 mg twice daily to be gradually increased to 100 mg three times a day if required and tolerated. As an alternative treatment, aripiprazole is suggested. The patient was given a follow-up appointment in 3 months' time.

Acknowledgments V.C. Brandt was supported by the Else Kröner-Fresenius-Stiftung

References

1. Paszek J, Pollok B, Biermann-Ruben K, Muller-Vahl K, Roessner V, Thomalla G, et al. Is it a tic?–Twenty seconds to make a diagnosis. Mov Disord. 2010;25:1106–8.
2. Jankovic J. Tourette syndrome. Phenomenology and classification of tics. Neurol Clin. 1997;15:267–75.
3. Kompoliti K, Goetz CG. Hyperkinetic movement disorders misdiagnosed as tics in Gilles de la Tourette syndrome. Mov Disord. 1998;13:477–80.
4. Kwak C, Dat Vuong K, Jankovic J. Premonitory sensory phenomenon in Tourette's syndrome. Mov Disord. 2003;18:1530–3.
5. The Tourette Syndrome Classification Study Group. Definitions and classification of tic disorders. Arch Neurol. 1993;50:1013–6.
6. Cath DC, Hedderly T, Ludolph AG, Stern JS, Murphy T, Hartmann A, et al. European clinical guidelines for Tourette syndrome and other tic disorders. Part I: assessment. Eur Child Adolesc Psychiatry. 2011;20:155–71.
7. Shapiro AK, Shapiro ES, Young JG, Feinberg TE. Gilles de la Tourette syndrome. New York: Raven Press; 1988.
8. Cath DC, Hoogduin CAL, van de Wetering BJM, van Woerkom TCAM, Roos RAC, Rooymans HGM. Tourette Syndrome and obsessive-compulsive disorder: an analysis of associated phenomena. In: Chase TN FA, Cohen DJ, editors. Advances in neurology, vol. 58. New York: Raven Press; 1992. p. 33–41.
9. Kumar R, Lang AE. Tourette syndrome. Secondary tic disorders. Neurol Clin. 1997;15:309–31.
10. de la Tourette G. GEAB. Etude sur une affection nerveuse caracterisee par le l'incoordination motrice accompagnee d'echolalie et de coprolalie. Archives de Neurol. 1985;9:158–200.
11. First MB, Pincus HA. The DSM-IV Text Revision: rationale and potential impact on clinical practice. Psychiatr Serv. 2002;53:288–92.
12. Finis J, Moczydlowski A, Pollok B, Biermann-Ruben K, Thomalla G, Heil M, et al. Echoes from childhood–imitation in Gilles de la Tourette Syndrome. Mov Disord. 2012;27:562–5.
13. Silva RR, Munoz DM, Barickman J, Friedhoff AJ. Environmental factors and related fluctuation of symptoms in children and adolescents with Tourette's disorder. J Child Psychol Psychiatry. 1995;36:305–12.
14. Lin H, Katsovich L, Ghebremichael M, Findley DB, Grantz H, Lombroso PJ, et al. Psychosocial stress predicts future symptom severities in children and adolescents with Tourette syndrome and/or obsessive-compulsive disorder. J Child Psychol Psychiatry. 2007;48:157–66.
15. Conelea CA, Woods DW, Brandt BC. The impact of a stress induction task on tic frequencies in youth with Tourette Syndrome. Behav Res Ther. 2011;49:492–7.
16. Leckman JF. Phenomenology of tics and natural history of tic disorders. Brain Dev. 2003;25 Suppl 1:S24–8.

17. Reese HE, Scahill L, Peterson AL, Crowe K, Woods DW, Piacentini J, et al. The premonitory urge to tic: measurement, characteristics, and correlates in older adolescents and adults. Behav Ther. 2014;45:177–86.
18. Banaschewski T, Woerner W, Rothenberger A. Premonitory sensory phenomena and suppressibility of tics in Tourette syndrome: developmental aspects in children and adolescents. Dev Med Child Neurol. 2003;45:700–3.
19. Robertson MM. Gilles de la Tourette syndrome: the complexities of phenotype and treatment. Br J Hosp Med (Lond). 2011;72:100–7.
20. Leckman JF, Walker DE, Cohen DJ. Premonitory urges in Tourette's syndrome. Am J Psychiatry. 1993;150:98–102.
21. Ganos C, Kahl U, Schunke O, Kuhn S, Haggard P, Gerloff C, et al. Are premonitory urges a prerequisite of tic inhibition in Gilles de la Tourette syndrome? J Neurol Neurosurg Psychiatry. 2012;83:975–8.
22. Eddy CM, Cavanna AE. Premonitory urges in adults with complicated and uncomplicated Tourette Syndrome. Behav Modif. 2013;38(2):264–75.
23. Ganos C, Ogrzal T, Schnitzler A, Munchau A. The pathophysiology of echopraxia/echolalia: relevance to Gilles de la Tourette syndrome. Mov Disord. 2012;27:1222–9.
24. Munchau A. Luxie loxie-hannah hannah-anna…blume. Mov Disord. 2011;26:931–2.
25. Cohrs S, Rasch T, Altmeyer S, Kinkelbur J, Kostanecka T, Rothenberger A, et al. Decreased sleep quality and increased sleep related movements in patients with Tourette's syndrome. J Neurol Neurosurg Psychiatry. 2001;70:192–7.
26. Kirov R, Kinkelbur J, Banaschewski T, Rothenberger A. Sleep patterns in children with attention-deficit/hyperactivity disorder, tic disorder, and comorbidity. J Child Psychol Psychiatry. 2007;48:561–70.
27. Bloch MH, Peterson BS, Scahill L, Otka J, Katsovich L, Zhang H, et al. Adulthood outcome of tic and obsessive-compulsive symptom severity in children with Tourette syndrome. Arch Pediatr Adolesc Med. 2006;160:65–9.
28. Palermo SD, Bloch MH, Craiglow B, Landeros-Weisenberger A, Dombrowski PA, Panza K, et al. Predictors of early adulthood quality of life in children with obsessive-compulsive disorder. Soc Psychiatry Psychiatr Epidemiol. 2011;46:291–7.
29. Stewart SE, Illmann C, Geller DA, Leckman JF, King R, Pauls DL. A controlled family study of attention-deficit/hyperactivity disorder and Tourette's disorder. J Am Acad Child Adolesc Psychiatry. 2006;45:1354–62.
30. Bloch MH, Leckman JF, Zhu H, Peterson BS. Caudate volumes in childhood predict symptom severity in adults with Tourette syndrome. Neurology. 2005;65:1253–8.
31. Peterson BS, Pine DS, Cohen P, Brook JS. Prospective, longitudinal study of tic, obsessive-compulsive, and attention-deficit/hyperactivity disorders in an epidemiological sample. J Am Acad Child Adolesc Psychiatry. 2001;40:685–95.
32. Robertson MM. Tourette syndrome, associated conditions and the complexities of treatment. Brain. 2000;123(Pt 3):425–62.
33. Depboylu C, Oertel WH, Münchau A. Tourette-Syndrom und andere Tic-Erkrankungen. In: Oertel WH, Deuschl G, Poewe W, editors. Parkinson-Syndrome und andere Bewegungsstörungen. Stuttgart: Georg Thieme Verlag KG; 2012. p. 312–25.
34. Goetz CG, Pappert EJ, Louis ED, Raman R, Leurgans S. Advantages of a modified scoring method for the Rush Video-Based Tic Rating Scale. Mov Disord. 1999;14:502–6.
35. Robertson MM, Banerjee S, Kurlan R, Cohen DJ, Leckman JF, McMahon W, et al. The Tourette syndrome diagnostic confidence index: development and clinical associations. Neurology. 1999;53:2108–12.
36. Leckman JF, Riddle MA, Hardin MT, Ort SI, Swartz KL, Stevenson J, et al. The Yale Global Tic Severity Scale: initial testing of a clinician-rated scale of tic severity. J Am Acad Child Adolesc Psychiatry. 1989;28:566–73.
37. Goodman WK, Price LH, Rasmussen SA, Mazure C, Fleischmann RL, Hill CL, et al. The Yale-Brown Obsessive Compulsive Scale. I. Development, use, and reliability. Arch Gen Psychiatry. 1989;46:1006–11.

38. Woods DW, Piacentini J, Himle MB, Chang S. Premonitory Urge for Tics Scale (PUTS): initial psychometric results and examination of the premonitory urge phenomenon in youths with Tic disorders. J Dev Behav Pediatr. 2005;26:397–403.
39. Cavanna AE, Schrag A, Morley D, Orth M, Robertson MM, Joyce E, et al. The Gilles de la Tourette syndrome-quality of life scale (GTS-QOL): development and validation. Neurology. 2008;71:1410–6.
40. Storch EA, Murphy TK, Geffken GR, Sajid M, Allen P, Roberti JW, et al. Reliability and validity of the Yale Global Tic Severity Scale. Psychol Assess. 2005;17:486–91.
41. Walkup JT, Rosenberg LA, Brown J, Singer HS. The validity of instruments measuring tic severity in Tourette's syndrome. J Am Acad Child Adolesc Psychiatry. 1992;31:472–7.
42. Rössner V, Müller-Vahl K, Neuner I. PUTS - premonitory urge tics scale: Fragebogen für Kinder. In: Müller-Vahl K, editor. Tourette-Syndrom und andere Tic-Erkrankungen im Kindes- und Erwachsenenalter. Berlin: MWV Medizinische Wissenschaftliche Verlagsgesellschaft; 2010.
43. Eddy CM, Rizzo R, Gulisano M, Agodi A, Barchitta M, Cali P, et al. Quality of life in young people with Tourette syndrome: a controlled study. J Neurol. 2011;258:291–301.
44. Murphy KR, Adler LA. Assessing attention-deficit/hyperactivity disorder in adults: focus on rating scales. J Clin Psychiatry. 2004;65 Suppl 3:12–7.
45. Collett BR, Ohan JL, Myers KM. Ten-year review of rating scales. V: scales assessing attention-deficit/hyperactivity disorder. J Am Acad Child Adolesc Psychiatry. 2003;42:1015–37.
46. Taylor A, Deb S, Unwin G. Scales for the identification of adults with attention deficit hyperactivity disorder (ADHD): a systematic review. Res Dev Disabil. 2011;32:924–38.
47. Ward MF, Wender PH, Reimherr FW. The Wender Utah Rating Scale: an aid in the retrospective diagnosis of childhood attention deficit hyperactivity disorder. Am J Psychiatry. 1993;150:885–90.
48. Conners CK, Erhardt D, Sparrow E. CAARS adult ADHD rating scales: a technical manual. North Tonawanda: Multi Health Systems; 1999.
49. Steketee G, Frost R, Bogart K. The Yale-Brown Obsessive Compulsive Scale: interview versus self-report. Behav Res Ther. 1996;34:675–84.
50. Rosario-Campos MC, Miguel EC, Quatrano S, Chacon P, Ferrao Y, Findley D, et al. The Dimensional Yale-Brown Obsessive-Compulsive Scale (DY-BOCS): an instrument for assessing obsessive-compulsive symptom dimensions. Mol Psychiatry. 2006;11:495–504.
51. Abramowitz JS, Deacon BJ. Psychometric properties and construct validity of the Obsessive-Compulsive Inventory–Revised: replication and extension with a clinical sample. J Anxiety Disord. 2006;20:1016–35.
52. Foa EB, Coles M, Huppert JD, Pasupuleti RV, Franklin ME, March J. Development and validation of a child version of the obsessive compulsive inventory. Behav Ther. 2010;41:121–32.
53. Jones AM, De Nadai AS, Arnold EB, McGuire JF, Lewin AB, Murphy TK, et al. Psychometric properties of the obsessive compulsive inventory: child version in children and adolescents with obsessive-compulsive disorder. Child Psychiatry Hum Dev. 2013;44:137–51.
54. Berg CJ, Rapoport JL, Flament M. The Leyton obsessional inventory-child version. J Am Acad Child Psychiatry. 1986;25:84–91.
55. Cooper J. The Leyton obsessional inventory. Psychol Med. 1970;1:48–64.
56. Stewart SE, Ceranoglu TA, O'Hanley T, Geller DA. Performance of clinician versus self-report measures to identify obsessive-compulsive disorder in children and adolescents. J Child Adolesc Psychopharmacol. 2005;15:956–63.
57. Uher R, Heyman I, Turner CM, Shafran R. Self-, parent-report and interview measures of obsessive-compulsive disorder in children and adolescents. J Anxiety Disord. 2008;22:979–90.
58. Sukhodolsky DG, Landeros-Weisenberger A, Scahill L, Leckman JF, Schultz RT. Neuropsychological functioning in children with Tourette syndrome with and without attention-deficit/hyperactivity disorder. J Am Acad Child Adolesc Psychiatry. 2010;49:1155–64.
59. Jackson GM, Mueller SC, Hambleton K, Hollis CP. Enhanced cognitive control in Tourette Syndrome during task uncertainty. Exp Brain Res. 2007;182:357–64.

60. Roessner V, Becker A, Banaschewski T, Rothenberger A. Executive functions in children with chronic tic disorders with/without ADHD: new insights. Eur Child Adolesc Psychiatry. 2007;16 Suppl 1:36–44.
61. Yuen T, Bradshaw JL, Sheppard D, Lee P, Georgiou-Karistianis N. Inhibition of return in children with Tourette's syndrome and comorbid forms: a preliminary study. Child Neuro Psychol. 2005;11:393–411.
62. Shin MS, Choi H, Kim H, Hwang JW, Kim BN, Cho SC. A study of neuropsychological deficit in children with obsessive-compulsive disorder. Eur Psychiatry. 2008;23:512–20.
63. Robertson MM. The prevalence and epidemiology of Gilles de la Tourette syndrome. Part 1: the epidemiological and prevalence studies. J Psychosom Res. 2008;65:461–72.
64. Centers for Disease Control and Prevention. Prevalence of diagnosed Tourette syndrome in persons aged 6–17 years–United States, 2007. MMWR Morb Mortal Wkly Rep. 2009;58: 581–5.
65. Schlander M, Schwarz O, Rothenberger A, Roessner V. Tic disorders: administrative prevalence and co-occurrence with attention-deficit/hyperactivity disorder in a German community sample. Eur Psychiatry. 2011;26:370–4.
66. Robertson MM. The prevalence and epidemiology of Gilles de la Tourette syndrome. Part 2: tentative explanations for differing prevalence figures in GTS, including the possible effects of psychopathology, aetiology, cultural differences, and differing phenotypes. J Psychosom Res. 2008;65:473–86.
67. Mol Debes NM, Hjalgrim H, Skov L. Limited knowledge of Tourette syndrome causes delay in diagnosis. Neuropediatrics. 2008;39:101–5.
68. Leckman JF, Zhang H, Vitale A, Lahnin F, Lynch K, Bondi C, et al. Course of tic severity in Tourette syndrome: the first two decades. Pediatrics. 1998;102:14–9.
69. Hassan N, Cavanna AE. The prognosis of Tourette syndrome: implications for clinical practice. Funct Neurol. 2012;27:23–7.
70. Pappert EJ, Goetz CG, Louis ED, Blasucci L, Leurgans S. Objective assessments of longitudinal outcome in Gilles de la Tourette's syndrome. Neurology. 2003;61:936–40.
71. Paschou P. The genetic basis of Gilles de la Tourette Syndrome. Neurosci Biobehav Rev. 2013;37:1026–39.
72. Pauls DL, Raymond CL, Stevenson JM, Leckman JF. A family study of Gilles de la Tourette syndrome. Am J Hum Genet. 1991;48:154–63.
73. O'Rourke JA, Scharf JM, Yu D, Pauls DL. The genetics of Tourette syndrome: a review. J Psychosom Res. 2009;67:533–45.
74. Davis LK, Yu D, Keenan CL, Gamazon ER, Konkashbaev AI, Derks EM, et al. Partitioning the heritability of Tourette syndrome and obsessive compulsive disorder reveals differences in genetic architecture. PLoS Genet. 2013;9:e1003864.
75. Buse J, Schoenefeld K, Munchau A, Roessner V. Neuromodulation in Tourette syndrome: dopamine and beyond. Neurosci Biobehav Rev. 2013;37(6):1069–84.
76. Swedo SE, Leonard HL, Garvey M, Mittleman B, Allen AJ, Perlmutter S, et al. Pediatric autoimmune neuropsychiatric disorders associated with streptococcal infections: clinical description of the first 50 cases. Am J Psychiatry. 1998;155:264–71.
77. Kurlan R. The PANDAS hypothesis: losing its bite? Mov Disord. 2004;19:371–4.
78. Leckman JF. Tourette's syndrome. Lancet. 2002;360:1577–86.
79. Chao TK, Hu J, Pringsheim T. Prenatal risk factors for Tourette Syndrome: a systematic review. BMC Pregnancy Childbirth. 2014;14:53.
80. Steinberg T, Shmuel-Baruch S, Horesh N, Apter A. Life events and Tourette syndrome. Compr Psychiatry. 2013;54:467–73.
81. Leckman JF, Bloch MH, Smith ME, Larabi D, Hampson M. Neurobiological substrates of Tourette's disorder. J Child Adolesc Psycho Pharmacol. 2010;20:237–47.
82. Ganos C, Roessner V, Munchau A. The functional anatomy of Gilles de la Tourette syndrome. Neurosci Biobehav Rev. 2013;37(6):1050–62.
83. Alexander GE, DeLong MR, Strick PL. Parallel organization of functionally segregated circuits linking basal ganglia and cortex. Annu Rev Neurosci. 1986;9:357–81.

84. Alexander GE, DeLong MR. Microstimulation of the primate neostriatum. II. Somatotopic organization of striatal microexcitable zones and their relation to neuronal response properties. J Neurophysiol. 1985;53:1417–30.
85. Worbe Y, Gerardin E, Hartmann A, Valabregue R, Chupin M, Tremblay L, et al. Distinct structural changes underpin clinical phenotypes in patients with Gilles de la Tourette syndrome. Brain. 2010;133:3649–60.
86. Singer HS. Tourette's syndrome: from behaviour to biology. Lancet Neurol. 2005;4:149–59.
87. Crittenden JR, Graybiel AM. Basal Ganglia disorders associated with imbalances in the striatal striosome and matrix compartments. Front Neuroanat. 2011;5:59.
88. Mink JW. The Basal Ganglia and involuntary movements: impaired inhibition of competing motor patterns. Arch Neurol. 2003;60:1365–8.
89. Kalanithi PS, Zheng W, Kataoka Y, DiFiglia M, Grantz H, Saper CB, et al. Altered parvalbumin-positive neuron distribution in basal ganglia of individuals with Tourette syndrome. Proc Natl Acad Sci U S A. 2005;102:13307–12.
90. Kataoka Y, Kalanithi PS, Grantz H, Schwartz ML, Saper C, Leckman JF, et al. Decreased number of parvalbumin and cholinergic interneurons in the striatum of individuals with Tourette syndrome. J Comp Neurol. 2010;518:277–91.
91. Worbe Y, Malherbe C, Hartmann A, Pelegrini-Issac M, Messe A, Vidailhet M, et al. Functional immaturity of cortico-basal ganglia networks in Gilles de la Tourette syndrome. Brain. 2012;135:1937–46.
92. Wang Z, Maia TV, Marsh R, Colibazzi T, Gerber A, Peterson BS. The neural circuits that generate tics in Tourette's syndrome. Am J Psychiatry. 2011;168:1326–37.
93. Peterson BS, Choi HA, Hao X, Amat JA, Zhu H, Whiteman R, et al. Morphologic features of the amygdala and hippocampus in children and adults with Tourette syndrome. Arch Gen Psychiatry. 2007;64:1281–91.
94. Peterson BS, Staib L, Scahill L, Zhang H, Anderson C, Leckman JF, et al. Regional brain and ventricular volumes in Tourette syndrome. Arch Gen Psychiatry. 2001;58:427–40.
95. Church JA, Fair DA, Dosenbach NU, Cohen AL, Miezin FM, Petersen SE, et al. Control networks in paediatric Tourette syndrome show immature and anomalous patterns of functional connectivity. Brain. 2009;132:225–38.
96. Peterson BS, Thomas P, Kane MJ, Scahill L, Zhang H, Bronen R, et al. Basal Ganglia volumes in patients with Gilles de la Tourette syndrome. Arch Gen Psychiatry. 2003;60:415–24.
97. Neuner I, Kupriyanova Y, Stocker T, Huang R, Posnansky O, Schneider F, et al. Microstructure assessment of grey matter nuclei in adult tourette patients by diffusion tensor imaging. Neurosci Lett. 2011;487:22–6.
98. Makki MI, Behen M, Bhatt A, Wilson B, Chugani HT. Microstructural abnormalities of striatum and thalamus in children with Tourette syndrome. Mov Disord. 2008;23:2349–56.
99. Roessner V, Overlack S, Baudewig J, Dechent P, Rothenberger A, Helms G. No brain structure abnormalities in boys with Tourette's syndrome: a voxel-based morphometry study. Mov Disord. 2009;24:2398–403.
100. Sowell ER, Kan E, Yoshii J, Thompson PM, Bansal R, Xu D, et al. Thinning of sensorimotor cortices in children with Tourette syndrome. Nat Neurosci. 2008;11:637–9.
101. Thomalla G, Siebner HR, Jonas M, Baumer T, Biermann-Ruben K, Hummel F, et al. Structural changes in the somatosensory system correlate with tic severity in Gilles de la Tourette syndrome. Brain. 2009;132:765–77.
102. Cheng B, Braass H, Ganos C, Treszl A, Biermann-Ruben K, Hummel FC, et al. Altered intrahemispheric structural connectivity in Gilles de la Tourette syndrome. Neuro image Clin. 2013;4:174–81.
103. Baumer T, Thomalla G, Kroeger J, Jonas M, Gerloff C, Hummel FC, et al. Interhemispheric motor networks are abnormal in patients with Gilles de la Tourette syndrome. Mov Disord. 2010;25:2828–37.
104. Plessen KJ, Wentzel-Larsen T, Hugdahl K, Feineigle P, Klein J, Staib LH, et al. Altered interhemispheric connectivity in individuals with Tourette's disorder. Am J Psychiatry. 2004;161:2028–37.

105. Gilbert DL. Motor cortex inhibitory function in Tourette syndrome, attention deficit disorder, and obsessive compulsive disorder: studies using transcranial magnetic stimulation. Adv Neurol. 2006;99:107–14.
106. Orth M, Munchau A, Rothwell JC. Corticospinal system excitability at rest is associated with tic severity in tourette syndrome. Biol Psychiatry. 2008;64:248–51.
107. Heise KF, Steven B, Liuzzi G, Thomalla G, Jonas M, Muller-Vahl K, et al. Altered modulation of intracortical excitability during movement preparation in Gilles de la Tourette syndrome. Brain. 2010;133:580–90.
108. Jackson SR, Parkinson A, Jung J, Ryan SE, Morgan PS, Hollis C, et al. Compensatory neural reorganization in Tourette syndrome. Curr Biol. 2011;21:580–5.
109. Jung J, Jackson SR, Parkinson A, Jackson GM. Cognitive control over motor output in Tourette syndrome. Neurosci Biobehav Rev. 2013;37:1016–25.
110. Muller-Vahl KR, Grosskreutz J, Prell T, Kaufmann J, Bodammer N, Peschel T. Tics are caused by alterations in prefrontal areas, thalamus and putamen, while changes in the cingulate gyrus reflect secondary compensatory mechanisms. BMC Neurosci. 2014;15:6.
111. Ganos C, Kuhn S, Kahl U, Schunke O, Brandt V, Baumer T, et al. Prefrontal cortex volume reductions and tic inhibition are unrelated in uncomplicated GTS adults. J Psychosom Res. 2014;76:84–7.
112. Peterson BS, Skudlarski P, Anderson AW, Zhang H, Gatenby JC, Lacadie CM, et al. A functional magnetic resonance imaging study of tic suppression in Tourette syndrome. Arch Gen Psychiatry. 1998;55:326–33.
113. Draganski B, Martino D, Cavanna AE, Hutton C, Orth M, Robertson MM, et al. Multispectral brain morphometry in Tourette syndrome persisting into adulthood. Brain. 2010;133:3661–75.
114. Kwon HJ, Lim WS, Lim MH, Lee SJ, Hyun JK, Chae JH, et al. 1-Hz low frequency repetitive transcranial magnetic stimulation in children with Tourette's syndrome. Neurosci Lett. 2011;492:1–4.
115. Maia TV, Frank MJ. From reinforcement learning models to psychiatric and neurological disorders. Nat Neurosci. 2011;14:154–62.
116. Grace AA. The tonic/phasic model of dopamine system regulation: its relevance for understanding how stimulant abuse can alter basal ganglia function. Drug Alcohol Depend. 1995;37:111–29.
117. Minzer K, Lee O, Hong JJ, Singer HS. Increased prefrontal D2 protein in Tourette syndrome: a postmortem analysis of frontal cortex and striatum. J Neurol Sci. 2004;219:55–61.
118. Wong DF, Brasic JR, Singer HS, Schretlen DJ, Kuwabara H, Zhou Y, et al. Mechanisms of dopaminergic and serotonergic neurotransmission in Tourette syndrome: clues from an in vivo neurochemistry study with PET. Neuropsychopharmacology. 2008;33:1239–51.
119. Wolf SS, Jones DW, Knable MB, Gorey JG, Lee KS, Hyde TM, et al. Tourette syndrome: prediction of phenotypic variation in monozygotic twins by caudate nucleus D2 receptor binding. Science. 1996;273:1225–7.
120. Muller-Vahl KR, Berding G, Kolbe H, Meyer GJ, Hundeshagen H, Dengler R, et al. Dopamine D2 receptor imaging in Gilles de la Tourette syndrome. Acta Neurol Scand. 2000;101:165–71.
121. Steeves TD, Ko JH, Kideckel DM, Rusjan P, Houle S, Sandor P, et al. Extrastriatal dopaminergic dysfunction in tourette syndrome. Ann Neurol. 2010;67:170–81.
122. Singer HS, Szymanski S, Giuliano J, Yokoi F, Dogan AS, Brasic JR, et al. Elevated intrasynaptic dopamine release in Tourette's syndrome measured by PET. Am J Psychiatry. 2002;159:1329–36.
123. Nikolaus S, Antke C, Muller HW. In vivo imaging of synaptic function in the central nervous system: II. Mental and affective disorders. Behav Brain Res. 2009;204:32–66.
124. Roessner V, Plessen KJ, Rothenberger A, Ludolph AG, Rizzo R, Skov L, et al. European clinical guidelines for Tourette syndrome and other tic disorders. Part II: pharmacological treatment. Eur Child Adolesc Psychiatry. 2011;20:173–96.
125. Verdellen C, van de Griendt J, Hartmann A, Murphy T, Group EG. European clinical guidelines for Tourette syndrome and other tic disorders. Part III: behavioural and psychosocial interventions. Eur Child Adolesc Psychiatry. 2011;20:197–207.

126. Muller-Vahl KR, Cath DC, Cavanna AE, Dehning S, Porta M, Robertson MM, et al. European clinical guidelines for Tourette syndrome and other tic disorders. Part IV: deep brain stimulation. Eur Child Adolesc Psychiatry. 2011;20:209–17.
127. Muller-Vahl K, Grotenhermen F. Cannabis therapy. Dtsch Arztebl Int. 2013;110:144.
128. Dutta N, Cavanna AE. The effectiveness of habit reversal therapy in the treatment of Tourette syndrome and other chronic tic disorders: a systematic review. Funct Neurol. 2013;28:7–12.
129. Debes N, Hjalgrim H, Skov L. The presence of attention-deficit hyperactivity disorder (ADHD) and obsessive-compulsive disorder worsen psychosocial and educational problems in Tourette syndrome. J Child Neurol. 2010;25:171–81.
130. Scahill L, Erenberg G, Berlin Jr CM, Budman C, Coffey BJ, Jankovic J, et al. Contemporary assessment and pharmacotherapy of Tourette syndrome. NeuroRx. 2006;3:192–206.
131. Pringsheim T, Marras C. Pimozide for tics in Tourette's syndrome. Cochrane Database Syst Rev. 2009;(2):CD006996.
132. Weisman H, Qureshi IA, Leckman JF, Scahill L, Bloch MH. Systematic review: pharmacological treatment of tic disorders–efficacy of antipsychotic and alpha-2 adrenergic agonist agents. Neurosci Biobehav Rev. 2013;37:1162–71.
133. Muller-Vahl KR, Krueger D. Does Tourette syndrome prevent tardive dyskinesia? Mov Disord. 2011;26:2442–3.
134. Ludolph AG, Roessner V, Munchau A, Muller-Vahl K. Tourette syndrome and other tic disorders in childhood, adolescence and adulthood. Dtsch Arztebl Int. 2012;109:821–288.
135. Ho CS, Chen HJ, Chiu NC, Shen EY, Lue HC. Short-term sulpiride treatment of children and adolescents with Tourette syndrome or chronic tic disorder. J Formos Med Assoc. 2009;108:788–93.
136. Robertson MM, Stern JS. Gilles de la Tourette syndrome: symptomatic treatment based on evidence. Eur Child Adolesc Psychiatry. 2000;9 Suppl 1:I60–75.
137. George MS, Trimble MR, Robertson MM. Fluvoxamine and sulpiride in comorbid obsessive–compulsive disorder and gilles de la tourette syndrome. Hum Psychopharmacol Clin Exp. 1993;8:327–34.
138. Gaffney GR, Perry PJ, Lund BC, Bever-Stille KA, Arndt S, Kuperman S. Risperidone versus clonidine in the treatment of children and adolescents with Tourette's syndrome. J Am Acad Child Adolesc Psychiatry. 2002;41:330–6.
139. Tourette's Syndrome Study G. Treatment of ADHD in children with tics: a randomized controlled trial. Neurology. 2002;58:527–36.
140. Du YS, Li HF, Vance A, Zhong YQ, Jiao FY, Wang HM, et al. Randomized double-blind multicentre placebo-controlled clinical trial of the clonidine adhesive patch for the treatment of tic disorders. Aust N Z J Psychiatry. 2008;42:807–13.
141. Spencer TJ, Sallee FR, Gilbert DL, Dunn DW, McCracken JT, Coffey BJ, et al. Atomoxetine treatment of ADHD in children with comorbid Tourette syndrome. J Atten Disord. 2008; 11:470–81.
142. Porta M, Sassi M, Cavallazzi M, Fornari M, Brambilla A, Servello D. Tourette's syndrome and role of tetrabenazine: review and personal experience. Clin Drug Investig. 2008;28:443–59.
143. Singer HS, Wendlandt J, Krieger M, Giuliano J. Baclofen treatment in Tourette syndrome: a double-blind, placebo-controlled, crossover trial. Neurology. 2001;56:599–604.
144. Smith-Hicks CL, Bridges DD, Paynter NP, Singer HS. A double blind randomized placebo control trial of levetiracetam in Tourette syndrome. Mov Disord. 2007;22:1764–70.
145. van Wattum PJ, Chappell PB, Zelterman D, Scahill LD, Leckman JF. Patterns of response to acute naloxone infusion in Tourette's syndrome. Mov Disord. 2000;15:1252–4.
146. Howson AL, Batth S, Ilivitsky V, Boisjoli A, Jaworski M, Mahoney C, et al. Clinical and attentional effects of acute nicotine treatment in Tourette's syndrome. Eur Psychiatry. 2004;19:102–12.
147. Silver AA, Shytle RD, Philipp MK, Wilkinson BJ, McConville B, Sanberg PR. Transdermal nicotine and haloperidol in Tourette's disorder: a double-blind placebo-controlled study. J Clin Psychiatry. 2001;62:707–14.

148. Curtis A, Clarke CE, Rickards HE. Cannabinoids for Tourette's Syndrome. Cochrane Database Syst Rev. 2009;(4):CD006565.
149. Marras C, Andrews D, Sime E, Lang AE. Botulinum toxin for simple motor tics: a randomized, double-blind, controlled clinical trial. Neurology. 2001;56:605–10.
150. Kwak CH, Hanna PA, Jankovic J. Botulinum toxin in the treatment of tics. Arch Neurol. 2000;57:1190–3.
151. McGuire JF, Piacentini J, Brennan EA, Lewin AB, Murphy TK, Small BJ, et al. A meta-analysis of behavior therapy for Tourette Syndrome. J Psychiatr Res. 2014;50:106–12.
152. Rizzo R, Gulisano M, Cali PV, Curatolo P. Tourette Syndrome and comorbid ADHD: current pharmacological treatment options. Eur J Paediatr Neurol. 2013;17:421–8.
153. Pringsheim T, Steeves T. Pharmacological treatment for Attention Deficit Hyperactivity Disorder (ADHD) in children with comorbid tic disorders. Cochrane Database Syst Rev. 2011;(4):CD007990.

Chapter 12
Wilson's Disease

Vladimir S. Kostić, Marina Svetel, Aleksandra Tomić, and Nikola Kresojević

Abbreviations

BG	Basal ganglia
MMSE	Mini-Mental State Examination
NPI	Neuropsychiatric Inventory
OLT	Orthotopic liver transplantation
QoL	Quality of life
SERT	Serotonin transporters
WD	Wilson's disease

Introduction

Wilson's disease (WD) is a rare autosomal-recessive disease caused by mutation in the *ATP7B* gene on chromosome 13, coding for a copper-transporting P-type ATPase important for copper transport and the elimination of excess copper from the body [1–3]. Since the mutated gene prevents the transport protein to function properly, copper preferentially accumulates in liver and brain but also in the kidneys, eyes, skeletal

V.S. Kostić, MD, PhD (✉) • M. Svetel, MD, PhD
Movement Disorders Department, Institute of Neurology CCS, School of Medicine, University of Belgrade, Ul. Dr Subotića 6, Belgrade 11000, Serbia
e-mail: vladimir.s.kostic@gmail.com; marinasvetel@gmail.com

A. Tomić, MD • N. Kresojević, MD
Movement Disorders Department, Institute of Neurology CCS, Belgrade, Serbia
e-mail: alexandra_tomic@yahoo.co.uk; nikola_kresojevic@yahoo.com

H. Reichmann (ed.), *Neuropsychiatric Symptoms of Movement Disorders*, Neuropsychiatric Symptoms of Neurological Disease,
DOI 10.1007/978-3-319-09537-0_12

system, etc. Although not the first to recognize the disease process, S.A.K. Wilson was the first who gave detailed clinical and pathological characterization of the entity that bears his name (also, *hepatolenticular degeneration*) in 1912 in *Brain*, where he published the seminal paper on more than 200 pages: "Progressive lenticular degeneration: A familial nervous disease associated with cirrhosis of the liver" [4]. A year later, Rumpel identified excess copper in the liver of a patient who died from WD [5].

The worldwide prevalence of WD ranges from 1 in 5,000 to 1 in 30,000, with an incidence from 15 to 30 per million [6]. The carrier frequency is approximately 1 in 90 (~1 % of the population). Consanguinity, common in some isolated populations, increases the prevalence of WD. Most symptoms initially appear in the second or third decade of life [7], and without treatment WD relentlessly progresses to fatal outcome, mainly due to a liver failure or complications of neurological disorders. Roberts and Schilsky [8] provided formal guidelines for diagnosis of WD.

Genetics and Molecular Pathogenesis of Wilson's Disease

ATP7B, the gene responsible for WD, is highly expressed in the liver, kidney, and placenta [1]. The Human Gene Mutation Database lists more than 750 different mutations in *ATP7B*. Therefore, systemic genetic testing for WD is difficult and expensive. Fortunately, in different ethnic groups a few mutations may be particularly prevalent (i.e., H1069Q in patients of European origin), and specific strategies (i.e., selection of exons) for initial screening can be chosen in the respective population groups. Most patients are compound heterozygotes. Interestingly enough, even affected homozygous twins may express wide variability in clinical features of WD, which suggests an operational role of additional factors (i.e., environmental, genetic, and epigenetic factors) [9]. In general, no consistent genotype-phenotype correlations have been established [10].

Dietary copper, absorbed in the stomach and duodenum and delivered into the circulation, reaches the liver complexed to albumin. In hepatocytes, a specific chaperone, ATOX1, delivers copper to the ATP7B, a 1411-amino acid, copper-transporting, P-type transmembrane ATPase. This WD protein is responsible for (a) incorporation of copper into apoceruloplasmin with subsequent delivery of the copper-ceruloplasmin complex into the serum and for (b) delivering excess copper to biliary canaliculi for excretion. Since the normal mechanism for elimination of excess copper is excretion in the bile and further loss in the stool, the impaired function of the ATP7B protein fails to adequately incorporate copper into apoceruloplasmin and, also, decreases its hepatocellular excretion into bile with subsequent copper accumulation and deleterious effects [7]. Simplified, a positive copper balance is established (~0.25 mg/day). When hepatic storage capacity for copper is exceeded, copper is released into the blood, followed by a compensatory dramatic increase in the urinary copper excretion. Unfortunately, such increase is unable to fully compensate for dysfunctional biliary excretion, and copper that escapes from the liver is further deposited in other organs (brain, kidney, cornea, skeletal system). The level of highly toxic circulating free copper also rises [11].

As an inborn error of copper metabolism, WD is pathologically manifested primarily as hepatic cirrhosis and the brain basal ganglia (BG) damage. In the brain, copper deposits cause brownish discoloration of the lenticular nucleus, with affection of the thalamus, brainstem, cerebellum, and cerebral cortex to various degrees. Necrosis, gliosis, and cystic changes in the BG are characteristic for advanced stages of WD [12].

Clinical Manifestations of Wilson's Disease

The initial manifestations of WD comprise neurological signs and symptoms in approximately 40 % of patients (usually after the age of 12 years), various forms of hepatic dysfunction in also about 40 % of patients (usually at an earlier age), or psychiatric features in approximately 15–20 % of patients [13]. What influences these individual variations in clinical presentation has yet not been elucidated.

As early as in his initial manuscript, Wilson [4] recognized behavioral/psychiatric changes in 8 out of 12 WD patients, which he addressed as "psychical." However, in the 1950s and 1960s it became clear that almost every WD patient would suffer from psychiatric problems at one point in the course of the disease [14]. It took even longer to recognize that psychiatric problems did not always present jointly with neurological symptoms. In 307 patients with WD, registered over 30 years, Prashanth et al. [15] detected diagnostic errors by referring physicians in 192 patients (62.5 %): among them, psychiatric diagnosis was given to 12 patients, ranging from schizophrenia to bipolar disorder, depression, mania, anxiety, and paranoid psychosis [16].

About a third of patients with WD present initially with only psychiatric features, while two thirds to almost all of them eventually develop psychiatric symptoms in the course of the disease [16]. Previous estimates of lifetime prevalence of psychiatric manifestations in WD ranged from 30 to 100 % [6, 17, 18]. The most common psychiatric manifestations in WD include behavioral (incongruous behavior and irritability) or personality changes and mood disturbances, particularly depression [17]. Psychoses are rare. Antisocial and criminal behavior, sexual preoccupation, and disinhibition, as well as anxiety, phobias, attention-deficit hyperactivity disorder, impulsivity, delusions, substance abuse, obsessive-compulsive behavior, catatonia, schizophrenia, and bipolar disorder, have also been reported. In children, psychiatric abnormalities may be subtle and include nonspecific situations such as unexplained deterioration in schoolwork [12]. Psychiatric manifestations in WD appear to be more common in association with neurologic involvement, while they are relatively rare in isolated hepatic form of WD [19].

In general, psychiatric symptoms may present with, predominate or even precede the other, mainly neurological symptoms. The diagnosis of WD is rarely established during the period in which psychiatric symptoms are the only manifestations [19].

Therefore, useful advice is that WD should always be considered in any young subject with unexplained psychiatric symptoms, particularly if accompanied by neurologic or hepatic dysfunction. Wilson's disease should also be suspected in younger patients with unexplained poor school performance, especially if associated with abdominal symptoms [20]. Pfeiffer [11] added the third situation to prompt consideration of WD in young persons suspected of drug abuse, since the symptoms can be similar [21].

Psychiatric manifestations associated with WD may be a consequence of brain tissue damage due to copper accumulation, but also may be a real comorbidity or, particularly in late appearance, side effects of specific treatment for WD. In general, they can be categorized into five groups: cognitive impairment, personality changes, affective disorders, psychosis, and others [22].

Cognitive Changes in Wilson's Disease

Cognitive decline in WD, observed even in the original manuscript by Wilson [4], has been considered by Cummings [23] as the first description of subcortical dementia. Early studies were not consistent in memory evaluation [24, 25] or in the significance of impact of motor dysfunction to cognitive deficits [26]. No correlation has been found between the degree of cognitive impairment and the severity of neurological symptoms [27]. The conclusion from these studies was that cognitive impairment in WD is generally subtle, affecting less than 25 % of patients, getting worse with increased disease duration, and predominantly associated with neurological manifestations [16]. Some authors ascribed at least a part of cognitive deterioration in WD to depression and hepatic encephalopathy, but it appeared even in their absence. Initially, cognitive impairment was broadly classified in two main, not mutually exclusive, categories: (a) the frontal lobe syndrome (characterized by executive dysfunction, attention deficits, poor planning, and decision making, with apathy, impaired social judgment, impulsivity, emotional lability, etc.) and (b) the subcortical dementia (characterized by executive dysfunction, slowness of thinking, and memory loss, but without cortical signs such as aphasia, apraxia, and agnosia) [25, 28]. The earliest studies interpreted cognitive deficit as a consequence of cortical involvement [29], but it can also appear in the absence of detectable cortical affection or hepatic encephalopathy, suggesting a role of the BG and subcortical structures [7, 27, 30].

More recent studies using extensive batteries of neuropsychological tests consistently found the presence of mild multidomain cognitive deficits in patients with neurological form of WD (the most dysfunctional being the executive domain), even in those with only subtle symptoms, long-term treatment course, and lack of depressive or anxiety symptoms [31–34]. In contrast, the cognitive deficits seem to be minimal or absent in asymptomatic patients. However, limitations in some of these studies include the small sample sizes and recruitment bias (i.e., exclusion of patients with depression and more severe motor impairment) and can be hardly extrapolated to the population level.

Portala et al. [35] reported that symptomatic WD patients had lower performance than the norms on the short-term memory task, while the results on the executive tests were within the normal range. Yet, the authors observed that their patients had significant difficulties when handling more than one task simultaneously. In contrast, Wenisch et al. [34] found remarkably preserved verbal intelligence and episodic memory abilities in WD patients with neurological signs when compared to those without them. Seniow et al. [36] reported a range of cognitive dysfunctions, such as frontal executive ability, memory, and visuospatial processing, in neurologically symptomatic vs. asymptomatic patients with WD. Although the lesions of the BG were "accused" to have the main role when attempts to explain cognitive changes in these patients were made, the multifocal pathology revealed by imaging examinations was associated with more severe cognitive decline than the selective BG lesions. In a study including only 12 patients, neuropsychological assessment revealed deficits in the sustained and focused attention, mental speed, verbal working memory, category fluency, and set-shifting abilities (all executive measures) but also in the verbal and visual learning and memory, suggesting both the frontal and subcortical involvements [31]. Impaired motor speed (73 % of patients) did not influence the performance on other neuropsychological tests. Frota et al. [32] also highlighted the role of executive dysfunction in WD: only 10 % of patients did not show any deficit in tests that evaluate executive function, while 80 % displayed an altered performance in ≥2 tests. In this study, 45 % of patients had the Mini-Mental State Examination (MMSE) scores below 1.5 SD in relation to healthy controls. Five percent of the sample fulfilled criteria for dementia, even when patients with severe motor impairment were excluded. The presence and severity of hyperintensities and brain atrophy on MRI strongly correlated with cognitive impairment related to WD. Finally, decision-making deficits may be present in WD patients, probably due to impairment in the frontostriatal loops involved in executive functions and feedback processing [33]. Diffusion tensor imaging revealed widespread alterations in the white matter of drug-naive WD patients [37], which can be associated with various neuropsychological abnormalities observed in WD.

The cognitive changes in WD may hypothetically influence activities of daily living and quality of life (QoL). In a multivariate analysis, higher scores of the Global Assessment Scale for WD tier 1 – cognitive and behavior domain – and lower MMSE scores were the most significant factors contributing to impaired health-related QoL in WD [38]. In accordance with previous reports [18], the MMSE scores were within the normal range. Interestingly, some studies observed a positive effect of penicillamine and zinc treatment on cognitive functioning in WD [39, 40].

Personality and Behavioral Changes in Wilson's Disease

Personality changes (including an antisocial personality), irritability, aggression, bizarre behavior, low threshold to anger, and disinhibition, occasionally extending to criminal behavior, were frequently used to describe patients with WD [17, 18, 41]. Lauterbach et al. [16] reported that the lifetime prevalence of persistent personality or behavioral changes varied between 46 and 71 %. Majority of studies concluded that predominant manifestations include irritability and aggression [6, 17, 18, 41], which was in accordance with common complaints of family members on increased aggression in these patients [22]. A case of a 16-year-old adolescent girl with WD was referred to psychiatry clinic due to self-mutilation (chest skin scratching) [42]. Svetel et al. [43] found that irritability and disinhibition were present in approximately one quarter of treated WD patients. Personality and behavioral changes often co-occurred with neurological symptoms in WD and correlated with lesions of the putamen and pallidum [30]. Irritability and incongruous behavior were more often associated with dystonia and bulbar features than with tremor [17]. Approximately 5 % of patients with WD exhibited increased sexual preoccupation and reduced sexual inhibition [6, 18], sometimes associated with psychosis. Successful treatment of paraphilic hypersexuality was noticed with antiandrogen cyproterone acetate in a psychotic patient with WD [44].

Surprisingly, in a study of personality traits using the Karolinska Scales of Personality, a self-report inventory [45], treated WD patients scored significantly lower than healthy controls on aggressiveness-hostility-related scores, and patients with predominantly neurological symptoms had the lowest irritability. It meant that aggression and hostility levels were low when determined by self-reports. In contrast, aggression and irritability were quite prevalent in studies were family members were interviewed or when interviews were conducted by experts [46]. Although in a small number of patients, Portala et al. [47] showed a trend toward a genotype/phenotype correlation regarding psychopathological symptoms and personality traits in treated WD patients.

Personality and behavioral changes in WD were at least partially explained with the existence of an abnormal metabolism of neurotransmitters, particularly dopamine, noradrenaline, and serotonin [45, 48, 49]. Goldstein et al. [50] observed beneficial effects on the Minnesota Multiphasic Personality Inventory during the long-term de-coppering treatment of WD.

Psychiatric Symptoms in Wilson's Disease

In a study that used the Neuropsychiatric Inventory (NPI) in order to characterize psychiatric symptoms in 50 consecutive, treated, and clinically stable patients with WD, 18 % had one, 14 % had two, and 40 % had ≥ three neuropsychiatric symptoms present [43]. The most prevalent symptoms were anxiety (62 % of patients), depression (26 %), as well as disinhibition and apathy (24 % each). Since the scores 1 and 2 on the NPI items may be clinically trivial, the analysis focused on those with a score ≥4 on each NPI item, and 44 % of patients had such a score on at least one of the following items: anxiety (34 %), depression (26 %), and apathy (18 %) [43].

Psychiatric Manifestations as the Initial Manifestation of Wilson's Disease

In 10–15 % of patients with WD, psychiatric disorders (personality changes, incongruous behavior, irritability, anxiety, mood disorders, psychosis) are the first and, at least initially, sole symptoms. They may occur alone for years before hepatic and/or neurologic involvement appears, and such a "scenario" is likely to influence the diagnostic and treatment delay [10]. This is particularly true for cases when, after appearance of psychiatric symptoms, neuroleptic therapy is introduced, and subsequent development of neurological symptoms in a natural course of WD is ascribed to complications of such treatment. Brewer [51] suggested that if behavioral/psychiatric symptoms precede neurological symptoms for more than 5 years, they are probably not due to WD. Another possibility is that psychiatric disturbances may be a part of joint initial presentation with hepatic or neurological symptoms in 30–64 % of WD patients [17, 22]. Severity of psychiatric manifestations may warrant psychiatric intervention in about half of such patients [22].

However, the results of available studies are not completely consistent. For instance, in a large series of 307 patients [15], the psychiatric presenting symptoms were rare: behavioral problems in 4.6 % and poor performance in school in 1.9 % of patients. Also, in a study with 282 patients, "pure" psychiatric presentation was reported in only seven patients (2.4 %) [52]. Conversely, Akil et al. [22] reported a series of 37 patients who presented primarily with neurological manifestation, where about two thirds had psychiatric problems prior to the diagnosis of WD. Analysis of 50 patients from 44 unrelated families in a study with a suggestive title "WD: a great masquerader" [53] revealed deterioration in school performance as one of the first manifestations in five patients but also depression (four patients), abnormal behavior (three patients), irritability (two patients), and impaired judgment in one patient. Inappropriate laughing and crying was the isolated initial manifestation in a 19-year-old girl.

Unfortunately, most of our knowledge is based on anecdotal case reports. Recently, Zumbrean and Schilsky [14] have summarized 36 case reports from the literature in which psychiatric manifestations were an initial presentation of WD. They found that psychosis was the most common description (36 %), followed by depression (22 %), personality changes, and learning problems (8.3 %, each). The mean latency from the first psychiatric symptoms and diagnosis of WD was 2.4 years. Interestingly, the majority of patients were males (75 %), while the age at onset varied between 5 and 59 years (mean, 22.6 years). Initial psychiatric manifestations in WD published as case reports also include attention-deficit hyperactivity disorder [54], catatonia [55], obsessive-compulsive disorder [56], alcohol abuse, delusions of jealousy [57], etc.

Psychiatric Manifestations During the Course of Wilson's Disease

Scheinberg and Sternlieb [6] stated that every patient with WD, in addition to persistence of the presenting psychiatric symptoms, will eventually develop psychiatric manifestations at some point during the course of the disease. Since the severity of psychiatric symptoms correlates more strongly with the extent of neurological findings than with the liver disease, it is more probable that the psychiatric manifestations reflect brain damage than that simply of a psychological reaction to the debilitating disease [58]. In a series of 350 WD patients, in 15 cases psychiatric manifestations were the predominant symptoms and include bipolar affective disorder, schizophrenia, and psychosis with cognitive decline [59]. With de-coppering therapy some improvement of psychiatric symptoms occurred in five patients, while seven of them needed additional symptomatic treatment [59]. However, psychiatric symptoms may not be only an inherent part of the clinical expression of WD but also a consequence of chelating therapy [14].

According to some authors, psychiatric symptoms in WD render poorer QoL [38] and a worse prognosis [60], while Brewer and Yuzbasiyan-Gurkan [61] stated that those patients who present with neurological or psychiatric symptoms had a better prognosis than those who present with liver disease.

Depression has been estimated to occur in 20–30 % of patients with WD, although some estimates are as high as 30–60 % [18, 62]. Depression in WD negatively influences the health-related QoL. A significant inverse correlation was obtained between depression scores and the QoL domains, even after stabilization of symptoms and disability [38]. Recently, Zimbrean and Schilsky [14] identified a total of 20 case series and cohort studies dealing with psychiatric symptoms in WD and reported the prevalence of major depression varying between 4 and 47 % and between 18 and 39 % for bipolar disorder. Using a structured clinical interview for DSM-IV Axis I disorders (SCID), Shanmugiah et al. [63] found that 24 % of patients fulfilled the diagnostic criteria for syndromic psychiatric diagnosis: bipolar affective disorder (18 %), major depression (4 %), and dysthymia (2 %). These results were almost identical to the results of Svetel et al. [43], who used the same diagnostic tools and found 14 % of WD patients to fulfill the criteria for bipolar affective disorder, 6 % for major depression, and 4 % for dysthymia. In the first study to use standardized epidemiological case-control design and standardized diagnostic instruments (DSM-IV SCID-ANTAS), Costa et al. [64] reported that, compared to controls, WD patients had a higher lifetime prevalence of major depression (OR = 5.7) and bipolar disorders (OR = 12.9). The authors reported an association between lower QoL and bipolar disorder.

The high prevalence of depression in WD highlights the problem of suicide. The estimates of suicidal behavior in literature on WD ranged between 4 and 16 % [16]. Walshe [65] did not mentioned suicide in the list of causes of death in 67 patients with WD. In a recent series of 164 patients with WD, Czlonkowska et al. [66]

reported suicide in only 1 out of 20 patients who died during the mean observation period of 12 years. However, among the causes of death in 30 patients from an initial cohort of 142 patients followed for a mean period of 11 years, four patients (13.3 %) committed suicide (major depression was diagnosed in two of them) [67]. According to these findings, the risk of suicide may not be trivial, as the mortality rate due to a suicide was 1.7 (95 % CI 0.1–3.3) times higher than expected in the age-matched Serbian population. Therefore, physicians treating WD patients should be aware of the risk.

Depressive symptomatology in WD has been related to an alteration of presynaptic serotonin transporters' (SERT) availability in the hypothalamus [62]. Significant negative correlation was found between depression severity scores and SERT density in the thalamus-hypothalamus, but not in the midbrain-pons [68].

Other affective disorders have also been reported in WD such as hypomania and mania [52, 69]. Anxiety was the presenting psychiatric symptom in 13 % of neurologically symptomatic WD patients [61] and the most prevalent symptom in treated, stable patients [43]. Although it may be isolated, anxiety is associated with depression in the majority of WD patients, as in some other diseases of the BG. Svetel et al. [43] reported correlation between depression and apathy, although apathy may occur in the absence of depression, suggesting that certain frontal-subcortical systems putatively involved in apathy (e.g., anterior cingulate-mesial frontal cortex) might be disrupted in a number of WD patients (24 %).

Schizophrenia-like disorders, catatonia, and hallucinations that can occur at various points in the course of WD are probably no more common in WD than in the general population [17, 41]; still, psychosis and catatonia are more frequent in neurological forms of the disease [61]. Delusions are rare, occur mainly in neurologically affected patients, and predominantly have persecutory structure. Dening and Berrios [17] identified only 2 out of 195 WD patients to express delusions and only one with hallucinations.

Clinical wisdom, based more on random experience collected from case reports than on thorough studies, suggests that diagnosis of WD should be considered in psychotic patients, particularly those with atypical features. Bidaki et al. [70] described a patient with WD presented with psychotic manifestations, who was erroneously treated as schizophrenia for almost 10 years. Stiller et al. [71] suggested some useful clinical cues. For instance, while disturbances of thinking, affect, and motion are typical for schizophrenia, dysarthria is not (i.e., dysarthria may be a red flag). Also, although hypersomnia may occur with major depression, it is more common in organic disorders and has been reported in WD [72].

Previous hypothetical connection of copper metabolism and schizophrenia [73] has been more recently highlighted by the findings that patients with schizophrenia had increased serum levels of copper and ceruloplasmin compared to healthy subjects (23 and 20 %, respectively) [74]. One of the plausible explanations for such a relationship may be a possible effect of increased serum copper on dopaminergic mechanisms through copper-dependent enzymes (monoamine oxidase, dopa-decarboxylase, beta-hydrolase) [75, 76].

Treatment

Wilson's disease, before the introduction of specific therapy considered as inevitably fatal within 5–10 years, is a treatable condition. The mainstay of treatment includes cupriuretic copper chelators (penicillamine and trientine) and copper-depleting agents (zinc and tetrathiomolybdate) (for details on therapy in WD, see [77]). In general, as Pfeiffer [11] stated, "treatment is a lifelong necessity, and compliance must be zealously monitored."

Unfortunately no guidelines for the treatment of psychiatric manifestations in WD have been adopted. Specific de-coppering therapy for WD can be itself beneficial in controlling psychiatric and behavioral manifestations [78], without parallel application of neuroleptic medication [79]. Early studies revealed that incongruous behavior and cognitive impairment improved better than irritability and depression during the specific treatment for WD [17]. Other psychiatric manifestations that were reported to improve on such a therapy include memory deficits and dementia, psychosis, aggression, hypersexuality, and disinhibition [16]. However, as for the neurological symptoms, the bulk of improvement occurs between 6 months and 2 years of adequate copper control [80]. Psychiatric manifestations of WD have a good response after administration of tetrathiomolybdate, without symptomatic exacerbations [81]. However, neurological exacerbations may occur with zinc and trientine [16], but are particularly common with penicillamine (10–50 %) [77], and in addition to neurological worsening, they may induce neuropsychiatric manifestations, such as psychosis [82]. Simply, either disease- or treatment-induced brain overload with copper can generate both neurological and psychiatric involvement [79]. Moreover, these exacerbations may be irreversible, and about 50 % of those who deteriorate never recovered to the level before penicillamine initiation [83].

Sometimes it is necessary to introduce psychotropic agents for control of various psychiatric presentations in parallel with the specific treatment for WD. The main concern is that patients with WD are particularly sensitive to extrapyramidal side effects of antipsychotics [84, 85], hypothetically due to lenticular degeneration in this disease. A patient with WD on antipsychotic drugs was described who developed neuroleptic malignant syndrome [86]. Aschermann et al. [87] suggested that persistent akinetic-rigid side effects of neuroleptic treatment in young patients required diagnostic tests to exclude WD even in "unsuspected" cases. Among atypical antipsychotics applied due to their fewer extrapyramidal side effects, clozapine [88], quetiapine [89], and olanzapine [85] were effective in treating psychiatric manifestations in WD. Caution is necessary, especially with clozapine, since patients with WD are more vulnerable to agranulocytosis due to hypersplenism.

Lithium, as a mood stabilizer, proved useful in WD, even in patients who do not respond to antipsychotics [14]. An advantage is that lithium is not metabolized by the liver and is excreted through the kidneys, but a disadvantage is that it may induce/exacerbate tremor. In a patient whose mania was resistant to quetiapine monotherapy, symptom control was achieved with addition of lithium [90].

Electroconvulsive therapy (ECT) has been used to treat psychiatric symptoms in WD [91–93]. ECT used to treat delusional depression in WD led to 3-min seizures followed by development of mania [91]. Still, Vaishnav and Gandhi [94] suggest that ECT is an encouraging option for the management of acute psychosis in WD, especially in patients who develop extrapyramidal symptoms along with psychosis.

Reports on the impact of liver transplantation on psychiatric symptoms were not consistent and varied from case reports of improvement [78, 95], through observation that behavioral and personality disorders remained unaffected, to severe worsening of psychiatric problems after transplantation [96]. In a series of 55 WD patients who received orthotopic liver transplantation (OLT), four out of seven patients who had neuropsychiatric manifestations improved after transplantation [97]. Also, in an analysis of 37 transplanted patients, Medici et al. [98] found that patients with neuropsychiatric symptoms had a significantly shorter survival even though neurological symptoms improved after the transplantation. Therefore, OLT cannot be recommended for patients with WD associated with psychiatric manifestations in the absence of liver disease [14]. Moreover, Ala et al. [7] stated that among other contraindications, WD patients with severe psychiatric disease with suicidal ideations are also not suitable candidates for transplantation under any circumstances.

Psychiatric manifestations in WD are not rare and account for an important part of the clinical presentation. They may occur isolated, not associated with neurological and hepatic manifestations, leading to delays in appropriate treatment or appropriate diagnosis. Since they adversely affect the QoL, it is necessary to be aware of their clinical heterogeneity in order to maintain the necessary level of suspicion to be able to promptly establish the diagnosis of WD and initiate adequate treatment accordingly. Unfortunately, no evidence-based guidelines for the treatment of psychiatric manifestations in WD have yet been proposed.

References

1. Bull PC, Thomas GR, Rommens JM, Forbes JR, Cox DW. The Wilson disease gene is a putative copper transporting P-type ATPase similar to the Menkes gene. Nat Genet. 1993;5:327–37.
2. Petrukhin K, Fischer SG, Pirastu M, et al. Mapping, cloning and genetic characterization of the region containing the Wilson disease gene. Nat Genet. 1993;5:338–43.
3. Tanzi RE, Petrukhin K, Chernov I, et al. The Wilson disease gene is a copper transporting P-type ATPase with homology to the Menkes gene. Nat Genet. 1993;5:344–50.
4. Wilson SAK. Progressive lenticular degeneration: a familial nervous disease associated with cirrhosis of the liver. Brain. 1912;34:295–509.
5. Rumpel A. Uber das Wesen und die Bedeutung der Leberveraderungen und der Pigmentierunen bei den damit verbundenen Fallen von Pseudosklerose, zugleich ein Beitrag zur Lehre von der Pseudosklerose (Westphal-Strumpell). Dtsch Z Nervenheilkd. 1913;49:54–73.
6. Scheinberg IH, Sternlieb I. Wilson's disease. Major Probl Int Med. 1984;23:1–24.
7. Ala A, Walker AP, Ashkan K, Dooley JS, Schilsky ML. Wilson's disease. Lancet. 2007; 369:397–408.
8. Roberts EA, Schilsky ML. A practise guideline on Wilson disease. Hepatology. 2003;37:1475–92.

9. Senzolo M, Loreno M, Fagiuoli S, et al. Different neurological outcome of liver transplantation for Wilson's disease in two homozygotic twins. Clin Neurol Neurosurg. 2007;109:71–5.
10. Lorincz MT. Neurologic Wilson's disease. Ann N Y Acad Sci. 2010;1184:173–87.
11. Pfeiffer RF. Wilson's disease. Semm Neurol. 2007;27:123–32.
12. Kumar N. Wilson disease. In: Galvez-Jimenez N, Tuite P, editors. Uncommon causes of movement disorders. Cambridge: Cambridge University Press; 2011. p. 46–61.
13. Fahn S, Jankovic J, Hallett M. Principles and practice of movement disorders. 2nd ed. Edinburgh: Elsevier Sauders; 2011. p. 507–12.
14. Zimbrean PC, Schilsky ML. Psychiatric aspects of Wilson disease: a review. Gen Hosp Psychiatry. 2014;36:53–62.
15. Prashanth LK, Taly AB, Sinha S, Arunodaya GR, Swamy HS. Wilson's disease: diagnostic errors and clinical implications. J Neurol Neurosurg Psychiatry. 2004;75:907–9.
16. Lauterbach EC, Cummings JL, Duffy J, et al. Neuropsychiatric correlates and treatment of lenticulostriatal diseases: a review of the literature and overview of research opportunities in Huntington's, Wilson's, and Fahr's disease. J Neuropsychiatry Clin Neurosci. 1998;10:249–66.
17. Dening TR, Berrios GE. Wilson's disease: psychiatric symptoms in 195 cases. Arch Gen Psychiatry. 1989;46:1126–34.
18. Akil M, Brewer GJ. Psychiatric and behavioral abnormalities in Wilson's disease. Adv Neurol. 1995;65:171–8.
19. Lorincz MT. Recognition and treatment of neurologic Wilson's disease. Semin Neurol. 2012;32:538–43.
20. Gronlund J, Nanto-Salonen K, Venetoklis J, Holmberg RL, Heinonen A, Stahlberg MR. Poor cognitive development and abdominal pain: Wilson's disease. Scand J Gastroenterol. 2006;41:361–4.
21. Brewer GJ. Recognition, diagnosis, and management of Wilson's disease. Proc Soc Exp Biol Med. 2000;223:39–46.
22. Akil M, Schwartz JA, Dutchak D, et al. The psychiatric presentations of Wilson's disease. J Neuropsychiatry Clin Neurosci. 1991;3:377–82.
23. Cummings JL. Subcortical dementia. Neuropsychology, neuropsychiatry, and pathophysiology. Br J Psychiatry. 1986;149:682–97.
24. Medalia A, Isaacs-Globerman K, Scheinberg H. Neuropsychological impairment in Wilson's disease. Arch Neurol. 1988;45:502–4.
25. Lang C. Wilson's disease: a dementing condition? J Clin Exp Neuropsychol. 1989;14:569–70.
26. Litman E, Medalia A, Semior G, Scheinberg IH. Rate of information processing in patients with Wilson's disease. J Neuropsychiatry Clin Neurosci. 1995;7:68–71.
27. Medalia A, Galynker I, Scheinberg H. The interaction of motor, memory, and emotional dysfunction in Wilson's disease. Biol Psychiatry. 1992;31:823–6.
28. Lang C, Muller D, Claus D, Druschky KF. Neuropsychological findings in treated Wilson's disease. Acta Neurol Scand. 1990;81:75–81.
29. Knehr CA, Bearn AG. Psychological impairment in Wilson's disease. J Nerv Ment Disord. 1956;156:251–5.
30. Oder W, Prayer L, Bremm G, Spatt J. Wilson's disease: evidence of subgroups derived from clinical findings and brain lesions. Neurology. 1993;43:120–4.
31. Hegde S, Sinha S, Rao SL, Taly AB. Cognitive profile and structural findings in Wilson's disease: a neuropsychological and MRI-based study. Neurol India. 2010;58:708–13.
32. Frota NAF, Barbosa ER, Porto CS, et al. Cognitive impairment and magnetic resonance imaging correlations in Wilson's disease. Acta Neurol Scand. 2013;127:391–8.
33. Ma H, Ly X, Han Y, et al. Decision-making impairments in patients with Wilson's disease. J Clin Exp Neuropsychol. 2013;35:472–9.
34. Wenisch E, De Tassigny A, Trocello JM, Beretti J, Girardot-Tinant N, Woimant F. Cognitive profile in Wilson's disease: a case series of 31 patients. Rev Neurol (Paris). 2013;169:944–9.
35. Portala K, Levander S, Westermark K, Ekselius L, von Knorring L. Pattern of neuropsychological deficits in patients with treated Wilson's disease. Eur Arch Psychiatry Clin Neurosci. 2001;251:362–8.

36. Seniow J, Bak T, Gajda J, Poniatowska R, Czlonkowska A. Cognitive functioning in neurologically symptomatic and asymptomatic forms of Wilson's disease. Mov Disord. 2002;17:1077–83.
37. Jadav R, Saini J, Sinha S, Bagepally B, Rao S, Taly AB. Diffusion tensor imaging (DTI) and its clinical correlates in drug naive Wilson's disease. Metab Brain Dis. 2013;28:455–62.
38. Svetel M, Pekmezović T, Tomić A, et al. Quality of life in patients with treated and clinically stable Wilson's disease. Mov Disord. 2011;26:1503–8.
39. Hach B, Hartung ML. Wirkung des Penicillamins auf die psychopathologischen Veranderungen der hepatozerebralen degeneration. Nervenarzt. 1979;50:115–20.
40. Rosselli M, Lorenzana P, Rosselli A, Vergara I. Wilson's disease, a reversible dementia: case report. J Clin Exp Neuropsychol. 1987;9:399–406.
41. Oder W, Grimm G, Kollegger H, Ferenci P, Schneider B, Deecke L. Neurological and neuropsychiatric spectrum of Wilson's disease: a prospective study of 45 cases. J Neurol. 1991;238:281–7.
42. Ozer O, Selimoglu MA. Self-injury behavior in an adolescent with Wilson's disease. Eur Child Adolesc Psychiatry. 2009;18:761–2.
43. Svetel M, Potrebić A, Pekmezović A, et al. Neuropsychiatric aspects of treated Wilson's disease. Parkinsonism Relat Disord. 2009;15:772–5.
44. Volpe FM, Tavares A. Cyproterone for hypersexuality in a psychotic patient with Wilson's disease. Prog Neuropsychopharmacol Biol Psychiatry. 2008;32:1994–5.
45. Portala K, Westermark K, Ekselius L, von Knorring L. Personality traits in treated Wilson's disease determined by means of the Karolinska Scales of Personality (KSP). Eur Psychiatry. 2001;16:362–71.
46. Portala K, Westermark K, van Knorring L, Ekselius L. Psychopathology in treated Wilson's disease determined by means of CPRS expert and self-ratings. Acta Psychiatr Scand. 2000;101:104–9.
47. Portala K, Waldenstrom E, van Knorring L, Westermark K. Psychopathology and personality traits in patients with treated Wilson's disease grouped according to gene mutations. Ups J Med Sci. 2008;113:79–94.
48. Horoupian DS, Sternlieb I, Scheinberg IH. Neuropathological findings in penicillamine-treated patients with Wilson's disease. Clin Neuropathol. 1988;7:62–7.
49. Nyberg P, Gottfries C-G, Holmgren G, Persson S, Roos B-E, Winblad B. Advanced catecholaminergic disturbances in the brain in case of Wilson's disease. Acta Neurol Scand. 1982;65:71–5.
50. Goldstein NP, Ewert JC, Randall RV, Gross JB. Psychiatric aspects of Wilson's disease (hepatolenticular degeneration): results of psychometric tests during long-term therapy. Am J Psychiatry. 1968;124:1155–61.
51. Brewer GJ. Neurologically presenting Wilson's disease: epidemiology, pathophysiology and treatment. CNS Drugs. 2005;19:185–92.
52. Taly AB, Meenakshi-Sundaram S, Sinha S, Swamy HS, Arunodaya GR. Wilson's disease: description of 282 patients evaluated over 3 decades. Medicine (Baltimore). 2007;86:112–21.
53. Soltanzadeh A, Soltanzadeh P, Nafissi S, Ghorbani A, Sikaroodi H, Lotfi J. Wilson's disease: a great masquerader. Eur Neurol. 2007;57:80–5.
54. Lin JJ, Lin KL, Wang HS, Wong MC. Psychological presentations without hepatic involvement in Wilson's disease. Pediatr Neurol. 2006;35:284–6.
55. Nayak RB, Shetageri VN, Bhogale GS, Patil NM, Chate SS, Chatopadhyay S. Catatonia: a rare presenting symptom of Wilson's disease. J Neuropsychiatry Clin Neurosci. 2012;24:E34–5.
56. Duggal HS, Nizamie SH. Wilson's disease presenting with obsessive-compulsive disorder. Indian J Psychiatry. 2000;42:312–6.
57. Spyridi S, Diakogiannis I, Michaelides M, Sokolaki S, Iacovides A, Kaprinis G. Delusional disorder and alcohol abuse in a patient with Wilson's disease. Gen Hosp Psychiatry. 2008;30:585–6.
58. Walshe JM, Yealland M. Wilson's disease: the problem of delayed diagnosis. J Neurol Neurosurg Psychiatry. 1992;55:692–6.
59. Srinivas K, Sinha S, Taly AB, et al. Dominant psychiatric manifestations in Wilson's disease: a diagnostic and therapeutic challenge. J Neurol Sci. 2008;266:104–8.
60. Rathbun JK. Neuropsychological aspects of Wilson's disease. Int J Neurosci. 1996;85(3–4):221–9.

61. Brewer GJ, Yuzbasiyan-Gurkan V. Wilson's disease. Medicine (Baltimore). 1992;71:139–64.
62. Hesse S, Barthel H, Hermann W, et al. Regional serotonin transporter availability and depression are correlated in Wilson's disease. J Neural Transm. 2003;110:923–33.
63. Shanmugiah A, Sinha S, Taly AB, et al. Psychiatric manifestations in Wilson's disease: cross-sectional analysis. J Neuropsychiatry Clin Neurosci. 2008;20:81–5.
64. Costa MG, Sorbello O, Moro MF, et al. Bipolar disorders and Wilson's disease. BMC Psychiatry. 2012;12:52.
65. Walshe JM. Cause of death in Wilson's disease. Mov Disord. 2007;22:2216–20.
66. Czlonkowska A, Tarnacka B, Litwin T, Gajela J, Rodo M. Wilson's disease-cause of mortality in 164 patients during 1992–2003 observation period. J Neurol. 2005;252:698–703.
67. Svetel M, Pekmezović T, Petrović I, et al. Long-term outcome in Serbian patients with Wilson's disease. Eur J Neurol. 2009;16:852–7.
68. Eggers B, Hermann W, Barthel H, Sabri O, Wagner A, Hesse S. The degree of depression in Hamilton rating scale is correlated with the density of presynaptic serotonin transporters in 23 patients with Wilson's disease. J Neurol. 2003;250:576–80.
69. Chien HF, Deguti MM, Cancado E, Azevedo RS, Scaff M, Barbosa ER. Neurological manifestations in Wilson's disease: report of 119 cases. Mov Disord. 2006;21:2192–6.
70. Bidaki R, Zarei M, Mahdy Mirhosseini SM, et al. Mismanagement of Wilson's disease as psychotic disorder. Adv Biomed Res. 2012;1:61.
71. Stiller P, Kassubek J, Schonfeldt-Lecuona C, Connemann BJ. Wilson's disease in psychiatric patients. Psychiatry Clin Neurosci. 2002;56:649.
72. Firneisz G, Szalay F, Halasz P, Komoly S. Hypersomnia in Wilson's disease: an unusual symptom in an unusual case. Acta Neurol Scand. 2000;101:286–8.
73. Bowman MB, Lewis MS. The copper hypothesis of schizophrenia: a review. Neurosci Biobehav Rev. 1982;6:321–8.
74. Jeon B, Kim JM, Jeong JM, et al. Dopamine transporter imaging with [^{123}I]-beta-CIT demonstrates presynaptic nigrostriatal dopaminergic damage in Wilson's disease. J Neurol Neurosurg Psychiatry. 1998;65:60–4.
75. Wolf TL, Kotun J, Meador-Woodruff JH. Plasma copper, iron, ceruloplasmin and ferroxidase activity in schizophrenia. Schizophr Res. 2006;86:167–71.
76. Herring NK, Konradi C. Myelin, copper, and the cuprizone model of schizophrenia. Front Biosci. 2011;3:23–40.
77. Roberts EA, Schilsky ML. Diagnosis and treatment of Wilson's disease: a Wilson's disease: an update. Hepatology. 2008;47:2089–111.
78. Sorbello O, Riccio D, Sini M, Carta M, Demelia L. Resolved psychosis after liver transplantation in a patient with Wilson's disease. Clin Pract Epidemiol Ment Health. 2011;7:182–4.
79. Loudianos G, Gitlin JD. Wilson's disease: Wilson's disease. Semm Liver Dis. 2000;20:353–64.
80. Brewer GJ. Wilson's disease: a clinician's guide to recognition, diagnosis, and management. Boston: Kluwer; 2001.
81. Brewer GJ, Johnson V, Dick RD, Kluin KJ, Fink JK, Brunberg JA. Treatment of Wilson's disease with ammonium tetrathiomolybdate. II Initial therapy in 33 neurologically affected patients and follow-up with zinc therapy. Arch Neurol. 1996;53:1017–25.
82. McDonald JV, Lake CR. Psychosis in an adolescent patient with Wilson's disease: effects of chelation therapy. Psychosom Med. 1995;57:202–4.
83. Brewer GJ, Terry CA, Aisen AM, Hill GM. Worsening of neurologic syndrome in patients with Wilson's disease with initial penicillamine therapy. Arch Neurol. 1987;44:490–3.
84. Hoogenraad TU. Wilson's disease. London: WB Saunders; 1996.
85. Chroni E, Lekka NP, Tsibri E, et al. Acute progressive akinetic-rigid syndrome induced by neuroleptics in a case of Wilson's disease. J Neuropsychiatry Clin Neurosci. 2001;13:531–2.
86. Kontaxakis V, Stefanis C, Markidis M, et al. Neuroleptic malignant syndrome in a patient with Wilson's disease. J Neurol Neurosurg Psychiatry. 1988;51:1001–2.
87. Aschermann Z, Szalay F, Schmidt E, Komoly S, Illes Z. Persistent akinetic-rigid side effects of neuroleptics may indicate Wilson's disease. Ideggyogy Sz. 2007;30:404–5.

88. Krim E, Barroso B. Psychiatric disorders treated with clozapine in a patient with Wilson's disease. J Neuropsychiatry Clin Neurosci. 2001;13:521–32.
89. Chakor RT, Santhosh NS. Severe neuropsychiatric presentation of Wilson's disease. Indian J Psychiatry. 2011;53:170–1.
90. Kulaksizoglu IB, Polat A. Quetiapine for mania with Wilson's disease. Psychosomatics. 2003;44:438–9.
91. Negro Jr PJ, Louza Neto MR. Results of ECT for a case of depression in Wilson's disease. J Neuropsychiatry Clin Neurosci. 1995;7:384.
92. Rodrigues AC, Dalgalarrondo P, Banzato CE. Successful ECT in a patient with a psychiatric presentation of Wilson's disease. J ECT. 2004;20:55.
93. Sahoo MK, Avasthi A, Sahoo M, Modi M, Biswas P. Psychiatric manifestations of Wilson's disease and treatment with electroconvulsive therapy. Indian J Psychiatry. 2010;52:66–8.
94. Vaishnav P, Gandhi HA. Electroconvulsive therapy in psychiatric manifestations in Wilson's disease. Indian J Psychiatry. 2013;35:206–8.
95. Geissler I, Heinemann K, Rohm S, Hauss J, Lamesch P. Liver transplantation for hepatic and neurological Wilson's disease. Transplant Proc. 2003;35:1445–6.
96. Kassam N, Witt N, Kneteman N, Bain VG. Liver transplantation for neuropsychiatric Wilson's disease. Can J Gastroenterol. 1998;12:65–8.
97. Schilsky MI, Scheinberg IH, Sternlieb I. Liver transplantation for Wilson's disease: indications and outcome. Hepatology. 1994;19:583–7.
98. Medici V, Mirante VG, Fassati LR, et al. Liver transplantation for Wilson's disease: the burden of neurological and psychiatric disorders. Liver Transplant. 2005;11:1056–63.

Chapter 13
Ataxia

Ludger Schöls and Thomas Klockgether

Classification and Genetics of Ataxia

Ataxia is characterized by lack of precision in metric and power of voluntary movements. This leads to increased variability in repetitive movements and impaired coordination. In everyday life, ataxia primarily manifests as unsteadiness of gait and stance, impaired dexterity, slurred speech, and diplopia. Although involvement of afferent somatosensory pathways and vestibular system contributes to ataxia, dysfunction of the cerebellum is the main cause.

According to causative factors, ataxias are divided into primary and secondary ataxias, the latter arising from malformation, vascular, inflammatory, immune-mediated, neoplastic, physical, or toxic causes. This chapter focuses on primary ataxias including hereditary and sporadic degenerative ataxias.

Hereditary ataxias are differentiated according to their mode of inheritance into autosomal recessive ataxias; autosomal dominant ataxias, also named spinocerebellar ataxias (SCAs); and X-linked ataxias.

In autosomal recessive ataxias, there is no generally accepted systematic disease nomenclature. Autosomal recessive ataxias are variably named according to the first describer, characteristic clinical features, or the responsible gene. The most common recessive ataxia in the Western world is Friedreich's ataxia (FRDA). Table 13.1 gives a list of the most relevant recessive ataxias.

L. Schöls, MD
Department of Neurology, University Hospital Tübingen,
Hoppe-Seyler Str. 3, Tübingen 72076, Germany
e-mail: ludger.schoels@uni-tuebingen.de

T. Klockgether, MD (✉)
Department of Neurology, University Hospital Bonn,
Sigmund-Freud-Str. 25, Bonn 53105, Germany
e-mail: klockgether@uni-bonn.de; Thomas.Klockgether@ukb.uni-bonn.de

H. Reichmann (ed.), *Neuropsychiatric Symptoms of Movement Disorders*,
Neuropsychiatric Symptoms of Neurological Disease,
DOI 10.1007/978-3-319-09537-0_13

Table 13.1 Autosomal recessive ataxias

Subtype	Gene	Age of onset (years)	Characteristic features	Cognitive deficits
Friedreich's ataxia	FXN	7–25 (extremes: 2–70)	Afferent ataxia, sensory neuropathy, corticospinal tract affection, variable scoliosis, cardiomyopathy, diabetes	Focal deficits
Ataxia with vitamin E deficiency	TTPA	2–50	Similar to Friedreich's ataxia, retinitis pigmentosa, head tremor	Unknown
Ataxia telangiectasia (AT)	ATM	<5 in most cases	Cerebellar ataxia and atrophy, chorea, dystonia, oculocephalic dissociation, telangiectasias, susceptibility to infections and cancer	Focal deficits
Ataxia with oculomotor apraxia type 1 (AOA1)	APTX	1–20	Cerebellar ataxia and atrophy, neuropathy, variable oculocephalic dissociation, chorea, dystonia	Frequent
Ataxia with oculomotor apraxia type 2 (AOA2)	SETX	7–25	Cerebellar ataxia and atrophy, neuropathy, variable oculocephalic dissociation	Unknown
Sensory ataxic neuropathy, dysarthria, and ophthalmoparesis (SANDO)	POLG1	Up to 50	Cerebellar and afferent ataxia, ophthalmoplegia, neuropathy, variable myoclonus and epilepsy	Frequent
Infantile-onset spinocerebellar ataxia (IOSCA)	C10orf2	Infancy	Ataxia, ophthalmoplegia, sensory neuropathy, variable optic atrophy, athetosis, pyramidal signs	Mental retardation
Cayman cerebellar ataxia	ATCAY	Infancy	Prominent but nonprogressive cerebellar dysfunction	Mental retardation
Autosomal recessive spastic ataxia of Charlevoix-Saguenay (ARSACS)	SACS	<20	Spasticity and cerebellar ataxia, neuropathy, MRI: T2-hypointense stripes of the central pons	Unknown
Autosomal recessive ataxia with SYNE1 mutations	SYNE1	17–46	Cerebellar ataxia and atrophy, variable spasticity	None

(continued)

Table 13.1 (continued)

Subtype	Gene	Age of onset (years)	Characteristic features	Cognitive deficits
Ataxia with coenzyme Q10 deficiency	ADCK3	1–11	Ataxia, variable myoclonus, epilepsy, stroke-like condition, exercise intolerance	Frequent
Cerebrotendinous xanthomatosis	CYP27A1	Up to 45	Ataxia, spasticity, diarrhea, early cataracts, tendon xanthomas	Dementia
Niemann-Pick type C	NPC1+2	2–30	Cerebellar ataxia, vertical supranuclear palsy, variable dystonia, splenomegaly	Dementia
GM2 gangliosidosis Tay-Sachs	HEXA	15–45	Cerebellar ataxia and atrophy, variable spasticity, dystonia, epilepsy	Dementia, psychosis
Congenital disorder of glycosylation type 1A	PMM2	Infancy	Cerebellar ataxia, neuropathy, retinitis pigmentosa	Mental retardation

In autosomal dominant cerebellar ataxias, genetic subtypes are numbered according to the order of first descriptions under the acronym SCA for spinocerebellar ataxia. Currently, more than 30 SCAs are known. The most common X-linked ataxia is the fragile X-associated tremor/ataxia syndrome (FXTAS).

Sporadic degenerative ataxias are characterized by sporadic occurrence of progressive ataxia that is not secondary to one of the etiologies listed above and for which no genetic cause could be established. The most common subtype is multiple system atrophy (MSA).

For all ataxias, variable age of onset and phenotypic variability have been described, and the full spectrum of associated phenotypes still remains to be discovered. This is especially true for neuropsychiatric manifestations of ataxias as they are much less systematically explored than motor affection.

The Cerebellar Cognitive-Affective Syndrome

The prominent clinical feature of ataxias is progressively impaired precision in metric and power of voluntary movements due to cerebellar degeneration. The motor function of the cerebellum is enabled by its dense connections with other parts of the nervous system that are involved in motor control. Although the cerebellar cortex has a remarkably homogeneous microanatomical structure, there is evidence for subdivision of the cerebellar cortex into functionally distinct compartments that emerge as a consequence of specific afferent and efferent connections.

Vestibular afferents strongly project to the flocculonodular lobe, spinal afferents to anterior and posterior parts of the vermis and the paravermal hemispheric regions of the anterior lobe, and cortical afferents via the pontine nuclei to the cerebellar hemispheres. With respect to efferent connections, the cerebellar cortex is divided into three sagittal zones, the vermis projecting via the fastigial nucleus to brainstem and spinal targets, an intermediate zone projecting via the interposed nucleus to the red nucleus and thalamus, and a lateral zone projecting via the dentate nucleus to the thalamus. In addition, the flocculonodular lobe projects to the vestibular nuclei.

As a consequence of these anatomical connections, lesions of the flocculonodular lobe and caudal vermis typically result in truncal and gait ataxia, lesions of the rostral vermis in gait ataxia, and hemispheric lesions in limb ataxia. Similar symptoms may occur as a result of lesions in the cerebellar nuclei and in different anatomical structures and tracts that project to the cerebellar compartments or are targets of them.

The unique anatomy of the cerebellar cortex characterized by a uniform microarchitecture and a complex but highly precise input-output organization suggests that the differential functions of the various cerebellar cortical subregions are due to uniform operations performed by the cerebellar cortex on diverse input information. Thus, the specific functions result from specific anatomical connections rather than from differential actions of these subregions. The precise nature of the operations performed by the cerebellum has not yet been finally defined. Currently preferred feedforward models of cerebellar function hypothesize that the cerebellum has internal experience-based models of movements that are permanently compared with the intended and actually performed movements. Error signals detected by the inferior olives are sent to the cerebellar cortex via the climbing fiber system and lead to modification of intended and ongoing movements. Cerebellar action thus results in an optimization of movements by dampening oscillations, defining the optimal metrics of movements, and coordinating different body parts.

In their 1998 landmark paper, Schmahmann and Sherman, based on clinical observations on 20 patients with acute or chronic lesion confined to the cerebellum, defined the cognitive-affective cerebellar syndrome. This syndrome is characterized by (1) disturbances of executive function, which includes deficient planning, set-shifting, abstract reasoning, working memory, and decreased verbal fluency; (2) impaired spatial cognition, including visual-spatial disorganization and impaired visual-spatial memory; (3) personality change characterized by flattening or blunting of affect and disinhibited or inappropriate behavior; and (4) linguistic difficulties, including dysprosodia, agrammatism, and mild anomia [1].

The anatomical substrate of the cognitive-affective function of the cerebellum is its connections with nonmotor areas of the cerebral cortex. As outlined above, each lobule of the cerebellar hemispheres receives cortical input via the pontine nuclei and projects back to the cerebral cortex via the dentate nucleus and thalamus. Thus, the cerebrocerebellar interactions are organized as multiple, parallel closed-loop circuits. Recent anatomical studies demonstrate that the output of the cerebellum targets not only motor cortical areas, as was previously assumed, but also nonmotor cortical areas in the prefrontal and posterior parietal cortex that are involved in cognitive functions. The cerebellum is thus in a position to permanently monitor, update, and optimize activity of the frontal and posterior parietal cortex, as it is known to do for the motor cortex [2].

Friedreich's Ataxia (FRDA)

Disease Definition

Friedreich's ataxia (FRDA) is the most frequent type of ataxia in the Western world with a prevalence of about 1/50,000 but is rare in Japan and sub-Saharan Africa. Frequency of mutation carriers is estimated to be about 1:90 in Germany [3].

Already the original description by Nikolaus Friedreich 150 years ago was impressively detailed and comprehensive: Progressive ataxia is typically starting around puberty. In typical cases, muscle stretch reflexes are abolished due to sensory axonal neuropathy, and Babinski's sign is positive indicating corticospinal tract involvement leading to slowing of movements and a central distribution of weakness especially of hip abduction and foot dorsiflexion. Dysarthria may develop only later in the disease and is most likely due to affection of the dentate nucleus of the cerebellum in combination with sensory deficits [4, 5]. After discovery of the disease-causing gene and broad availability of genetic diagnostics, the spectrum of the FRDA phenotype became clear to include also late-onset cases with onset up to 40 years and in rare cases even up to 70 years. All FRDA patients present with predominantly afferent ataxia with positive Romberg's sign, pyramidal tract affection, and at most mild cerebellar atrophy on MRI [6, 7]. Especially in its early-onset forms, FRDA is frequently associated with cardiomyopathy with thickening of the interventricular septum and diabetes that frequently requires administration of insulin.

Genetically, FRDA is caused by the expansion of a GAA trinucleotide repeat in intron 1 of the *FXN gene* [8]. More than 96 % of patients are homozygous for such a repeat expansion, and the remaining 4 % carry an expansion on one allele and a point mutation on the other. The expansion impairs translation and consecutively leads to reduced levels of the *FXN* gene product frataxin. Residual frataxin levels depend on the repeat length with larger repeats resulting in smaller amounts of protein and consecutively earlier onset and more severe course of disease.

The functional role of frataxin is still not fully understood. Frataxin is a mitochondrial protein that is involved in iron-sulfur cluster synthesis. As such, it is essential for the function of respiratory chain complexes I–III. Oxidative stress due to impaired handling of intramitochondrial iron is thought to play a role in pathogenesis, but results from animal models as well as measurements in human samples were equivocal.

From a pathological point of view, there is degeneration of the dorsal columns and corticospinal tracts in the spinal cord as well as degeneration of the dentate nucleus in the cerebellum. An increase of iron content in the dentate nucleus has been proposed from early MRI studies but has not been confirmed by detailed neuropathological studies and recent high-tesla MRI [9, 10].

Neuropsychiatric Symptoms

The cognitive profile in ataxias is difficult to assess as many tests may be confounded by impaired motor function and cognitive capacities have rarely been studied systematically in FRDA. In a series of 13 FRDA patients with a mean age of 23.7 and at average 9.7 years at school, Mantovan and colleagues found a global IQ of 93 ± 11 using the Wechsler Intelligence Scale (revised). The intelligence profile of FRDA patients was characterized by concrete thinking and poor capacity in concept formation and visuospatial reasoning. Additionally, FRDA patients showed reduced speed of information processing, and the learning effect seen in controls was notably absent in patients with FRDA [11].

In a larger series of 36 Spanish patients, Nieto and colleagues confirmed that FRDA patients have no global cognitive impairment and do not develop frank dementia. In the Mini-Mental Status Examination (MMSE), patients reached 28.8 ± 1.3 out of 30 points. However, despite absence of dementia, focal neuropsychological deficits have been observed indicative of executive problems and parietotemporal dysfunction. Patients showed decreased mental speed, problems in conceptual thinking, diminished verbal fluency, deficits in acquisition of verbal information, visuoperceptive and visuoconstructive problems, and poor action naming [12].

The influence of age of onset on cognitive performance in FRDA has been studied in 29 patients with early-onset (<25 years of age) FRDA in comparison to 7 patients with late-onset forms (25–39 years of age). Both patient groups shared slowed motor processing speed and impaired conceptual thinking and verbal fluency. However, only early-onset patients showed a diminished cognitive processing speed and impaired visuoperceptive and visuoconstructive abilities [13].

Since the dentate nucleus is the only severely affected part of the cerebellum in FRDA, it may be speculated that the cognitive deficits in FRDA represent the part of the cerebellar cognitive syndrome that is more or less specifically mediated by defects of the dentate nucleus. However, an alternative explanation for cognitive deficits in FRDA may derive from cerebral atrophy which has recently been reported in FRDA patients [14, 15].

Concerning depression, scores in the Beck Depression Inventory (BDI) were only slightly higher in a group of 36 patients with Friedreich's ataxia than in controls [11]. However, in another series of 22 FRDA patients, about one third (8/22) fulfilled the criteria of major depression [16]. There was no correlation between BDI score and age of onset, age of examination, severity of ataxia, and duration of disease. This imaging study suggests that depression in FRDA is not a simply reactive phenomenon but rather associated to structural abnormalities with reduction of gray matter volume in the depressive group. Regression analyses found BDI scores to be inversely correlated with gray matter volume at the right superior frontal gyrus. A recent approach using diffusion tensor imaging observed significant changes in diffusivity characteristics in the dentatothalamic and thalamocortical tracts, suggesting extensive white matter degeneration in FRDA. Correlation of white matter changes in the dentatorubral tract with the cognitive assessment suggested that this tract is an important contributor to cognitive disturbances in FRDA [17].

Other Recessive Ataxias

Disease Definition

In autosomal recessive forms of ataxia, the disease manifests in only one generation, whereas the parents are healthy. Therefore, especially in smaller families, recessive ataxias frequently occur as sporadic cases with a negative family history. Early onset (<30 years of age) and consanguineous parents are suggestive of recessive ataxias but not obligatory factors. Late-onset variants are increasingly recognized for many subtypes.

Due to rapid progress in genetic characterization, many new genes for recessive ataxias have been described during the last few years [18]. At present, more than 30 genotypes are defined and can be increasingly differentiated with improved genetic techniques which allow parallel sequencing of virtually all ataxia genes in a similar time frame and at approximately the same costs as one single gene before. All of these genotypes appear to be extremely rare (<1/100,000), but systematic studies of frequency distribution of recessive ataxias are widely missing [19]. Among the relatively more frequent forms are ataxia telangiectasia (AT), ataxia with oculomotor apraxia type 1 (AOA1) and type 2 (AOA2), autosomal recessive spastic ataxia of Charlevoix-Saguenay (ARSACS), and ataxia with polymerase gamma mutations (POLG) [20] (See Table 13.1).

The classification of recessive ataxias is frequently revised due to new genes discovered. Some mutations are found in genes involved in metabolic pathways like alpha-tocopherol transfer protein (TTPA) responsible for ataxia with primary vitamin E deficiency, microsomal triglyceride transfer protein (MTP) causing abetalipoproteinemia, and aarF domain-containing kinase 3 (ADCK3) mutations resulting in ataxia with coenzyme Q10 deficiency. Whereas these diseases are classified as autosomal recessive ataxia genes, other autosomal recessive genes causing ataxia are counted as hereditary neurometabolic disorders like cerebrotendinous xanthomatosis (CTX), Niemann-Pick disease type C (NPC), Tay-Sachs disease (GM2 gangliosidosis type 1), metachromatic leukodystrophy (MLD), Krabbe disease (globoid cell leukodystrophy), and congenital disorder of glycosylation type Ia (CDG1a).

Neuropsychiatric Symptoms

Neuropsychiatric symptoms have been reported especially in autosomal recessive ataxias due to hereditary neurometabolic disorders like Tay-Sachs disease, NPC, MLD, Krabbe, CTX, and CDG1 [21]. These disorders show a highly variable phenotype not only in age of onset but also in neuropsychiatric manifestations. For example, CDG1a may manifest as infantile-onset multisystemic disease with axial hypotonia, developmental delay, and impaired growth. Neurologic manifestations include psychomotor retardation and cerebellar hypoplasia in infancy followed by neuropathy and retinitis pigmentosa in childhood. The childhood form of CDG1a starts between age 3 and 10 years and is characterized by ataxia, severely delayed language and motor development, inability to walk, and intellectual disability with IQ 40–70. In the adult variant of CDG1a, intellectual ability is stable [22].

Neuropsychiatric symptoms are frequent in neurometabolic ataxias. Correspondingly, neurometabolic diseases are frequently found as the cause of ataxia in patients who present with the combination of ataxia and cognitive decline and/or psychiatric manifestations. A screen for neurometabolic disorders in a series of 105 patients with cryptic adult-onset ataxia found underlying neurometabolic diseases in six patients including two with NPC, one Tay-Sachs, one CTX, one MLD, and one LBSL. Interestingly, all but the LBSL case had cognitive deficits and three had psychiatric manifestations like paranoid-hallucinatory psychosis. In the subgroup of patients with ataxia in combination with cognitive deficits and psychiatric manifestations, a neurometabolic cause was found in 50 % [23].

Among the "classical" autosomal recessive ataxias, neuropsychological deficits are reported to be rather frequent in AOA1 [24], IOSCA, POLG [25, 26], and early childhood cases of Q10 deficiency/ADCK3 [27], but larger series and systematic studies assessing neuropsychiatric symptoms are missing. In ataxia telangiectasia, mild to moderate intellectual impairment has been described with focal neuropsychological deficits in attention, (non)verbal memory, and verbal fluency [28]. In ARSACS, IQ levels tend to be in the lower range of normal, but most affected individuals are able to cope well with daily living tasks and cognitive skills tend to be preserved into late adult life [29].

Fragile X-Associated Tremor/Ataxia Syndrome (FXTAS)

Disease Definition

The fragile X-associated tremor/ataxia syndrome (FXTAS) mostly manifests among male carriers of a so-called premutation in the *fragile X mental retardation 1 (FMR1) gene*. The premutation consists of a trinucleotide repeat expansion of 55–200 CGG triplets in the 5′UTR of *FMR1*. In comparison, normal alleles in healthy controls carry up to 54 CGG triplets, and so-called full mutations have >200 CGG repeats and cause fragile X syndrome, the most common cause of inherited mental retardation in boys. The premutation is unstable during maternal meiosis with a tendency to expand further to a full mutation. Consequently, female carriers of a premutation are at risk of having children with fragile X syndrome.

Patients with FXTAS primarily present with cerebellar ataxia and tremor, especially intention tremor but also action or rest tremor. Other common symptoms include cognitive decline, parkinsonism, and peripheral neuropathy. On MRI, increased signals in the middle cerebellar peduncle and in the deep white matter of the cerebellum and also the cerebrum are characteristic but not specific findings in FXTAS.

FXTAS shows age-related penetrance, but not all older male carriers become symptomatic. Penetrance of ataxia and tremor is estimated to be 17 % with 50–59 years of age, 38 % in 60–69, 47 % in 70–79, and 75 % in >80-year-old premutation carriers [30]. *FMR1* premutations have a prevalence of 1/800 in males and 1/300 in females [31, 32] indicating that FXTAS may be underdiagnosed and related cognitive problems may be a relevant factor for cognitive impairment in the general population.

Neuropsychiatric Symptoms

Older male carriers of FXTAS premutation have been reported with cognitive impairment involving executive dysfunction, selective attention, inhibition, and working as well as declarative memory. Cornish and colleagues described age-dependent cognitive changes especially in response inhibition in male carriers of the *FMR1* premutation [33]. In females, cognitive deficits have been infrequently reported [34]. Cognitive impairment and dementia may precede motor symptoms and may represent the most debilitating symptom of premutation carriers.

Sevin and colleagues compared cognitive function in 35 premutation carriers and 39 intrafamilial controls with age >50 years. Using the Mattis Dementia Rating Scale, they found performance to decrease gradually from controls to carriers of short premutations (55–69 CGG) and carriers of larger premutations (70–200 CGG) with more severe deficits in the latter group. Cognition was impaired especially in three subscores: semantic fluency, abstract reasoning, and visuospatial performance. After adjustment for age (63.5 years) and education (9.7 years), the penetrance for marked cognitive impairment was 33 % for larger premutation carriers compared to 5 % in controls and 6 % in carriers of small premutations indicating that the penetrance of cognitive impairment increases with the CGG repeat size [35]. Cognitive decline was not restricted to patients with motor signs of FXTAS but may occur independently.

Additionally, FMR1 premutation carriers were found to have an increased risk of psychiatric phenotypes with a lifetime prevalence for mood disorders of 65 % and for anxiety of 52 % according to DSM-IV criteria [36]. Neuropsychiatric assessment with the neuropsychiatric inventory revealed significantly higher scores on the agitation/aggression ($p<0.004$), depression ($p<0.004$), apathy ($p<0.004$), disinhibition ($p<0.004$), and irritability ($p<0.004$) scales in males with FXTAS compared with controls. Cognitive performances on the Mini-Mental State Examination did not correlate with severity of symptoms on the neuropsychiatric inventory [37].

Spinocerebellar Ataxias (SCAs)

Disease Definition

The spinocerebellar ataxias (SCAs) are a genetically heterogeneous group of more than 30 autosomal dominantly inherited progressive ataxia disorders. Genetically, they can be subdivided into three groups. SCA1, SCA2, SCA3, SCA6, SCA7, and

SCA17 are caused by translated CAG repeat expansion mutations coding for an elongated polyglutamine tract within the respective proteins. These disorders belong to a larger group of polyglutamine disorders that also include Huntington's disease. Whereas SCA1, SCA2, SCA3, SCA7, and SCA17 are multisystemic disorders that affect not only the cerebellum but have significant extracerebellar pathology; involvement in SCA6 is almost exclusively confined to the cerebellum. The second group comprises SCA8, SCA10, SCA12, SCA31, and SCA36 which are caused by untranslated repeat mutations. A third group comprises SCAs which are due to conventional non-repeat mutations, mainly point mutations. A number of SCAs have been linked to a chromosomal locus, but the disease gene and causative mutations have not yet been found [38]. Detailed information on all spinocerebellar ataxias can be found on http://neuromuscular.wustl.edu/ataxia/recatax.html.

An epidemiological study performed in the Netherlands found a prevalence of SCAs of 0.8–3.0:100,000 [39]. A study from Norway found a prevalence of 4.2:100,000 [40]. However, regional prevalence rates may be much higher due to founder effects.

The distribution among the various genetic subtypes varies from region to region. Worldwide, SCA1, SCA2, SCA3, and SCA6 are the most common SCAs and account for the disease in more than half of all SCA families [41].

Neuropsychiatric Symptoms

In general, SCA patients have no global cognitive impairment and do not develop dementia. However, although this general rule applies to most genetic forms, there are some notable exceptions. SCA17 is due to CAG repeat expansion in the TATA-binding protein (TBP) gene. Clinical descriptions of SCA17 patients consistently report cognitive decline finally resulting in dementia [42, 43]. Cognitive decline in SCA17 may start both before and after the onset of motor problems and often shows rapid progression. Cognitive decline may be associated with psychiatric symptoms including depression, mania, hallucinations, paranoia, and aggressive behavior. A morphometric MRI study showed an association of psychiatric symptoms with gray matter loss in the frontal and temporal lobes, the cuneus and cingulum, and of cognitive dysfunction with gray matter loss of the nucleus accumbens. On the other hand, motor problems were related to morphometric changes in the cerebellum and basal ganglia [44]. Mental retardation and nonprogressive intellectual impairment have been observed in SCAs which are due to non-repeat mutation, in particular in SCA13 [45].

Several studies using different assessment instruments including the Wisconsin Card Sorting Test and Stroop test consistently found impaired executive functions in SCA patients. The first reports came from Kish et al. who studied patients with dominantly inherited ataxia, before genetic testing became available [46, 47]. With discovery of the causative mutations, studies were published that described executive impairment in genetically defined SCA. Deficits were specifically found in polyglutamine SCAs with multisystemic involvement, including SCA1 [48], SCA2 [49], and SCA3 [50, 51] but also SCA8 [52], SCA19 [53], and SCA27 [54]. More recently, studies comparing executive functions in several SCAs were published. Bürk et al. [55] found more pronounced deficits in SCA1 compared to SCA2 and SCA3 [55], whereas others did not find major differences between SCA1, SCA2, and SCA3 [56, 57]. Abnormalities of executive function in SCA6, which is considered a purely cerebellar disorder, are less obvious. Nevertheless, two studies definitely found such deficits in SCA6 [56, 58]. Another consistent finding emerging from available studies is impaired verbal fluency which like executive impairment is thought to result from frontal dysfunction. Definite deficits were not only found in SCA1, SCA2, and SCA3 but also SCA6 [49, 51, 57, 59].

SCA patients do not have general memory problems. However, a number of studies reported impaired verbal memory, particularly in SCA1 and SCA2, whereas SCA6 patients performed normally in respective tests. Whether SCA patients have problems with working memory and attention is not quite clear. Available studies give inconsistent results. However, when deficits were found, they were mild and mainly observed in multisystemic SCAs.

There is no indication that there are language deficits in SCA patients [60, 61], whereas visuospatial deficits were reported in some studies [51, 52], but not in others [49].

Depression is frequently reported in studies investigating neuropsychiatric abnormalities in SCA patients. However, as in similar studies in other chronic brain diseases, such as Parkinson's disease, prevalence rate is highly disparate between different studies. One problem of several of these studies is the reliance on self-assessment scales. One study reported depressive symptoms in 20–30 % of SCA1, SCA2, and SCA6 patients but 60 % of SCA3 patients [62]. In another study, the SCA1 and SCA2 had higher scores on the Hamilton Depression Scale, but only 5 % reached scores above the cutoff for depression [57]. In one of the largest studies encompassing 79 SCA3 patients, moderate to severe Beck Depression Inventory (BDI) scores were found in 33.5 %. Increased BDI scores were more frequent in patients than in caregivers and at-risk persons but less frequent than in multiple sclerosis patients [63]. In contrast, a study of 526 SCA1, SCA2, SCA3, and SCA6 patients that used the Patient Health Questionnaire for assessment of depression found a prevalence of only 17 % which is not higher than that of primary care patients [64] or attendees of neurology clinics in general. There were no differences between the genetic subtypes. A small subset of these patients underwent an interview-based psychiatric assessment which yielded a similar prevalence of depression [65]. Interestingly, however, the same group of authors reported that in those who had depression, this had a significant impact on health-related quality of life [66].

In conclusion, SCA patients have unambiguous deficits of executive functions and verbal fluency, whereas all other cognitive domains including memory, language, and visuospatial abilities appear to be intact or only marginally affected. Interestingly, the brain region implicated in executive control and verbal fluency is the frontal cortex which according to recent anatomical evidence reviewed above is connected to the cerebellar hemisphere via the dentate nucleus. Deficits in these domains could therefore be attributed to cerebellar dysfunction. Alternatively, they could be the consequence of neurodegeneration of the frontal cortex itself or of connection between the cerebellum and frontal cortex. The observation that SCA6 patients, who suffer from a purely cerebellar degeneration, have deficits of executive control shows that cerebellar degeneration alone is sufficient to cause frontal-like neuropsychological deficits. However, deficits are more pronounced in multisystemic SCAs showing that impairment is stronger in diseases in which degeneration goes beyond the cerebellum even if there is no evidence that there is specific degeneration of the frontal cortex in these SCAs. Instead, it is conceivable that degeneration of fiber connections including those arising from the dentate nucleus and of the thalamus contributes to the stronger involvement in these SCAs.

Sporadic Degenerative Ataxias

Disease Definition

In the majority of patients suffering from adult-onset, progressive ataxia, ataxia manifests without an obvious familial background. There is a wide range of potentially acquired causes resulting in secondary ataxia. However, a considerable part of sporadic ataxia patients suffer from a "nongenetic" sporadic degenerative disease, such as multiple system atrophy of cerebellar type (MSA-C) or sporadic adult-onset ataxia of unknown etiology (SAOA) [67] that is not due to an acquired cause. MSA-C is a neuropathologically well-defined category. Currently used clinical diagnostic criteria allow making an in vivo diagnosis with high specificity but limited sensitivity [68]. The nosological status of SAOA, on the other hand, is less clear. This category that was previously named idiopathic cerebellar ataxia (IDCA) may comprise patients with unrecognized gene mutations or acquired disease causes [69, 70]. It is also conceivable that some SAOA indeed have a mild form of MSA. Nevertheless, degeneration in most SAOA patients is usually confined to the cerebellum, whereas degeneration in MSA is typically multisystemic and often involves the basal ganglia.

Neuropsychiatric Symptoms

In contrast to SCAs, the information about neuropsychiatric deficits in sporadic degenerative ataxias is much more limited. Interpretation of some studies in MSA is made difficult by the fact that they were performed in patients with the parkinsonian type of MSA, MSA-P, or did not differentiate between the MSA-C and MSA-P.

In a group of MSA patients, Robbins et al. [71] found deficits in tests shown to be sensitive to frontal lobe dysfunction without evidence for a general intellectual deterioration. However, the group comprised mainly MSA patients with a parkinsonian predominance (MSA-P) [71]. Nevertheless, a study of 20 MSA-C patients reported similar deficits with impaired verbal memory and verbal fluency [72]. Another study confirmed the presence of cognitive deficits in MSA but found them more pronounced in MSA-P than in MSA-C. Deficits in MSA-C were confined to impaired visuospatial abilities [73]. In contrast, a recent study that tested 61 MSA patients found frontal deficits measured with the Frontal Assessment Battery in 41 % of patients without differences of cognitive performance between MSA-P and MSA-C [74].

In the study that initially defined IDCA, Harding (1981) found 28 % of her patients demented [4]. This comparably high rate was not confirmed in subsequent studies. In a detailed study of cognitive function of 67 SAOA patients, only mild and unspecific cognitive disturbances were found [75]. In a group of 27 SAOA patients, reported Mini-Mental State Examination scores ranging from 25 to 30 with a median of 29 [70].

References

1. Schmahmann JD, Sherman JC. The cerebellar cognitive affective syndrome. Brain. 1998; 121(Pt 4):561–79.
2. Strick PL, Dum RP, Fiez JA. Cerebellum and nonmotor function. Annu Rev Neurosci. 2009;32:413–34.
3. Epplen C, Epplen JT, Frank G, Miterski B, Santos EJ, Schols L. Differential stability of the (GAA)n tract in the Friedreich ataxia (STM7) gene. Hum Genet. 1997;99(6):834–6.
4. Harding AE. "Idiopathic" late onset cerebellar ataxia. A clinical and genetic study of 36 cases. J Neurol Sci. 1981;51:259–71.
5. Schulz JB, Boesch S, Burk K, Durr A, Giunti P, Mariotti C, et al. Diagnosis and treatment of Friedreich ataxia: a European perspective. Nat Rev Neurol. 2009;5(4):222–34.
6. Durr A, Cossee M, Agid Y, Campuzano V, Mignard C, Penet C, et al. Clinical and genetic abnormalities in patients with Friedreich's ataxia. N Engl J Med. 1996;335(16):1169–75.
7. Schols L, Amoiridis G, Przuntek H, Frank G, Epplen JT, Epplen C. Friedreich's ataxia. Revision of the phenotype according to molecular genetics. Brain J Neurol. 1997;120(Pt 12):2131–40.
8. Campuzano V, Montermini L, Molto MD, Pianese L, Cossee M, Cavalcanti F, et al. Friedreich's ataxia: autosomal recessive disease caused by an intronic GAA triplet repeat expansion. Science. 1996;271(5254):1423–7.
9. Koeppen AH, Michael SC, Knutson MD, Haile DJ, Qian J, Levi S, et al. The dentate nucleus in Friedreich's ataxia: the role of iron-responsive proteins. Acta Neuropathol. 2007;114(2): 163–73.
10. Rabe K, Kraff O, Minnerop M, Beck A, Schöls L, Gizewski E, et al. Cerebellar pathology in Friedreich's ataxia: atrophied dentate nuclei with normal iron content. Neuroimage 2014, in press.
11. Mantovan MC, Martinuzzi A, Squarzanti F, Bolla A, Silvestri I, Liessi G, et al. Exploring mental status in Friedreich's ataxia: a combined neuropsychological, behavioral and neuroimaging study. Eur J Neurol. 2006;13(8):827–35.
12. Nieto A, Correia R, de Nobrega E, Monton F, Hess S, Barroso J. Cognition in Friedreich ataxia. Cerebellum. 2012;11(4):834–44.
13. Nieto A, Correia R, de Nobrega E, Monton F, Barroso J. Cognition in late-onset Friedreich ataxia. Cerebellum. 2013;12(4):504–12.
14. Della Nave R, Ginestroni A, Tessa C, Salvatore E, Bartolomei I, Salvi F, et al. Brain white matter tracts degeneration in Friedreich ataxia. An in vivo MRI study using tract-based spatial statistics and voxel-based morphometry. Neuroimage. 2008;40(1):19–25.
15. Franca Jr MC, D'Abreu A, Yasuda CL, Bonadia LC, Santos da Silva M, Nucci A, et al. A combined voxel-based morphometry and 1H-MRS study in patients with Friedreich's ataxia. J Neurol. 2009;256(7):1114–20.

16. Silva CB, Yasuda CL, D'Abreu A, Cendes F, Lopes-Cendes I, Franca Jr MC. Neuroanatomical correlates of depression in Friedreich's ataxia: a voxel-based morphometry study. Cerebellum. 2013;12(3):429–36.
17. Akhlaghi H, Yu J, Corben L, Georgiou-Karistianis N, Bradshaw JL, Storey E, et al. Cognitive deficits in Friedreich ataxia correlate with micro-structural changes in dentatorubral tract. Cerebellum. 2014;13(2):187–98.
18. Anheim M, Tranchant C, Koenig M. The autosomal recessive cerebellar ataxias. N Engl J Med. 2012;366(7):636–46.
19. Anheim M, Fleury M, Monga B, Laugel V, Chaigne D, Rodier G, et al. Epidemiological, clinical, paraclinical and molecular study of a cohort of 102 patients affected with autosomal recessive progressive cerebellar ataxia from Alsace, Eastern France: implications for clinical management. Neurogenetics. 2010;11(1):1–12.
20. Schulte C, Synofzik M, Gasser T, Schols L. Ataxia with ophthalmoplegia or sensory neuropathy is frequently caused by POLG mutations. Neurology. 2009;73(11):898–900.
21. Debs R, Froissart R, Aubourg P, Papeix C, Douillard C, Degos B, et al. Krabbe disease in adults: phenotypic and genotypic update from a series of 11 cases and a review. J Inherit Metab Dis. 2013;36(5):859–68.
22. Sparks SE, Krasnewich DM. Congenital disorders of N-linked glycosylation pathway overview. In: Pagon RA, Adam MP, Bird TD, Dolan CR, Fong CT, Smith RJH, Stephens K (eds). GeneReviews(R). Seattle: University of Washington; 1993.
23. Muller Vom Hagen J, Synofzik M, Schicks J, Krageloh-Mann I, Schols L. Leukodystrophies in idiopathic adult-onset ataxia: frequency and phenotype in 105 patients. Mov Disord. 2013;28(14):2033–5.
24. Le Ber I, Moreira MC, Rivaud-Pechoux S, Chamayou C, Ochsner F, Kuntzer T, et al. Cerebellar ataxia with oculomotor apraxia type 1: clinical and genetic studies. Brain J Neurol. 2003;126(Pt 12):2761–72.
25. Horvath R, Hudson G, Ferrari G, Futterer N, Ahola S, Lamantea E, et al. Phenotypic spectrum associated with mutations of the mitochondrial polymerase gamma gene. Brain J Neurol. 2006;129(Pt 7):1674–84.
26. Gramstad A, Bindoff LA, Lillebo A, Tzoulis C, Engelsen BA. Neuropsychological performance in patients with POLG1 mutations and the syndrome of mitochondrial spinocerebellar ataxia and epilepsy. Epilepsy Behav Epilepsy Behav. 2009;16(1):172–4.
27. Horvath R, Czermin B, Gulati S, Demuth S, Houge G, Pyle A, et al. Adult-onset cerebellar ataxia due to mutations in CABC1/ADCK3. J Neurol Neurosurg Psychiatry. 2012;83(2):174–8.
28. Vinck A, Verhagen MM, Gerven M, de Groot IJ, Weemaes CM, Maassen BA, et al. Cognitive and speech-language performance in children with ataxia telangiectasia. Dev Neurorehabil. 2011;14(5):315–22.
29. Vermeer S, van de Warrenburg BP, Kamsteeg EJ. Arsacs. In: Pagon RA, Adam MP, Bird TD, Dolan CR, Fong CT, Smith RJH, Stephens K (eds). GeneReviews(R). Seattle: University of Washington; 1993.
30. Jacquemont S, Hagerman RJ, Leehey MA, Hall DA, Levine RA, Brunberg JA, et al. Penetrance of the fragile X-associated tremor/ataxia syndrome in a premutation carrier population. JAMA. 2004;291(4):460–9.
31. Rousseau F, Rouillard P, Morel ML, Khandjian EW, Morgan K. Prevalence of carriers of premutation-size alleles of the FMRI gene–and implications for the population genetics of the fragile X syndrome. Am J Hum Genet. 1995;57(5):1006–18.
32. Dombrowski C, Levesque S, Morel ML, Rouillard P, Morgan K, Rousseau F. Premutation and intermediate-size FMR1 alleles in 10572 males from the general population: loss of an AGG interruption is a late event in the generation of fragile X syndrome alleles. Hum Mol Genet. 2002;11(4):371–8.
33. Cornish KM, Li L, Kogan CS, Jacquemont S, Turk J, Dalton A, et al. Age-dependent cognitive changes in carriers of the fragile X syndrome. Cortex; a journal devoted to the study of the nervous system and behavior. 2008;44(6):628–36.

34. Hagerman RJ, Leavitt BR, Farzin F, Jacquemont S, Greco CM, Brunberg JA, et al. Fragile-X-associated tremor/ataxia syndrome (FXTAS) in females with the FMR1 premutation. Am J Hum Genet. 2004;74(5):1051–6.
35. Sevin M, Kutalik Z, Bergman S, Vercelletto M, Renou P, Lamy E, et al. Penetrance of marked cognitive impairment in older male carriers of the FMR1 gene premutation. J Med Genet. 2009;46(12):818–24.
36. Bourgeois JA, Seritan AL, Casillas EM, Hessl D, Schneider A, Yang Y, et al. Lifetime prevalence of mood and anxiety disorders in fragile X premutation carriers. J Clin Psychiatry. 2011;72(2):175–82.
37. Bacalman S, Farzin F, Bourgeois JA, Cogswell J, Goodlin-Jones BL, Gane LW, et al. Psychiatric phenotype of the fragile X-associated tremor/ataxia syndrome (FXTAS) in males: newly described fronto-subcortical dementia. J Clin Psychiatry. 2006;67(1):87–94.
38. Durr A. Autosomal dominant cerebellar ataxias: polyglutamine expansions and beyond. Lancet Neurol. 2010;9:885–94.
39. van de Warrenburg BP, Sinke RJ, Verschuuren-Bemelmans CC, et al. Spinocerebellar ataxias in the Netherlands: prevalence and age at onset variance analysis. Neurology. 2002;58:702–8.
40. Erichsen AK, Koht J, Stray-Pedersen A, Abdelnoor M, Tallaksen CM. Prevalence of hereditary ataxia and spastic paraplegia in southeast Norway: a population-based study. Brain. 2009;132:1577–88.
41. Schols L, Bauer P, Schmidt T, Schulte T, Riess O. Autosomal dominant cerebellar ataxias: clinical features, genetics, and pathogenesis. Lancet Neurol. 2004;3:291–304.
42. Rolfs A, Koeppen AH, Bauer I, et al. Clinical features and neuropathology of autosomal dominant spinocerebellar ataxia (SCA17). Ann Neurol. 2003;54:367–75.
43. Mariotti C, Alpini D, Fancellu R, et al. Spinocerebellar ataxia type 17 (SCA17): oculomotor phenotype and clinical characterization of 15 Italian patients. J Neurol. 2007;254:1538–46.
44. Lasek K, Lencer R, Gaser C, et al. Morphological basis for the spectrum of clinical deficits in spinocerebellar ataxia 17 (SCA17). Brain. 2006;129:2341–52.
45. Waters MF, Minassian NA, Stevanin G, et al. Mutations in voltage-gated potassium channel KCNC3 cause degenerative and developmental central nervous system phenotypes. Nat Genet. 2006;38:447–51.
46. Kish SJ, el Awar M, Schut L, Leach L, Oscar Berman M, Freedman M. Cognitive deficits in olivopontocerebellar atrophy: implications for the cholinergic hypothesis of Alzheimer's dementia. Ann Neurol. 1988;24:200–6.
47. Kish SJ, El-Awar M, Stuss D, et al. Neuropsychological test performance in patients with dominantly inherited spinocerebellar ataxia: relationship to ataxia severity. Neurology. 1994;44:1738–46.
48. Burk K, Bosch S, Globas C, et al. Executive dysfunction in spinocerebellar ataxia type 1. Eur Neurol. 2001;46:43–8.
49. Burk K, Globas C, Bosch S, et al. Cognitive deficits in spinocerebellar ataxia 2. Brain. 1999;122:769–77.
50. Zawacki TM, Grace J, Friedman JH, Sudarsky L. Executive and emotional dysfunction in Machado-Joseph disease. Mov Disord. 2002;17:1004–10.
51. Braga-Neto P, Pedroso JL, Alessi H, et al. Cerebellar cognitive affective syndrome in Machado Joseph disease: core clinical features. Cerebellum. 2012;11:549–56.
52. Lilja A, Hamalainen P, Kaitaranta E, Rinne R. Cognitive impairment in spinocerebellar ataxia type 8. J Neurol Sci. 2005;237:31–8.
53. Schelhaas HJ, van de Warrenburg BP, Hageman G, Ippel EE, van Hout M, Kremer B. Cognitive impairment in SCA-19. Acta Neurol Belg. 2003;103:199–205.
54. Brusse E, de Koning I, Maat-Kievit A, Oostra BA, Heutink P, van Swieten JC. Spinocerebellar ataxia associated with a mutation in the fibroblast growth factor 14 gene (SCA27): a new phenotype. Mov Disord. 2006;21:396–401.
55. Burk K, Globas C, Bosch S, et al. Cognitive deficits in spinocerebellar ataxia type 1, 2, and 3. J Neurol. 2003;250:207–11.

56. Klinke I, Minnerop M, Schmitz-Hubsch T, et al. Neuropsychological features of patients with Spinocerebellar Ataxia (SCA) Types 1, 2, 3, and 6. Cerebellum. 2010;9(3):433–42.
57. Fancellu R, Paridi D, Tomasello C, et al. Longitudinal study of cognitive and psychiatric functions in spinocerebellar ataxia types 1 and 2. J Neurol. 2013;260:3134–43.
58. Cooper FE, Grube M, Elsegood KJ, et al. The contribution of the cerebellum to cognition in Spinocerebellar Ataxia type 6. Behav Neurol. 2010;23:3–15.
59. Suenaga M, Kawai Y, Watanabe H, et al. Cognitive impairment in spinocerebellar ataxia type 6. J Neurol Neurosurg Psychiatry. 2008;79:496–9.
60. Kawai Y, Takeda A, Abe Y, Washimi Y, Tanaka F, Sobue G. Cognitive impairments in Machado-Joseph disease. Arch Neurol. 2004;61:1757–60.
61. Gambardella A, Annesi G, Bono F, et al. CAG repeat length and clinical features in three Italian families with spinocerebellar ataxia type 2 (SCA2): early impairment of Wisconsin Card Sorting Test and saccade velocity. J Neurol. 1998;245:647–52.
62. McMurtray AM, Clark DG, Flood MK, Perlman S, Mendez MF. Depressive and memory symptoms as presenting features of spinocerebellar ataxia. J Neuropsychiatry Clin Neurosci. 2006;18:420–2.
63. Cecchin CR, Pires AP, Rieder CR, et al. Depressive symptoms in Machado-Joseph disease (SCA3) patients and their relatives. Community Genet. 2007;10:19–26.
64. Spitzer RL, Kroenke K, Williams JB. Validation and utility of a self-report version of PRIME-MD: the PHQ primary care study. Primary Care Evaluation of Mental Disorders. Patient Health Questionnaire. JAMA. 1999;282(18):1737–44.
65. Schmitz-Hubsch T, Coudert M, du Tezenas MS, et al. Depression comorbidity in spinocerebellar ataxia. Mov Disord. 2011;26:870–6.
66. Schmitz-Hubsch T, Coudert M, Giunti P, et al. Self-rated health status in spinocerebellar ataxia-results from a European multicenter study. Mov Disord. 2010;25(5):587–95.
67. Klockgether T. Sporadic ataxia with adult onset: classification and diagnostic criteria. Lancet Neurol. 2010;9:94–104.
68. Gilman S, Wenning GK, Low PA, et al. Second consensus statement on the diagnosis of multiple system atrophy. Neurology. 2008;71:670–6.
69. Harding AE. Friedreich's ataxia: a clinical and genetic study of 90 families with an analysis of early diagnostic criteria and intrafamilial clustering of clinical features. Brain J Neurol. 1981;104(3):589–620.
70. Abele M, Minnerop M, Urbach H, Specht K, Klockgether T. Sporadic adult onset ataxia of unknown etiology: a clinical, electrophysiological and imaging study. J Neurol. 2007;254:1384–9.
71. Robbins TW, James M, Lange KW, Owen AM, Quinn NP, Marsden CD. Cognitive performance in multiple system atrophy. Brain. 1992;115(Pt 1):271–91.
72. Burk K, Daum I, Rub U. Cognitive function in multiple system atrophy of the cerebellar type. Mov Disord. 2006;21:772–6.
73. Kawai Y, Suenaga M, Takeda A, et al. Cognitive impairments in multiple system atrophy: MSA-C vs MSA-P. Neurology. 2008;70:1390–6.
74. Siri C, Duerr S, Canesi M, et al. A cross-sectional multicenter study of cognitive and behavioural features in multiple system atrophy patients of the parkinsonian and cerebellar type. J Neural Transm. 2013;120:613–8.
75. Berent S, Giordani B, Gilman S, et al. Patterns of neuropsychological performance in multiple system atrophy compared to sporadic and hereditary olivopontocerebellar atrophy. Brain Cogn. 2002;50:194–206.

Index

H. Reichmann (ed.), *Neuropsychiatric Symptoms of Movement Disorders*, Neuropsychiatric Symptoms of Neurological Disease,
DOI 10.1007/978-3-319-09537-0

O

P

MIX
Papier aus verantwortungsvollen Quellen
Paper from responsible sources
FSC® C105338

If you have any concerns about our products,
you can contact us on
ProductSafety@springernature.com

In case Publisher is established outside the EU,
the EU authorized representative is:
Springer Nature Customer Service Center GmbH
Europaplatz 3, 69115 Heidelberg, Germany

Printed by Libri Plureos GmbH
in Hamburg, Germany